Handbook of
Liver
Disease

To my wife, Mary Jo, and son, Matthew (L.S.F.)
To my wife, Melenie, and children,
Emmet III, Brian and Meghan (E.B.K)

For Churchill Livingstone

Commissioning Editor: Sheila Khullar
Project Editor: Antonia Seymour
Copy Editor: Graham Wild
Project Controller: Sarah Lowe
Indexer: Hilary Tarrant
Design Direction: Jeannette Jacobs

Handbook of Liver Disease

Edited by

Lawrence S. Friedman MD

Associate Professor of Medicine, Harvard Medical School;
Associate Physician, Gastrointestinal Unit, Massachusetts
General Hospital, Boston, Massachusetts, USA

Emmet B. Keeffe MD

Professor of Medicine; Medical Director, Liver Transplant
Program; Chief of Clinical Gastroenterology, Stanford
University Medical Center, Stanford, California, USA

Foreword by

Willis C. Maddrey MD

Professor of Internal Medicine, Executive Vice President for
Clinical Affairs, The University of Texas, Southwestern
Medical Center, Dallas, Texas, USA

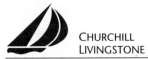

CHURCHILL
LIVINGSTONE

EDINBURGH LONDON NEW YORK PHILADELPHIA SAN FRANCISCO SYDNEY TORONTO
1998

CHURCHILL LIVINGSTONE
A Division of Harcourt Brace and Company Limited

© Harcourt Brace and Company Limited 1998
D is a registered trademark of Harcourt Brace and Company Limited

ISBN   0 443 05520 3

British Library Cataloguing in Publication Data
A catalogue record for this book is available from the British Library.

Library of Congress Cataloging in Publication Data
A catalog record for this book is available from the Library of Congress.

Medical knowledge is constantly changing. As new information becomes available, changes in treatment, procedures, equipment and the use of drugs become necessary. The editors and contributors and the publishers have, as far as it is possible, taken care to ensure that the information given in the text is accurate and up to date. However, readers are strongly advised to confirm that the information, especially with regard to drug usage, complies with latest legislation and standards of practice.

Produced by Longman Asia Ltd. Hong Kong
SP/01

Contents

Contributors

Helen M. Ayles BSc MBBS MRCP
Registrar, Hospital for Tropical Diseases, London, UK

Bruce R. Bacon MD
Professor of Internal Medicine; Director, Division of Gastroenterology and Hepatology, Saint Louis University School of Medicine, St Louis, Missouri, USA

William F. Balistreri BA MD
Director, Division of Pediatric Gastroenterology and Nutrition; Dorothy M. M. Kersten Professor of Pediatrics; Medical Director, Pediatric Liver Transplantation, Children's Hospital Medical Center, Cincinnati, Ohio, USA

Martin Black MD
Professor of Medicine, Temple University Hospital, Philadelphia, Pennsylvania, USA

Laurence M. Blendis MD FRCP FRCP(C)
Professor of Medicine, University of Toronto, The Toronto Hospital, Toronto, Canada; Institute of Gastroenterology, Ichilo Hospital, Tel Aviv, Israel

Srinivas Channapragada MD
Attending Physician, John F Kennedy Hospital, Edison; Muhlenberg Medical Center, Plainfield, New Jersey, USA

Sanjiv Chopra MD
Director of Clinical Hepatology, Beth Israel Deaconess Medical Center; Associate Professor of Medicine, Harvard Medical School, Boston, Massachusetts, USA

Raymond T. Chung MD
Assistant in Medicine, Massachusetts General Hospital; Instructor in Medicine, Harvard Medical School, Boston, Massachusetts, USA

Albert J. Czaja MD
Professor of Medicine, Mayo Medical School; Consultant in Gastroenterology, Mayo Clinic, Rochester, Minnesota, USA

Kevin De Cock MD FRCP DTM+H
Senior Lecturer, London School of Hygiene and Tropical Medicine, London, UK

Adrian M. Di Bisceglie MD
Professor of Internal Medicine; Associate Chairman, Department of Internal Medicine, Saint Louis University School of Medicine, St Louis, Missouri, USA

Anna Mae Diehl MD
Professor of Medicine, Johns Hopkins University School of Medicine, Baltimore, Maryland, USA

Lorna Dove MD
Research Fellow, University of California San Francisco, San Francisco, California, USA

Lawrence S. Friedman MD
Associate Professor of Medicine, Harvard Medical School; Associate Physician, Gastrointestinal Unit, Massachusetts General Hospital, Boston, Massachusetts, USA

Gabriel Garcia AB MD
Associate Professor of Medicine, Stanford University School of Medicine, Stanford, California, USA

John L. Gollan MD PhD FRACP FRCP
Associate Professor of Medicine, Harvard Medical School; Director, Gastroenterology Division, Brigham & Women's Hospital, Boston, Massachusetts, USA

Norman D. Grace MD FACP FACG
Professor of Medicine, Tufts University School of Medicine; Chief of Gastroenterology, Faulkner Hospital, Boston, Massachusetts, USA

Susan Greenbloom BSc MD FRCP(C)
Gastroenterologist, Etobicoke General Hospital, Etobicoke, Ontario, Canada

James H. Grendell MD
Professor of Medicine, Cornell University Medical College; Chief, Division of Digestive Diseases, Department of Medicine, New York Hospital–Cornell Medical Center, New York, New York, USA

Donald J. Hillebrand MD
Assistant Professor of Medicine, Associate Medical Director of Liver Transplantation, Transplantation Institute, Loma Linda University Medical Center, Loma Linda, California, USA

Joanne C. Imperial MD
Assistant Professor of Medicine, Stanford University School of Medicine, Stanford, California, USA

Ira M. Jacobson MD FACP PC
Clinical Associate Professor of Medicine, Cornell University Medical College; Associate Attending Physician, New York Hospital, New York, New York, USA

Marshall M. Kaplan MD
Professor of Medicine, Tufts University School of Medicine; Chief, Division of Gastroenterology, New England Medical Center, Boston, Massachusetts, USA

Emmet B. Keeffe MD
Professor of Medicine; Medical Director, Liver Transplant Program; Chief of Clinical Gastroenterology, Stanford University Medical Center, Stanford, California, USA

Michelle S. Kennedy MD
Research Fellow, Division of Pediatric Gastroenterology and Nutrition, Children's Hospital Medical Center, Cincinnati, Ohio, USA

Raymond S. Koff MD
Chairman, Department of Medicine, Columbia MetroWest Medical Center, Framingham; Professor of Medicine, University of Massachusetts Medical School, Boston, Massachusetts, USA

Kris V. Kowdley MD FACP
Associate Professor of Medicine, University of Washington School of Medicine, Seattle, Washington, USA

Young-Mee Lee MD
Assistant Professor, Tufts University School of Medicine, New England Medical Center, Boston, Massachusetts, USA

Jay H. Lefkowitch MD
Professor of Clinical Pathology, Columbia University College of Physicians and Surgeons, New York, New York, USA

Keith D. Lillemoe MD FACS
Professor of Surgery, The Johns Hopkins Medical Institutions, Baltimore, Maryland, USA

Peter F. Malet MD
Associate Professor of Internal Medicine, Liver Unit, Department of Internal Medicine, University of Texas Southwestern Medical Center, Dallas, Texas, USA

Paul Martin MD
Associate Professor of Medicine; Director, Hepatology, Division of Digestive Diseases and Dumont-UCLA Transplant Program, Los Angeles, California, USA

Mack C. Mitchell Jr MD FACP FACG
Clinical Professor of Medicine, University of North Carolina; Chairman, Department of Internal Medicine, Carolinas Medical Center, Charlotte, North Carolina, USA

Timothy R. Morgan MD
Associate Professor of Medicine, University of California, Irvine, California; Chief, Hepatology, VA Medical Center, Long Beach, California, USA

Kevin D. Mullen MB FRCPI
Consultant Gastroenterologist/Hepatologist and Associate Professor of Medicine, Case Western Reserve School of Medicine, MetroHealth Medical Center, Cleveland, Ohio, USA

Santiago J. Muñoz MD
Associate Professor of Medicine, Temple School of Medicine; Director, Center for Liver Diseases; Head, Hepatology Section, Albert Einstein Medical Center, Philadelphia, Pennsylvania, USA

Brent A. Neuschwander-Tetri MD
Associate Professor of Internal Medicine, Saint Louis University, St Louis, Missouri, USA

Catherine Ann Petruff MD
Instructor in Medicine, Harvard Medical School, Boston; Physician, Beth Israel Deaconess Medical Center, Boston, Massachusetts, USA

José Proenza MD
Senior Fellow in Gastroenterology, Albert Einstein Medical Center, Philadelphia, Pennsylvania, USA

James V. Puleo MD
Teaching Fellow in Medicine, Tufts University School of Medicine; Fellow in Gastroenterology, Faulkner Hospital, Boston, Massachusetts, USA

John W. Pyne MD
Senior Gastroenterology Fellow, University of California Irvine, Irvine, California, USA

K. Rajender Reddy MD FACP
Professor of Medicine, Division of Hepatology, University of Miami School of Medicine, Miami, Florida, USA

Hugo R. Rosen MD
Assistant Professor of Medicine, Division of Gastroenterology/Hepatology and Liver Transplantation Program, Oregon Health Sciences University, Portland, Oregon, USA

Kenneth D. Rothstein MD
Associate Director, Center for Liver Diseases, Albert Einstein Medical Center; Assistant Professor of Medicine, Temple School of Medicine, Philadelphia, Pennsylvania, USA

Bruce A. Runyon MD
Professor of Medicine, Director of Hepatology, Medical Director of Liver Transplantation, Transplantation Institute, Loma Linda University Medical Center, Loma Linda, California, USA

Thomas D. Schiano MD
Temple University Hospital Liver Unit, Philadelphia, Pennsylvania, USA

Anthony S. Tavill MD FRCP FACP
Mathile and Morton Stone Professor, Friedman Center for Digestive and Liver Disorders, Mount Sinai Medical Center, Case Western Reserve University School of Medicine, Cleveland, Ohio, USA

Russell H. Wiesner MD
Professor of Medicine, Mayo Medical School, Medical Director, Liver Transplantation, Mayo Clinic, Rochester, Minnesota, USA

Jacqueline L. Wolf MD
Assistant Professor of Clinical Medicine, Harvard Medical School; Physician, Brigham & Women's Hospital, Boston, Massachusetts, USA

Florence Wong MD FRACP FRCP(C)
Assistant Professor, University of Toronto, Toronto, Ontario, Canada

Teresa L. Wright MD
Associate Professor of Medicine, University of California San Francisco; Chief, Gastroenterology Section, Veterans Affairs Medical Center, San Francisco, California, USA

Wisam F. Zakko MD
Senior Fellow in Gastroenterology, Brigham & Women's Hospital, Boston, Massachusetts, USA

Gillian Ann D'Adamo Zeldin MD
Fellow, Division of Gastroenterology, Johns Hopkins University School of Medicine, Baltimore, Maryland, USA

Foreword

Stunning achievements in hepatology have stimulated many clinicians and investigators to take a new and, in some cases renewed, interest in the liver and the diseases that affect it. *Handbook of Liver Disease* provides a concise overview in each section of the present state of hepatology. Outlines regarding pathogenesis and natural history are interspersed with clinical clues and status reports regarding therapy for the major disorders affecting the liver. The risks of data reduction and the necessary assumptions imposed by the goal of brevity are more than offset by the advantages of carefully considered presentation of pertinent information in an accessible format.

These are new world times for hepatology, as is amply demonstrated throughout the handbook. Towering advances have been achieved in hepatic virology and in liver transplantation. The lessons learned from hepatic virology are many. Identification of the viruses that cause hepatitis A through E and the creation of readily available and reliable tests provided platforms for understanding the spectrum and natural history of these diverse disorders. The recognition that hepatitis viruses B and C are the major causes of chronic hepatitis and cirrhosis and are important precursors to the development of hepatocellular carcinoma justify the emphasis on these agents.

The story of the evolution of knowledge regarding hepatitis B is a triumph of modern medicine and is amply described in this volume. In a generation the hepatitis B virus has been discovered and cloned, along with delineation of the natural histories of the several diseases it causes, creation of an effective vaccine, and develop-

ment of therapies which are effective in some. The ever-widening use of the hepatitis B vaccine is beginning to have the hoped-for impact on the prevalence of hepatitis B in many settings with impressive reductions in the risk to a neonate born to a mother who has hepatitis B and the virtual elimination of transfusion and occupationally-acquired hepatitis B.

The 1990s might well be described as the decade of hepatitis C. Following the identification of the hepatitis C virus as the 1990s began, a cascade of observations led to the recognition that hepatitis C is *the* major cause of chronic hepatitis and cirrhosis in the United States and that the progression of the disease is often clinically silent. Hepatitis C has been an overriding interest of many who care for patients with liver diseases. There is a story within a story with the recognition that the injuries caused by the hepatitis C virus and alcohol are additive. These observations may explain in part why there appears to be a subset of alcoholics who progress to cirrhosis. Furthermore it is established that hepatitis C is present worldwide in many genotypic forms and that the virus rapidly changes under immune pressure. This has led to further understanding of the virus while thus far thwarting efforts to develop an effective vaccine. Lofty goals for hepatology include the development of a vaccine to prevent hepatitis C and more effective therapies for the millions of patients who are already infected.

The characterization of the hepatitis A virus rapidly led to the development of effective vaccines which offer protection for susceptible individuals thereby reducing reliance on the use of gamma globulin which is expensive, uncomfortable for the patient, and offers only short-term benefit.

In the late 1990s a new viral challenge has been identified. The virus designated hepatitis G appears to be transmitted by blood and is found in some patients who have liver disease. However, despite extensive study there is no evidence that the hepatitis G virus *causes* liver disease. There are expectations transmitted in a name. A hepatitis virus should cause hepatitis! Even with the present information it may prove difficult to be confident that hepatitis G virus does not ever cause hepatitis (or as yet anything else) and that its presence should not be part of the criteria for exclusion of blood offered by a donor. Issues regarding the dilemmas posed by these observations are developed throughout this volume.

The other achievement that has redirected and expanded hepatology has been the development of clinically effective liver transplantation. We find ourselves with access to ever-safer operations, smoother postoperative courses, and fewer complications through the development of effective immunosuppressive regimens and more successful approaches to the management of complications both before and after the transplant is placed. A (if not the) major limitation of application of liver transplantation is the need for rationing based on an inadequate supply of organs. Notable advances in assessing candidacy and outcome have added several major disorders - alcohol-induced liver disease, hepatitis B, and small hepatocellular carcinomas - to the list of patients who are considered. The quest for organs has led to innovative approaches using living related donors, split livers, auxiliary liver approaches and the search for effective liver support devices.

There is much more to hepatology than viral hepatitis and liver transplantation. The advances in management of the major complications of liver disease, including spontaneous sepsis, ascites, bleeding from gastroesophageal varices, hepatorenal syndrome and hepatic encephalopathy, are fully addressed. Alcohol-induced liver disease remains a major cause of cirrhosis and the quest continues for approaches to minimize or even reverse liver injury in these patients. The important advances in the understanding of the diagnosis and natural history of the major cholestatic disorders including primary biliary cirrhosis, primary sclerosing cholangitis and drug-induced cholestasis are well presented. Non-alcoholic steatohepatitis, a rather recently described disorder, affects many and has generated considerable interest. Other important areas, including the impressive spectrum of liver diseases caused by therapeutic drugs as well as the liver problems found in patients who have Wilson's disease, alpha-1 antitrypsin deficiency, hemochromatosis, Budd-Chiari syndrome, and a host of other disorders, are well covered. In addition the chapters regarding the effects of systemic disease including sepsis, heart failure and HIV as well as the effects of surgery and pregnancy on the liver are carefully documented. There is much in the *Handbook of Liver Disease* to remind us of where we are in hepatology and to direct us to important areas in need of clarification.

Willis C. Maddrey

Preface

Advances in the science and practice of hepatology have been explosive in recent years. Among the recent developments in hepatology have been improved understanding of the molecular virology and epidemiology of the hepatitis viruses and new treatments for viral hepatitis, discovery of the genes that cause hereditary liver diseases, including the gene for Wilson's disease and a candidate gene for hemochromatosis, improved methods for the treatment of portal hypertension such as variceal band ligation and the transjugular intrahepatic portosystemic shunt, novel radiographic approaches to hepatobiliary imaging including magnetic resonance cholangiography, and widespread application of liver transplantation as routine treatment for acute and chronic liver failure.

These and other advances in the field of hepatology have been chronicled in a number of excellent encyclopedic textbooks. In the day-to-day practice of medicine, however, there is a need for access to the latest information at a moment's notice in a form that is concise, accurate and up-to-date. The aim of *Handbook of Liver Disease* is to provide such a resource to the busy practitioner. Using an outline format of focused paragraphs, short sentences, phrases and lists, accompanied by figures and tables, this book provides the clinician with concise, yet in-depth, summaries of the current practice of hepatology for each major disease entity. The purpose is not to provide just the bare essentials, but rather the whole story in an economical format, so that the richness and texture of the science that underlies current practice is readily apparent. While written with practicing gastroenterologists or hepatologists in mind, this book will also prove useful to primary care physicians, trainees in gastroenterology and internal medicine, and medical students rotating on a gastroenterology or hepatology service.

The list of contributors to this book reads like a "Who's Who" of hepatology, and we are grateful to each of them for their elegant and thoughtful contributions. We are particularly appreciative of Sheila Khullar and her colleagues at Churchill Livingstone for their outstanding support in helping us bring this book to fruition.

Lawrence S. Friedman
Emmet B. Keeffe

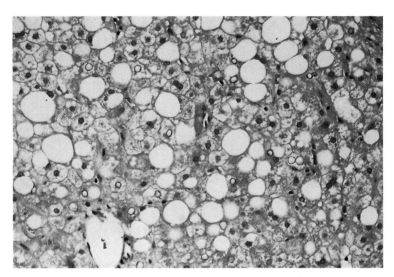

Fig. 6.1   Fatty liver (steatosis) in alcoholic liver disease. See page 90.

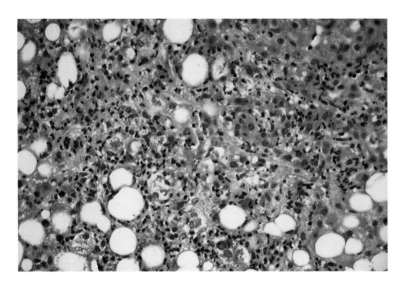

Fig. 6.2   Alcoholic hepatitis. See page 90.

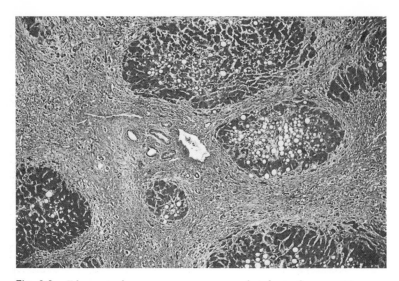

Fig. 6.3   Fibrogenic damage as a consequence of cirrhosis. See page 91.

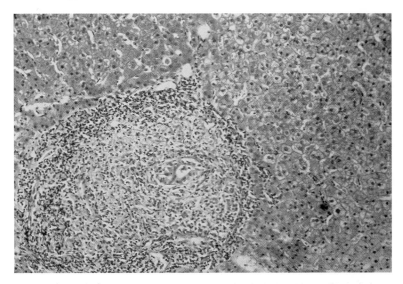

Fig. 14.3   Stage I florid bile duct lesion. A damaged bile duct is at the center of the lymphocytic granulomatous reaction (Masson trichrome, ×372). See page 202.

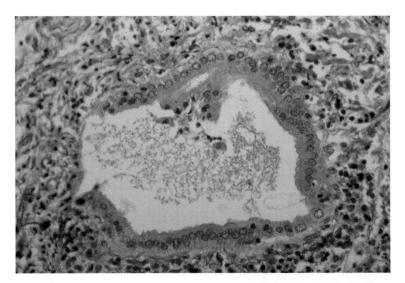

Fig. 14.4   Stage 1 florid bile duct lesion. The epithelial cell lining of a small duct is infiltrated with lymphocytes (H&E, ×930). See page 203.

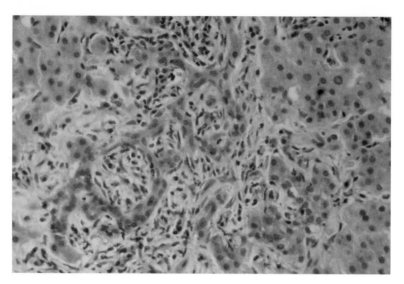

Fig. 14.5   Stage II primary biliary cirrhosis. Atypical bile duct hyperplasia is seen. There are tortuous bile ducts with inflammatory cell infiltrate consisting of primarily lymphocytes and few neutrophils (H&E, ×930). See page 203.

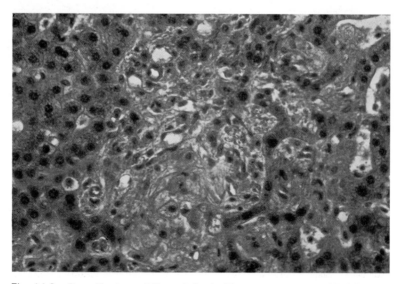

Fig. 14.6   Stage II primary biliary cirrhosis. There are no recognizable bile ducts in this portal triad (Masson trichrome, ×930). See page 204.

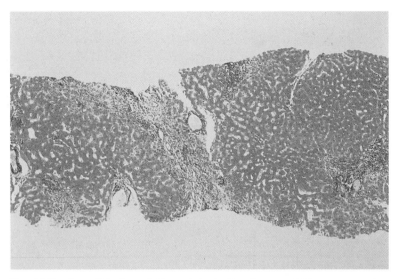

Fig. 14.7   Stage III primary biliary cirrhosis. Portal-to-portal fibrous septum is shown (Masson trichrome, ×162). See page 204.

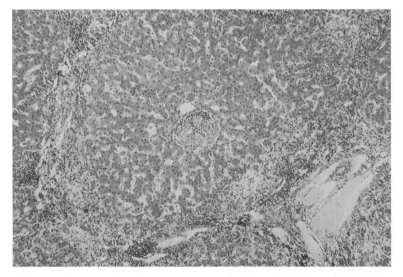

Fig. 14.8   Stage IV primary biliary cirrhosis. There is a noncaseating granuloma in the center of a nodule. Portal triads are linked by bands of connective tissue and inflammatory cells. (Masson trichrome, ×162). See page 205.

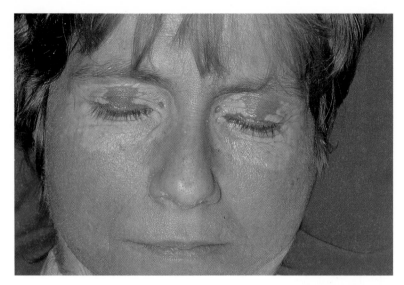

Fig. 14.9   Middle-aged woman with extensive bilateral xanthelasmas. See page 207.

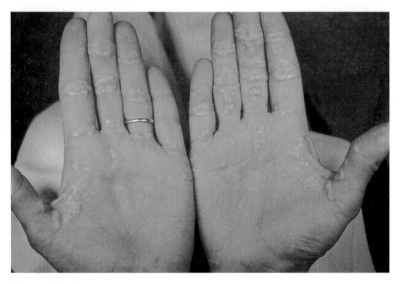

Fig. 14.10   Bilateral plantar xanthomas in the palms of a patient with PBC. See page 207.

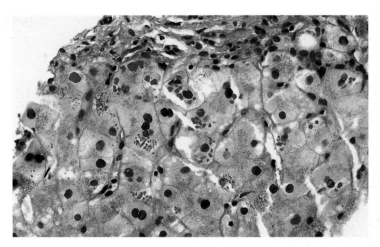

Fig. 18.1   Alpha-1 antitrypsin deficiency: periportal hepatocytes contain numerous eosinophilic, periodic acid–Schiff-positive, diastase-resistant globules (×110). See page 258.

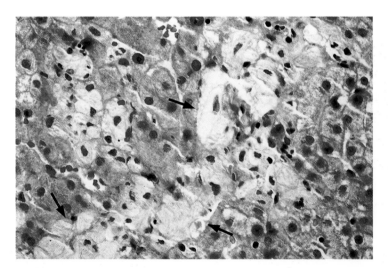

Fig. 18.2   Gaucher's disease: lipid-laden histiocytic cells (arrows) in the hepatic sinusoids (H&E, ×110). See page 261.

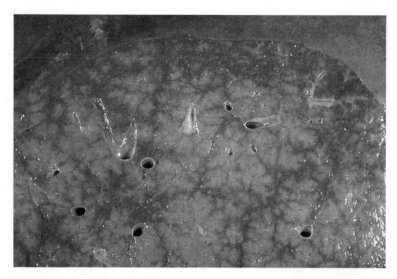

Fig. 20.3 Macroscopic appearance of the liver in congestive cardiac failure. See page 281.

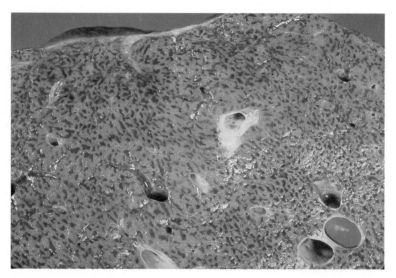

Fig. 20.4 Cut surface of the liver in congestive cardiac failure showing the "nutmeg appearance". See page 282.

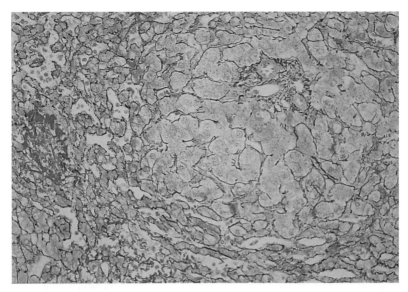

Fig. 20.5   Collapse of reticulin network around terminal hepatic veins and nodular transformation in congestive cardiac failure. See page 283.

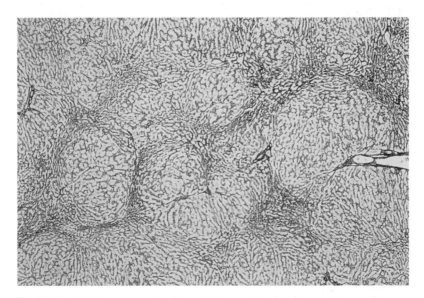

Fig. 20.6   Nodular regenerative hyperplasia associated with congestive cardiac failure. See page 284.

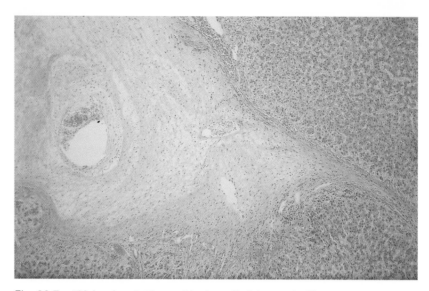

Fig. 20.7   Phlebosclerosis observed in the wall of the terminal hepatic vein in congestive cardiac failure. See page 284.

Assessment of liver function and diagnostic studies

PAUL MARTIN, M.D.   LAWRENCE S. FRIEDMAN, M.D.

Key Points

1 There is no ideal study or battery of studies to evaluate the many functions of the liver. The colloquial term "liver function tests" includes true tests of hepatic function (e.g., serum albumin), excretory function (e.g., bilirubin), and tests reflective of hepatic inflammatory activity (e.g., serum aminotransferases)

2 Abnormal liver function tests are often the first indication of liver disease. The widespread inclusion of liver function tests in routine blood work panels uncovers many patients with asymptomatic hepatic dysfunction

3 Normal or minimally abnormal liver function tests do not exclude serious liver disease, even advanced cirrhosis

4 Laboratory abnormalities may provide information about severity of liver damage and thus prognosis; sequential testing may allow assessment of the effectiveness of therapy

5 Liver biopsy remains the gold standard for detecting and determining the cause of liver disease. A variety of imaging studies are useful in detecting focal hepatic defects, the presence of portal hypertension, and abnormalities of the biliary tract

1   Routine Liver Function Tests

A   Serum bilirubin

1   Jaundice
- often first sign of liver disease
- clinically apparent when serum bilirubin exceeds 3 mg/dL

2   Metabolism
- breakdown product of hemoglobin and, to a lesser extent, heme-containing enzymes; 95% of bilirubin is derived from senescent red blood cells
- following red blood cell breakdown in reticuloendothelial system, heme is degraded by the enzyme heme oxygenase in endoplasmic reticulum
- bilirubin is released into blood and tightly bound to albumin; free or unconjugated bilirubin is lipid soluble, is not filtered by glomerulus, and does not appear in urine
- unconjugated bilirubin is taken up by the liver by a carrier-mediated process, attaches to intracellular storage proteins (ligands), and is conjugated by the enzyme uridine diphosphate (UDP)-glucuronyl transferase to form a diglucuronide and, to a lesser extent, a monoglucuronide. Conjugation makes bilirubin water soluble, and this form of bilirubin appears in urine. When serum bilirubin glucuronides are elevated, some binding to albumin occurs, leading to absence of bilirubinuria despite conjugated hyperbilirubinemia. This phenomenon explains delayed resolution of jaundice during recovery from acute liver disease
- conjugated bilirubin is excreted by active transport across the canalicular membrane into bile
- in bile, bilirubin enters the small intestine; in the distal ileum and colon bilirubin is hydrolyzed by beta-glucuronidases to form unconjugated bilirubin, which is then reduced by gut bacteria to colorless urobilinogens. A small amount is reabsorbed by the enterohepatic circulation and mostly excreted in the bile, with a smaller proportion undergoing urinary excretion
- urobilinogens or their colored derivatives urobilins are excreted in feces

3   Measurement of serum bilirubin
a   Van den Bergh reaction
- bilirubin molecule combines with diazotized sulfanilic acid to form chromogenic pyrrolase
- total serum bilirubin represents all bilirubin which reacts within 30 minutes in the presence of alcohol (an accelerating agent)
- direct serum bilirubin is the fraction which reacts with the diazo reagent in an aqueous medium within 1 minute and corresponds to conjugated bilirubin
- indirect serum bilirubin is determined by subtracting the direct reacting fraction from the total bilirubin level

b   More specific methods (e.g., high-pressure liquid chromatography) demonstrate that the van den Bergh reaction is imprecise and often overestimates conjugated

bilirubin. However, the van den Bergh method is the standard test employed by diagnostic laboratories

4 Classification of hyperbilirubinemia

  a Unconjugated (bilirubin always < 5 mg/dL)

  - overproduction: (presentation to liver of quantity of bilirubin which exceeds hepatic capacity for uptake and conjugation) – hemolysis, ineffective erythropoiesis, resorption of hematoma
  - defective uptake and storage of bilirubin: Gilbert's syndrome (idiopathic unconjugated hyperbilirubinemia)

  b Conjugated

  - hereditary: Dubin–Johnson, Rotor's syndromes
  - cholestasis (bilirubin is *not* a sensitive test of hepatic dysfunction)
    - intrahepatic: cirrhosis, hepatitis, primary biliary cirrhosis, drug induced
    - extrahepatic biliary obstruction: choledocholithiasis, stricture, neoplasm, biliary atresia, sclerosing cholangitis

  c Very high bilirubin levels

  - > 30 mg/100 mL: usually signifies hemolysis *plus* parenchymal liver disease or biliary obstruction; urinary excretion of conjugated bilirubin may help prevent even higher levels of hyperbilirubinemia
  - > 60 mg/100 mL: seen in patients with hemoglobinopathies (e.g., sickle cell anemia) who develop obstructive jaundice or acute hepatitis

5 Urine bilirubin and urobilinogen

  - bilirubinuria indicates an increase in serum conjugated (direct) bilirubin
  - urinary urobilinogen (rarely measured nowadays) is found in patients with hemolysis (increased production of bilirubin), gastrointestinal hemorrhage, or hepatocellular disease (impaired removal of urobilinogen from blood)
  - absence of urobilinogen from urine suggests interruption of enterohepatic circulation of bile pigments, as in complete bile duct obstruction
  - urobilinogen detection and quantification add little diagnostic information to evaluation of hepatic dysfunction

B   Serum aminotransferases

  1 Intracellular enzymes released from injured hepatocytes; most useful marker of hepatic injury (inflammation or cell necrosis)

  - aspartate aminotransferase (AST, SGOT (serum glutamic oxaloacetic transaminase))
    - found in cytosol and mitochondria
    - found in liver as well as skeletal muscle, heart, kidney, brain and pancreas
  - alanine aminotransferase (ALT, SGPT (serum glutamic pyruvic transaminase))
    - found in cytosol

– highest concentration in liver (more sensitive and specific than AST for liver inflammation and cell necrosis)

2 Clinical usefulness

- aminotransferase elevations are often the first biochemical abnormality detected in patients with viral or drug-induced hepatitis. Degree of elevation may correlate with extent of hepatic injury but is generally not of prognostic significance; in chronic hepatitis by convention elevated aminotransferase levels persist for longer than 6 months

- in alcoholic hepatitis AST is usually no more than 2–10 times the upper limit of normal and ALT is normal or near normal; relatively low ALT levels may result from a deficiency of pyridoxal 5-phosphate, a necessary cofactor for hepatic synthesis of ALT

- aminotransferase levels may be >3000 U/L in acute or chronic viral hepatitis or drug-induced liver injury; in fulminant hepatic failure or ischemic hepatitis (shock liver) higher values (>5000 U/L) may be found

- in obstructive jaundice, aminotransferase values are usually <500 U/L; rarely values may reach 3000 U/L in acute cholecystitis, followed by a rapid decline to normal

3 Low aminotransferase levels have been associated with uremia and possibly hemodialysis

C Serum alkaline phosphatase

1 Enzyme is bound to hepatic canalicular membrane; hepatic alkaline phosphatase is one of several alkaline phosphatase isoenzymes found in man. A variety of laboratory methods are available for measurement; thus, comparison of results obtained by different techniques may be inaccurate

2 Sensitive test for detection of biliary tract obstruction (a normal value is highly unusual in significant biliary obstruction); interference with bile flow may be intra- or extrahepatic

- increase in alkaline phosphatase appears to result from increased hepatic synthesis of the enzyme rather than leakage from bile duct cells or failure to clear circulating alkaline phosphatase. Because it is synthesized in response to obstruction, the level of alkaline phosphatase may be normal early in the course of acute suppurative cholangitis when the serum aminotransferases are already elevated

- increased bile acid concentrations may promote the synthesis of alkaline phosphatase

- serum alkaline phosphatase has a half-life of ~7 days; levels may remain elevated up to 1 week after relief of biliary obstruction and return of bilirubin to normal

3 Isolated elevation of alkaline phosphatase

a May indicate infiltrative liver disease: tumor, abscess, granulomas, amyloidosis

b Very high levels are associated with biliary obstruction, sclerosing cholangitis, primary biliary cirrhosis: evaluation generally includes hepatic ultrasonography, antimitochondrial antibody, and cholangiography

c Other sources of alkaline phosphatase: bone, intestine, kidney, placenta (different isoenzymes)

- striking elevations seen in Paget's disease of bone, osteoblastic bone metastases, small bowel obstruction, normal pregnancy
- hepatic origin of an elevated alkaline phosphatase level is suggested by simultaneous elevation of either serum 5'-nucleotidase or gamma-glutamyltranspeptidase (GGTP)
- hepatic alkaline phosphatase is more heat stable than bony alkaline phosphatase. Degree of overlap makes this test less useful than GGPT or 5'-nucleotidase

4 Mild elevations of alkaline phosphatase often seen in hepatitis and cirrhosis

5 Low levels of alkaline phosphatase may occur in hypothyroidism, pernicious anemia, zinc deficiency, congenital hypophosphatasia, and fulminant Wilson's disease.

D   Gamma glutamyltranspeptidase (GGTP)

1 Although present in many different organs, GGTP is found in particularly high concentrations in the epithelial cells lining biliary ductules

2 It is a very sensitive indicator of hepatobiliary disease but is not specific for hepatobiliary disease. Levels are elevated in other conditions, including renal failure, myocardial infarction, pancreatic disease, and diabetes mellitus

3 GGTP is inducible and thus levels may be elevated by ingestion of phenytoin or alcohol in the absence of other clinical evidence of liver disease

4 Because of its long half-life of 26 days, it is limited as a marker of surreptitious alcohol consumption

5 Its major clinical use is to exclude a bony source of an elevated serum alkaline phosphatase level

6 Many patients with an isolated serum GGTP elevation have no other evidence of liver disease; an extensive evaluation is usually not warranted

E   5'-Nucleotidase (5NT)

1 Found in the liver in association with canalicular and sinusoidal plasma membranes

2 Although 5NT is distributed in other organs, serum levels are felt to reflect hepatobiliary release by the detergent action of bile salts on plasma membranes

3 Serum 5NT levels correlate well with serum alkaline phosphatase levels. An elevated 5NT in association with an elevated alkaline phosphatase is specific for hepatobiliary dysfunction and is superior to GGTP in this regard

4 5NT measurement is useful in pediatric patients to differentiate physiologic elevation of serum alkaline phosphatase from hepatobiliary dysfunction

F   Lactate dehydrogenase (LDH)

Measurement of LDH and even the more specific isoenzyme (LDH5) adds little to evaluation of suspected hepatic dysfunction. High levels of LDH are seen in hepatocellular necrosis, shock liver, cancer, and hemolysis. The ALT : LDH ratio may have a role in differentiating acute viral hepatitis (>1.5) from shock liver and acetaminophen toxicity (<1.5)

G Serum proteins

Majority of proteins circulating in plasma are synthesized by the liver; levels indicate synthetic capability of the liver

1 **Albumin**
  - accounts for 65% of protein in serum
  - half-life of about 3 weeks
  - concentration in blood depends on albumin synthetic rate (normal = 12 g/day) and plasma volume
  - **hypoalbuminemia** may result from expanded plasma volume or decreased albumin synthesis. Frequently associated with ascites and expansion of extravascular albumin pool at expense of intravascular albumin pool. Common in chronic liver disease, indicator of severity; less common in acute liver disease. Not specific for liver disease; may also reflect glomerular, urinary, or gastrointestinal losses

2 **Globulins**
  - often increased in chronic liver disease but not specific for liver disease
  - pattern of elevation may suggest the etiology of underlying liver disease
    - elevated IgG: autoimmune hepatitis
    - elevated IgM: primary biliary cirrhosis

3 **Coagulation factors**
  a Most are synthesized by liver, including factors I (fibrinogen), II (prothrombin), V, VII, IX, and X and have much shorter half-lives than that of albumin. Factor VII decreases first due to its shortest half-life, followed by factors X and IX. Factor V is not vitamin K dependent, and measurement of it can help distinguish vitamin K deficiency from hepatocellular dysfunction in a patient with a prolonged prothrombin time. Serial measurement of factor V levels has been used to assess prognosis in fulminant hepatic failure; value less than 20% of normal portends a poor outcome without liver transplantation. Measurement of factor II (des-gamma-carboxyprothrombin) has also been used to assess liver function. Elevated levels are found in cirrhosis, hepatocellular carcinoma, and in patients on sodium warfarin (Coumadin), a vitamin K antagonist. Administration of vitamin K results in normalization of des-gamma-carboxyprothrombin in patients on Coumadin but not in those with cirrhosis

  b The prothrombin time is useful in assessing severity and prognosis of acute liver disease. The one-stage prothrombin time described by Quick measures the rate of conversion of prothrombin to thrombin after activation of the extrinsic coagulation pathway in the presence of a tissue extract (thromboplastin) and Ca^{++} ions. Deficiency of one or more of the liver-produced factors results in a prolonged prothrombin time.

  c Prolongation of the prothrombin time in cholestatic liver disease may result from vitamin K deficiency. Other explanations for a prolonged prothrombin time apart from hepatocellular disease or vitamin K deficiency include consumptive coagulopathies, inherited deficiencies of a coagulation factor, or medications that antagonize the prothrombin complex. Vitamin K deficiency as the cause of a prolonged prothrombin time can be determined by administration of Vitamin K

10 mg subcutaneously. Correction or improvement of the prothrombin time by at least 30% within 24 hours implies that hepatic synthetic function is intact

2   Assessment of Hepatic Metabolic Capacity

A variety of drugs which undergo purely hepatic metabolism and have predictable bio-availability have been used. Typically, a metabolite is measured in plasma, urine, or breath following intravenous or oral administration of the parent compound. These tests are not widely used in practice

A   Antipyrine clearance

1 Antipyrine is metabolized by cytochrome P-450 oxygenase with good absorption after oral administration and elimination entirely by the liver

2 It is not protein bound and thus unaffected by changes in serum proteins

3 In chronic liver disease there is good correlation between prolongation of the antipyrine half-life and disease severity as measured by the Child's class (see Ch. 9)

4 Its clearance is less impaired in acute liver disease and obstructive jaundice

5 Disadvantages of this test include its long half-life in serum, which requires multiple blood sampling, poor correlation with in vitro assessment of hepatic microsomal capacity, and alteration of antipyrine metabolism by increased age, diet, alcohol, smoking, and environmental exposure

B   Aminopyrine breath test

1 Based on detection of $^{14}CO_2$ in breath 2 hours after an oral dose of [^{14}C]dimethyl aminoantipyrine (aminopyrine), which undergoes hepatic metabolism

2 Excretion is diminished in patients with cirrhosis as well as acute liver disease

3 May be used as a prognosticator in patients with alcoholic hepatitis and in cirrhotics undergoing surgery

4 The enzymatic pathway of [^{14}C]aminopyrine is sensitive to deficiency of vitamin B_{12} and folate or amino acids as well as systemic infection or thyroid dysfunction

5 A limitation of the aminopyrine breath test is its lack of sensitivity in hepatic dysfunction due to cholestasis or extrahepatic obstruction

C   Caffeine clearance

1 Caffeine clearance after oral ingestion can be assessed by measuring levels in either saliva or serum; the accuracy appears similar to the [^{14}C]aminopyrine breath test without the need for a radioisotope

2 Results are clearly abnormal in clinically severe liver disease but the test is insensitive in mild hepatic dysfunction

3 Caffeine clearance decreases with age or cimetidine use and increases with cigarette smoking

D   Galactose elimination capacity

1 Galactose clearance from blood as a result of hepatic phosphorylation can be

determined following either intravenous or oral administration. Typically serial serum levels of galactose are obtained from 20 to 50 minutes after an intravenous bolus, with correction for urinary galactose excretion

2   Above a plasma concentration of 50 mg/dL removal of galactose reflects hepatic functional mass, whereas below this plasma level clearance reflects hepatic blood flow

3   [^{14}C]galactose is distributed in extracellular water and thus is affected by changes in volume

4   Galactose clearance is impaired in acute and chronic liver disease as well as metastatic hepatic neoplasms but is typically unaffected in obstructive jaundice

5   The oral galactose tolerance test incorporates [^{14}C]galactose with measurement of breath [^{14}C]O_2. The results of this breath test correlate with [^{14}C]aminopyrine testing

6   [^{14}C]galactose testing appears to be equivalent to the serum albumin in distinguishing healthy subjects from cirrhotics and is no more accurate than standard liver function tests in assessing prognosis in patients with chronic liver disease

7   Use of galactose elimination testing in one report was more accurate than the Mayo index in predicting a fatal outcome in patients with primary biliary cirrhosis

E   Lidocaine metabolite

1   Monoethylglycinexylidide (MEGX), a product of hepatic lidocaine metabolism, is easily measured by a fluorescence polarization immune assay 15 minutes after an intravenous dose of lidocaine

2   The test may offer prognostic information about the likelihood of life-threatening complications in cirrhotic patients

3   The test has also been used to assess the viability of donor liver allografts

4   Easy to use with few adverse reactions, although it may be unsuitable for some cardiac patients. Test results may be affected by simultaneous use of certain drugs metabolized by cytochrome P-450 3A4 and high bilirubin levels. Test results are affected by age and body mass and are higher in men than women

5   The role of the MEGX test remains an area of active investigation

3   Other Tests of Liver Function

A   Serum bile acids

1   Synthesized from cholesterol in the liver, conjugated to glycine or taurine, and excreted in the bile. They facilitate fat digestion and absorption within the small intestine. Bile acids recycle through the enterohepatic circulation; secondary bile acids form by the action of intestinal bacteria

2   Detection of an elevated level of serum bile acids is a sensitive marker of hepatobiliary dysfunction

3   A variety of methods are available to assay individual and total bile acids. Assaying an individual bile acid such as conjugated cholic acid is probably as useful as measuring total bile acid concentration

4   A number of different bile acid tests have been described, including fasting and

postprandial levels and determination of levels after a bile acid load, either oral or intravenous

5 The requirement for multiple specimens in dynamic tests of bile acid levels makes them cumbersome

6 Normal bile acid levels in the presence of hyperbilirubinemia suggests hemolysis or Gilbert's syndrome

B Urea synthesis

1 Hepatic metabolism of nitrogen from protein results in urea production. Urea is distributed in total body water and is excreted in urine or diffuses into the intestine, where urease-producing bacteria hydrolyze it to CO_2 and ammonia

2 The rate of urea synthesis can be calculated from the urinary urea excretion and blood urea nitrogen after estimation of body water, with correction for gastrointestinal hydrolysis of urea

3 An alternate kinetic method using ^{14}C-labeled urea has been described

4 The rate of urea synthesis is significantly reduced in cirrhosis and correlates with the Child score, although it is insensitive for detecting well-compensated cirrhosis

C Bromsulphalein (BSP)

Clearance of BSP after an intravenous bolus was used in the past as a measure of hepatic function. The most accurate information was obtained by the 45-minute retention test and initial fractional rate of disappearance. BSP testing has fallen out of favor due to reports of severe allergic reactions, lack of accuracy in distinguishing hepatocellular from obstructive jaundice, and the availability of simpler tests of liver function

D Indocyanine green

This dye is removed by the liver after intravenous injection. A blood level is obtained 20 minutes after administration. Compared with BSP its hepatic clearance is more efficient, and it is nontoxic. Its accuracy in assessing liver dysfunction is no better than standard Child scoring. Its major role is as a measure of hepatic blood flow

4 Liver Biopsy

Remains the definitive test to confirm the diagnosis of specific liver diseases such as Wilson's disease or hemochromatosis, assess prognosis in many forms of parenchymal liver disease such as chronic viral hepatitis, and evaluate allograft dysfunction in liver transplant recipients

A Indications for liver biopsy (Table 1.1)

B Contraindications to liver biopsy (Table 1.2)

A bleeding time should be obtained in patients with renal insufficiency to detect platelet dysfunction, which may require correction by infusion of arginine vasopressin (DDAVP) (0.3 μg/kg in 50 mL N saline i.v.) immediately prior to biopsy. Patients should be cautioned to avoid agents such as aspirin or nonsteroidal anti-inflammatory drugs, which may also produce platelet dysfunction, for 10–14 days prior to elective liver biopsy

Assessment of abnormal liver function tests
Diagnosis and prognosis of chronic hepatitis and/or cirrhosis
Confirmation and prognosis of alcoholic liver disease
Detection of systemic disorders involving the liver, including fever of unknown origin
Assessment and severity of drug-induced liver injury
Confirmation of suspected hepatic malignancy, primary or metastatic
Confirmation of multisystem infiltrative disorders
Screening of relatives of patients with familial diseases
Tissue for culture
Evaluation of response to therapies for liver diseases (e.g., Wilson's disease, hemochromatosis, autoimmune hepatitis, chronic viral hepatitis)
Exclusion of graft rejection, reinfection, or ischemia after liver transplant

(Table 1.1: Indications for liver biopsy)

Absolute	Relative

Severe coagulopathy
  Prothrombin time >3 seconds prolonged
  Platelets <60 000/mm³
  Abnormal bleeding time
	Large amount of ascites
	Infection in right pleural cavity
	Cholangitis, biliary obstruction

Suspected echinococcal disease	
Presumed hemangioma	
Uncooperative patient	

(Table 1.2: Contraindications to liver biopsy)

C   Technique

1 Liver biopsy can be safely performed as an outpatient if none of the contraindications noted above are present and the patient can be adequately observed for at least 6 hours following the procedure, with access to hospitalization if necessary (required in up to 5% of patients)

2 Local anesthetic is infiltrated subcutaneously and into the intercostal muscle and peritoneum. A short-acting sedative may be given to allay anxiety

3 A transthoracic approach is standard; a subcostal approach should only be attempted with ultrasound guidance

4 The biopsy is performed at end-expiration; a variety of needles can be used, including a biopsy "gun"

5 The biopsy site is tamponaded by having the patient lie on his or her right side or by pressure from a sandbag

6 When the standard approach is contraindicated, as by coagulopathy, a transjugular route may be feasible

7 Focal hepatic defects are best biopsied under radiologic guidance (see below)

D Complications

1 Postbiopsy pain with or without radiation to the right shoulder occurs in up to 15% of patients. Vasovagal reactions are also common. Severe complications are rare

2 Bleeding is the most serious complication. Increasing age, presence of hepatic malignancy, and the number of passes made are predictors of the likelihood of bleeding, as is the use of a cutting needle rather than a suction needle

3 Patients who have clinical evidence of hemodynamically significant bleeding, persistent pain unrelieved by acetaminophen, or other clinical evidence of a significant complication need hospital admission. Pneumothorax may require a chest tube, whereas serious bleeding may be controlled by selective embolization at angiography or, if necessary, ligation of the right hepatic artery or hepatic resection

5 Hepatic Imaging

A variety of sophisticated imaging modalities are now available to assess the hepatic parenchyma, vasculature, and biliary tree. The choice of initial and subsequent studies should be determined by the clinical scenario in consultation with a radiologist (Table 1.3)

A Plain abdominal x-rays and barium studies

1 Plain abdominal x-rays generally add little to the diagnostic evaluation of liver disease. However, on occasion calcification can be detected, due usually to gallstones, echinococcal cysts, or old lesions of tuberculosis or histoplasmosis. Tumors or vascular lesion may also be calcified

2 A barium swallow is significantly less sensitive than endoscopic evaluation to detect varices

B Ultrasound

The initial radiological study of choice for many hepatobiliary disorders. It is relatively inexpensive, does not require ionizing radiation, and is portable so it can be used at the bedside. Ultrasound depicts interfaces in tissue of different acoustic properties

1 With B-mode, or "gray-scale," ultrasound the reflection of high-frequency sound pulse is displayed as shades of gray, whereas with "real-time" ultrasound demonstration of physiologic events such as arterial pulsation is possible due to the rapidity of scanning

2 Ultrasound cannot penetrate gas or bone, which may preclude adequate examination of the viscera. Furthermore, increased resolution is generally at the expense of decreased tissue penetration

3 Ultrasound is better at detecting focal lesions than parenchymal disease

4 Hepatic masses as small as 1 cm may be detected by ultrasound and cystic lesions may be distinguished from solid ones

Clinical problem	Initial imaging study	Supplemental imaging studies (If necessary)
Jaundice	US	CT, if dilated ducts, to detect obstructing lesion or, if suspicious of a mass in the pancreas or porta hepatis, ERCP to determine site and exact cause of dilated ducts
Hepatic parenchymal disease	US MRI	Doppler US, color Doppler US, or MRI with flow sequences if a vascular abnormality is suspected and in some instances of portal hypertension
Screening for liver mass	US	
Characterizing known liver mass		
Suspicious malignancy	US- or CT-directed biopsy	CT portograms, MRI, intraoperative US
Suspicious benign lesion	Nuclear medicine scan (e.g., 99m Tc-labeled red blood cells scan for suspected hemangioma)	US- or CT-directed biopsy
Suspicious abscess	US or CT US- or CT-directed aspiration	Nuclear medicine abscess scan (gallium or ^{111}In-labeled white blood cell scan)
Suspected biliary duct abnormalities	US to detect biliary dilatation, stones, or mass ERCP or THC to define ductal anatomy	CT or endoscopic ultrasonography to detect stones or cause of extrinsic compression

US, ultrasound; CT, computed tomography; MRI, magnetic resonance imaging;
ERCP, endoscopic retrograde cholangiopancreatography; THC, transhepatic cholangiography

(Table 1.3: Approach to use of imaging studies)

5 Ultrasound can also facilitate percutaneous biopsy of solid hepatic masses, drainage of hepatic abscesses, or paracentesis of loculated ascites

6 Ultrasound with the Doppler technique is used to assess the patency of hepatic and portal vasculature in liver transplant candidates and recipients

C   Computed tomography (CT)

1 CT scanning is generally more accurate than ultrasound in defining hepatic anatomy, normal and pathological

2 Detects small differences in the attenuation of x-ray beams. Oral contrast to define bowel lumen and intravenous contrast to enhance vascular structures increases anatomical definition

3 Spiral or helical CT is a more recent refinement which allows faster imaging at the

peak of intravenous contrast enhancement. CT generally is limited by cost, radiation exposure, and lack of portability

4   CT with intravenous contrast is an excellent way to identify and characterize hepatic masses. Cystic and solid masses can be distinguished, as can abscesses. Contrast enhancement after an intravenous bolus may be accurate enough to identify cavernous hemangiomas, which have a characteristic appearance. Neoplastic vascular invasion may also be identified

5   CT portography with intravenous contrast administered via a catheter in the superior mesenteric artery enhances the sensitivity of lesion detection within the liver

6   Lipiodol is preferentially taken up and retained by hepatocellular carcinomas and can be used as a contrast agent to detect small neoplastic lesions ($\leq$5 mm)

7   CT can also suggest the presence of cirrhosis and portal hypertension as well as changes consistent with fatty liver or hemochromatosis

D   Magnetic resonance imaging (MRI)

1   Relies on the magnetic properties of protons present in various parts of the body. A T1 image measures the rate at which the protons realign themselves after a pulse of radiowaves, whereas a T2 image measures the rate at which the energy emitted by the radiowave declines. MRI does not require ionizing radiation and can provide images in a number of planes. MRI provides excellent resolution between tissues containing differing amounts of fat and water

2   MRI is an excellent method of evaluating blood flow and can detect hepatic iron overload

3   It is not portable, is currently expensive, and has a slow imaging time, so that physiologic events such as peristasis can result in blurred images. The magnetic field used precludes imaging in patients with pacemakers or other metallic devices

4   MRI is the imaging study of choice in confirming the presence of vascular lesions, notably hemangiomas. It is also useful in the differentiation of a regenerating nodule from hepatocellular carcinoma; on a T2-weighted image the nodule's signal intensity is equivalent to that of normal hepatic parenchyma, whereas that of carcinoma is higher

5   The role of MRI in assessing diffuse and focal liver disease continues to evolve MRI cholangiography is an alternative to diagnostic endoscopic cholangiopancreatography

E   Radioisotope scanning

1   Specific isotopes used are preferentially taken up by hepatocytes, Kupffer's cells, or neoplastic or inflammatory cells. Radioisotope scanning is particularly helpful in the assessment of suspected acute cholecystitis (see Ch. 32), although for parenchymal and focal liver disease, ultrasound and CT have largely superseded nuclear medicine studies

2   Technetium 99m-labeled sulfur colloid is used for anatomic evaluation of the liver and is taken up by Kupffer's cells. Any process such as a neoplasm, cyst, or abscess which replaces those cells results in a "cold" area. Lesions greater than 2 cm in diameter can usually be detected

3   Diffuse hepatic disease which leads to disrupted hepatic blood flow and reduced

reticuloendothelial function will result in diminished hepatic radioisotope uptake with diversion of isotope to bone marrow and spleen. Occasionally, the hepatic uptake can be patchy, resulting in false-positive mass effects

4 The caudate lobe of its liver, because of its independent venous drainage, may be unaffected by obstruction of the hepatic vein in Budd–Chiari syndrome (see Ch. 19) and may thus may have preferential uptake of isotope

5 Indium-labeled colloid is also taken up by Kupffer's cells but involves more radiation exposure than technetium. Newer techniques include single-photon emission computed tomography (SPECT), which allows visualization of the cross-sectional distribution of a radioisotope, and positron emission tomography (PET), which provides information about blood flow and tissue metabolism

References

1 Crawford JL, Gollan JL. *Bilirubin metabolism and pathophysiology of jaundice*. In: Schiff L, Schiff ER (eds). *Diseases of the Liver*. (Philadelphia: Lippincott, 1993) 42–84

2 Edelman RR, Warach S. *Magnetic resonance imaging*. (N Engl J Med 1993) 328: 785–91

3 Ferrucci JT. *Liver tumor imaging: current concepts*. (AJR 1990) 155: 473–84

4 Friedman LS, Martin P, Munoz SJ. *Liver function tests and the objective evaluation of the patient with liver disease*. In: Zakim D, Boyer TD (eds). *Hepatology: A Textbook of Liver Disease*. (Philadelphia: Saunders, 1996) 791–833

5 McGill DB, Rakela J, Zinmeister AR. *A 21 year experience with major hemorrhage after percutaneous liver biopsy*. (Gastroenterology 1990) 99: 1396–1400

6 Morgan DJ, Elliott SL, Ghabrial H, Smallwood RA. *Quantitative liver function tests: a realizable goal?* (Can J Gastroenterol 1991) 5: 77–85

7 Moseley RH. *Evaluation of abnormal liver function tests*. (Med Clin N Am 1996) 80: 887–906

8 Rubin RA, Mitchell DG. *Evaluation of the solid hepatic mass*. (Med Clin N Am 1996) 80: 907–28

9 Saini S. *Imaging of the hepatobiliary tract*. (N Engl J Med 1997) 336: 1889–94

10 Tygstrup N. *Assessment of liver function: principles and practice*. (J Gastroenterol Hepatol 1990) 5: 468–82

11 Zeman RK, Fox SH, Silverman PM, et al. *Helical (spiral) CT of the abdomen*. (AJR 1993) 160: 719–25

Acute liver failure

GABRIEL GARCIA, M.D.   EMMET B. KEEFFE, M.D.

▼

Key Points

1 Acute liver failure is a syndrome of rapidly evolving hepatic synthetic dysfunction that is complicated by coagulopathy and, in advanced stages, hepatic encephalopathy

2 Acute liver failure is commonly divided into two subgroups: (1) fulminant hepatic failure, with hepatic encephalopathy developing within 8 weeks of the onset of illness (or at least 2 weeks after the onset of jaundice); and (2) subfulminant hepatic failure, with hepatic encephalopathy developing 8 weeks to 6 months after the onset of illness (or 2 weeks to 3 months after the onset of jaundice)

3 Fulminant hepatic failure is most often caused by acute hepatitis A, acute hepatitis B or acetaminophen overdose, while subfulminant hepatic failure is more often caused by drug-induced hepatotoxicity or unknown factors (commonly designated as non-A, non-B hepatitis)

4 The major complications of acute liver failure that require preventive measures or specific therapy include cerebral edema, coagulopathy, renal failure, hypoglycemia, and infection

5 Management of acute liver failure is directed toward aggressive supportive care in an intensive care unit and determination of whether or not liver transplantation is indicated

6 Application of prognostic criteria associated with death from acute liver failure is critical in determining which patients are likely to recover and which are likely to die and should be considered for liver transplantation

▲

1 Definitions

A Acute liver failure[1,2]

This is a general term applied to the rapid development of hepatic synthetic dysfunction associated with significant coagulopathy, usually defined by a prothrombin time or factor V level less than 50% of normal. The designation severe acute liver failure is applied when hepatic encephalopathy develops

B Fulminant hepatic failure (FHF)

This is a term that was introduced by Trey and Davidson in 1970 for patients who met the following criteria:

> Acute onset of liver disease with coagulopathy
> Development of hepatic encephalopathy within 8 weeks of the onset of illness
> No prior evidence of liver disease

Other investigators[3] have based the definition of FHF on the interval between the first detection of jaundice, rather than hepatic illness, and the appearance of encephalopathy; they use a maximum of 2 weeks, rather than 8 weeks, as the time interval between the onset of jaundice and encephalopathy

C Subfulminant hepatic failure

This is used to designate a further subgroup of patients with acute liver failure characterized by the later development of hepatic encephalopathy, i.e., 2 weeks (or 8 weeks) to 3 months (or 6 months) after the onset jaundice (or illness). In this setting, there is a greater likelihood that the cause of liver failure is either drug-induced hepatotoxicity or indeterminate (commonly called non-A, non-B hepatitis), or that the apparent acute liver failure actually represents an acute presentation of a chronic liver disease, such as Wilson's disease or autoimmune hepatitis. In this subgroup of patients:

1 Sequelae of portal hypertension are more often present
2 Cerebral edema occurs less commonly
3 The prognosis is worse than that of FHF

D New terminology

More recently a new, but yet to be accepted, terminology was introduced by investigators at King's College Hospital[4] based on the interval between the onset of jaundice and encephalopathy:

1 **Hyperacute liver failure**, with an interval of less than 7 days
2 **Acute liver failure**, with an interval of between 8 and 28 days
3 **Subacute liver failure**, with an interval of between 4 and 12 weeks

This may be the best classification for distinguishing patients with a distinct clinical course characterized (paradoxically) by a greater frequency of cerebral edema but a better prognosis (shortest interval between jaundice and encephalopathy), as in acetaminophen hepato-toxicity or fulminant hepatitis A or B, from those with a worse prognosis (longest duration between jaundice and encephalopathy), as in patients with drug-induced liver injury or non-A, non-B hepatitis

2 Epidemiology

There are few reliable data on the incidence of acute liver failure or FHF because there is no standard ICD-9 code specific for FHF. Using data from deaths, hospitalizations with death certificates, and discharge diagnoses, the number of deaths from FHF is estimated to be 3.5 per million with a hospitalization rate of 31.2 per million. Based on the Centers for Disease Control and Prevention Viral Hepatitis Surveillance Program and Sentinel Counties Study data, the total number of annual deaths due to acute viral hepatitis in the United States is approximately 2000, of which approximately half are due to hepatitis B, one third to non-A, non-B hepatitis, and one sixth to hepatitis A

3 Causes

The most common causes of acute liver failure are viral hepatitis and drugs (Table 2.1). The list of reported causes of acute liver failure is considerably longer (Table 2.2). About 20–40% of cases do not have an identifiable etiology and may be due to viral or non-viral causes. The identification of the cause of acute liver failure is important because the etiology has a bearing on prognosis and management

	Frequency (%)
Hepatitis A	0–8
Hepatitis B	3–47
Acetaminophen overdose	2–56
Other drug or toxin	5–18
Other identified cause	1–14
Unidentified cause[a]	19–44

[a]Often designated non-A, non-B hepatitis
Adapted from Lidofsky (1995)[5]

(Table 2.1: Causes of fulminant hepatic failure)

4 Clinical Presentation

A   Viral hepatitis (see also Chs 3 and 4)

  1 **Hepatitis A.** Approximately 75,000 cases of icteric hepatitis A occur annually in the United States, with a case–fatality rate of 0.2–0.4%. FHF has particularly been

Viral hepatitis	Hepatitis A virus
	Hepatitis B virus
	Hepatitis C virus
	Hepatitis D virus
	Hepatitis E virus
Hepatitis due to other viruses	Herpesviruses 1, 2 and 6
	Adenovirus
	Epstein–Barr virus
	Cytomegalovirus
Drug-induced liver injury	Acetaminophen overdose
	Idiosyncratic drug reactions
Toxins	*Amanita phalloides*
	Organic solvents
	Phosphorus
Metabolic	Acute fatty liver of pregnancy
	Reye's syndrome
Vascular events	Acute circulatory failure
	Budd–Chiari syndrome
	Veno-occlusive disease
	Heat stroke
Miscellaneous	Wilson's disease
	Autoimmune hepatitis
	Massive infiltration with tumor
	Liver transplantation with primary graft nonfunction

Adapted from Keeffe (1996)[6]   *(Table 2.2: Causes of acute liver failure)*

observed in intravenous drug users and the elderly, with patients > age 50 years
having an overall mortality rate of 3%. This disease is now preventable with hepatitis
A vaccine

2 **Hepatitis B**. Approximately 100,000 cases of icteric hepatitis B occur annually in
the United States, with a case–fatality rate of 1.0–1.2%. Some cases may be negative
for hepatitis B surface antigen (HBsAg) because of infection by mutant strains of the
virus that cause infection and disease but do not produce HBsAg or hepatitis B e
antigen (HBeAg). It has been suggested that acute infection with the precore mutant
strain of hepatitis B virus (HBV) that is unable to synthesize HBeAg is more
frequently associated with a fulminant presentation than is acute wild-type HBV
infection. The detection in serum or liver of HBV DNA by polymerase chain reaction
tests may allow a diagnosis of fulminant HBV infection in patients infected with
mutant forms of the virus. Rapid withdrawal of immunosuppressive drugs or
chemotherapy may also precipitate FHF. Hepatitis B is preventable with vaccination

3 **Hepatitis C**. It has been difficult to implicate the hepatitis C virus (HCV) as a cause
of fulminant hepatitis; however, there has been a recently published, well-
characterized case of FHF following transfusion-associated hepatitis C. Patients with
non-A, non-B FHF only rarely have HCV RNA detectable in serum. Occasionally

chronic HCV infection has been implicated as a co-factor in fulminant HBV infection

4 **Hepatitis D** Hepatitis D virus (HDV), or the delta agent, is a defective virus which requires simultaneous infection with HBV for pathogenicity. Patients with HBV infection who are coinfected or superinfected with HDV more frequently present with fulminant hepatitis. Although HDV infection is present in <10% of all cases of acute hepatitis B, more than half of HBsAg-positive cases of FHF are due to HDV rather than HBV infection alone

5 **Hepatitis E.** This waterborne calcivirus is prone to cause fulminant hepatitis with death rates as high as 20% in pregnant women, particularly those infected during the third trimester. In the United States, occasional cases of hepatitis E have been seen in travelers returning from endemic areas

6 **Hepatitis G.** The newly discovered hepatitis G virus (HGV) has been linked with cases of fulminant hepatitis in Japan, but studies are limited and cause and effect have not been established between HGV and FHF

7 **Cytomegalovirus (CMV).** A rare cause of fulminant hepatitis, which may be seen in CMV-seronegative liver transplant recipients of CMV-positive organs when patients are heavily immunosuppressed. Ganciclovir therapy is appropriate and may be beneficial

8 **Herpes simplex and herpes zoster viruses.** Potential causes of fulminant hepatitis, particularly in immunosuppressed hosts. The presence of cutaneous lesions and profound disseminated intravascular coagulation are early signs of infection. Acyclovir therapy is indicated when the disease is recognized

9 **Parvovirus B19.** The presence of parvovirus B19-specific DNA sequences in patients with FHF, particularly those with associated aplastic anemia, suggests a causal role for this virus in fulminant non-A, non-B hepatitis

B   Drug or toxin-induced FHF (see also Ch. 8)

May occur because of intrinsic, predictable hepatotoxicity of a drug, such as acetaminophen, or as an idiosyncratic reaction to a prescribed drug, such as isoniazid. The pathologic spectrum of drug-induced hepatotoxicity is broad, but massive liver cell necrosis or microvesicular fatty change are the most common histopathologic findings in patients with FHF.

1 **The most common drug associated with FHF is acetaminophen, which causes a dose-related predictable liver injury**
   - FHF usually occurs from a massive ingestion of acetaminophen as a suicide attempt. In acute ingestion, acetaminophen-induced FHF usually requires a total dose of >15 g to cause a severe or fatal outcome
   - Acetaminophen hepatotoxicity may also occur without suicide intent secondary to chronic daily use of 3–8 g of acetaminophen in patients with alcoholism (a syndrome termed "therapeutic misadventure")
   - Acetaminophen toxicity is potentiated by substances such as alcohol or barbiturates which induce the microsomal P-450 drug-metabolizing enzymes and promote a greater fraction of acetaminophen to be metabolized to its toxic intermediate, N-acetyl-p-benzoquinoneimine (NAPQI). In addition, alcoholism with poor dietary intake may be associated with depleted hepatic stores of

glutathione, which conjugates NAPQI, and this mechanism also appears to be important in acetaminophen-induced hepatotoxicity in alcoholics

Following massive ingestion of acetaminophen in the setting of suicide intent, a characteristic clinical syndrome evolves:

- initial phase (0–24 hours):
  - anorexia, nausea, vomiting
- latent phase (24–48 hours):
  - resolution of gastrointestinal symptoms
  - elevated serum aminotransferase levels
- overt hepatocellular necrosis phase (>48 hours):
  - progressive abnormalities of liver function tests, jaundice, encephalopathy
  - renal failure may occur

> Acetaminophen hepatotoxicity should be considered in:
> - any patient following suicide gesture
> - any patient with acute liver injury
> - habitual users of alcohol who ingest "therapeutic" doses of acetaminophen
> - homeless alcoholics
> - malnourished patients

The history of ingestion, amount of ingestion, and timing of ingestion are often inaccurate or vague. It may be particularly difficult to make a diagnosis in emotionally disturbed patients who hide their ingestion during the latent phase.

Improvement of hepatic function often occurs within days of the onset of acetaminophen hepatotoxicity, but complete recovery may take weeks. Damage may be permanent to other organs, such as the kidneys

2 Many other toxins and drugs have been implicated in FHF; a partial list of specific interest follows:
- *Amanita* and *Galerina* species of mushrooms contain two toxins: phallotoxins (cyclic heptapeptide inhibitors of actin polymerization/depolymerization) and amatoxins (cyclic octapeptides that inhibit RNA polymerase II). The former toxins cause an early cholera-like diarrheal illness; the latter extensively damage liver, intestinal epithelium, and renal tubular cells. Amatoxins are filtered efficiently by the glomerulus and undergo extensive enterohepatic circulation
- chlorinated hydrocarbons such as trichloroethylene generally affect people working in manufacturing with heavy exposure to industrial cleaning solvents. The severity of the illness is related to the proximity and duration of exposure; mild hepatotoxicity improves on withdrawal from the industrial site
- dapsone causes a severe hypersensitivity reaction (the sulfone syndrome)

characterized by fever, exfoliative dermatitis, hemolytic anemia, atypical lymphocytosis, jaundice, and, rarely, FHF
- valproate and high-dose parenteral tetracyclines may cause severe microvesicular fatty liver
- other drugs that should be considered in cases of FHF: amiodarone, carbamazepine, disulfiram, flutamide, halothane, imipramine, isoniazid, lisinopril, niacin (particularly sustained-release preparations), phenytoin, propylthiouracil, and sulfonamides.

C   Autoimmune hepatitis (see Ch. 5)

Although the typical patient with autoimmune hepatitis presents with symptoms and signs of chronic liver disease, the rare fulminant presentation is important to recognize early so that stabilization of the disease with immunosuppressive drugs may be attempted. Hyperglobulinemia, the detection of serum autoantibodies (antinuclear and anti-smooth muscle antibodies), and a characteristic liver biopsy (when safe to obtain) showing severe chronic hepatitis are typical and can establish the diagnosis

D   Wilson's disease (see Ch. 17)

A fulminant presentation of Wilson's disease is characterized by very high serum bilirubin levels, due in part to hemolysis, and a low or normal alkaline phosphatase level. Kayser–Fleischer rings are usually present and are a key early diagnostic sign. Liver transplantation should be performed emergently once the patient is stable

E   Hepatic vein thrombosis or veno-occlusive disease (see Ch. 19)

Obstruction of the major hepatic veins can be related to an inferior vena caval web or thrombosis associated with a hypercoagulable state. Common causes of hepatic vein thrombosis include a myeloproliferative syndrome, which is often occult, and deficiencies of factor V Leyden, protein C, protein S, or antithrombin III. Veno-occlusive disease is most often related to the chemotherapeutic conditioning regimen used in preparation for bone marrow transplantation; radiation injury and herbal preparations (crotolaria tea) are uncommon causes

F   Ischemic hepatic injury (see Ch. 20)

Hepatic ischemia may be cardiogenic and associated with shock or secondary to chronic right heart or biventricular failure associated with coronary artery disease, valvular heart disease, or pericardial disease. Other rare causes of ischemic liver injury include extreme environmental heat (heat stroke) and status epilepticus

G   Reye's syndrome (see Ch. 23)

Reye's syndrome is an acute illness characterized by vomiting, increased intracranial pressure, and microvesicular fatty liver. Early aggressive therapy of cerebral edema is key to management

H   Acute fatty liver of pregnancy (see Ch. 21)

The sudden onset of jaundice, encephalopathy, and pre-eclampsia in the third trimester of pregnancy signals this potentially lethal disease

I   Indeterminate or non-A, non-B FHF

From 20% to 40% of cases of FHF are unexplained after clinical history and standard laboratory investigation. Sensitive tests HBV DNA may identify a few patients with HBsAg-negative "occult" HBV infection

5   Complications

The clinical syndrome of FHF is the result of hepatocellular injury and its effects on the physiology of multiple organs. Predictable effects include synthetic dysfunction (coagulation factors, albumin, glucose) and excretory failure (bilirubin, urea, drugs)

A   Encephalopathy (see Ch. 13)

This is the hallmark of FHF. Once grade 3 or 4 coma develops, the incidence of multiorgan failure and death is high. The prognosis is poor if the period of time between the onset of jaundice and encephalopathy exceeds 7 days

Withdrawal of dietary protein and blood from the gut, and lactulose therapy, may be beneficial in early stages of hepatic encephalopathy, but these measures are not helpful in grade 3 or 4 encephalopathy

The clinician must distinguish the abnormal mental status that results from hepatic encephalopathy from that caused by cerebral edema, since the management and prognosis are different

B   Cerebral edema

Cerebral edema is the most common identifiable cause of death in FHF. It occurs in >75% of FHF patients with grade 4 encephalopathy. This complication is seen more commonly in patients with rapid onset of liver failure and is unusual (<10%) in patients with late-onset or subfulminant hepatic failure

The pathogenesis of cerebral edema is unknown, but there is evidence for both a vasogenic and a cytotoxic mechanism of injury. The presence of cerebral edema can impair cerebral blood flow and cause an irreversible ischemic neurologic deficit

1 General measures to treat cerebral edema
- decrease tactile stimulation
- raise head of bed 10°
- avoid hypotension, hypoxia, hypercarbia

2 Specific measures to treat cerebral edema
- mannitol (0.4 g/kg i.v. bolus) every hour until ICP improves; ineffective in patient with renal failure unless coupled with continuous arteriovenous hemodialysis or ultrafiltration or in patients with a serum osmolarity >310 mosm/L
- hyperventilation (consider in stage 3 or 4 coma)
- corticosteroids are ineffective

Cerebral edema is diagnosed clinically by the presence of systemic hypertension, hyperventilation, abnormal pupillary reflexes, muscular rigidity, and, late in the course, decerebrate posturing. Papilledema is rare, and impairment of brain stem function is a late finding

In patients with grade 3 or 4 encephalopathy, intracranial pressure (ICP) may be monitored. Cerebral perfusion pressure (mean arterial pressure minus ICP) is the key measurement. Attempts should be made to raise the blood pressure and lower the ICP to maintain a cerebral perfusion pressure >50 mmHg.

C   Renal failure

Renal failure is common and early in severe acetaminophen hepatotoxicity, but late and usually preceded by moderate fluid retention in patients with FHF of other etiologies. **Early renal failure in patients with acetaminophen hepatotoxicity and FHF is associated with a 95% mortality without liver transplantation**

Current practice is to replace fluids if the patient is hypovolemic. Consider dopamine at a dose of 2–4 µg/kg/h and hemodialysis or continuous venovenous hemofiltration if the patient is being considered for transplantation. Infusions of prostaglandin E_1 do not improve patient survival but improve renal function

D   Metabolic disorders

1   Hypoglycemia: multifactorial, must be monitored and treated
2   Acidosis: early and associated with poor prognosis in patients with acetaminophen overdose
3   Alkalosis: most common acid–base abnormality and often accompanied by hypokalemia and central hyperventilation
4   Hypoxemia: consider atelectasis, aspiration, infection, acute respiratory distress syndrome (ARDS), and pulmonary hemorrhage

E   Coagulopathy

Bleeding generally occurs only in patients with profound prolongation of the prothrombin time and a platelet count <50,000/mm³. The usual source of upper gastrointestinal bleeding is erosive gastritis or esophagitis

Gastrointestinal bleeding can be prevented by H_2-receptor blocker therapy. Significant bleeding should be treated with platelet and plasma infusions. Whether patients should receive platelet transfusions and fresh frozen plasma in the absence of significant bleeding is controversial, since the resulting fluid overload may be deleterious

F   Sepsis

Common – seen in >80% of patients with advanced stages of coma, with approximately 20% having bloodborne bacterial or fungal infections. Patients with FHF are at risk because of the multiple invasive procedures required as part of ICU care. In addition, liver failure and multiple organ failure are accompanied by translocation of microorganisms through the gut wall and neutrophil dysfunction.

A careful search for infections should be made daily. Infection should be treated specifically when identified or empirically in the absence of a source. Consider infection in a patient who was improving and then suddenly decompensates

6   Management

1 **The overall goals of management are to support patients in whom the prognosis is good until they recover** (Table 2.3) **and to move quickly to liver transplantation in patients in whom the prognosis is poor**[7,8]

   Acetylcysteine therapy (loading oral dose: 140 mg/kg, followed by 70 mg/kg every 4 hours for 68 hours for a total of 17 doses) to restore glutathione stores should be given up to 36 hours after an acetaminophen overdose

---

Full hemodynamic monitoring (arterial line, pulmonary artery catheter)

Endotracheal intubation and intracranial pressure monitoring for stage 3 encephalopathy

Parenteral glucose (D10 or 20) to prevent hypoglycemia

Correct electrolyte and acid–base disorders

Parenteral H_2-receptor blocker infusion to minimize chance of gastrointestinal bleeding

Treat elevated intracranial pressure with mannitol

Treat fever with broad-spectrum antibiotics after cultures, and consider antifungal therapy

If acetaminophen poisoning is suspected, treat as follows:

   Gastric lavage with large-bore tube to remove any pills still present
   If no pills are present, give *N*-acetylcysteine 140 mg/kg per nasogastric tube stat and 70 mg/kg p.o. every 4 hours for 72 hours. An alternate parenteral approach is to give 150 mg/kg i.v. in 200 mL D5W over 15 minutes, followed by 50 mg/kg in 500 mL D5W over 4 hours and 100 mg/kg in 1000 mL D5W over 16 hours (total 20 hours therapy)
   If pills are present on lavage, give activated charcoal and parenteral N-acetylcysteine

---

(Table 2.3: General management of FHF)

2 The presence of easily obtained clinical data during the patient's course predicts severe liver failure with death rates >90%, as outlined in Table 2.4

3 A liver transplant team should be contacted and the patient transferred to a transplant facility; patients may decompensate quickly, and it is difficult to orchestrate liver transplantation for patients with FHF

4 When patients develop encephalopathy or agitation, they should be transferred to an ICU for aggressive supportive management

   • if viral hepatitis is suspected, it is important to screen family members or personal contacts for susceptibility (lack of immunity from prior exposure or vaccination). If appropriate, immune globulin and hepatitis A or B vaccination should be administered to prevent secondary cases among close contacts

   • for suspected mushroom poisoning, management includes forced diuresis with intravenous hydration and duodenal intubation and aspiration via a large-bore tube, if a patient is seen early. Penicillin G, 1 million units/h i.v., may reduce the concentration of amatoxins in bile, possibly by interrupting their enterohepatic circulation

- for suspected Wilson's disease, the patient should be stabilized with intravenous hydration and plasmapheresis, and immediately evaluated for liver transplantation. A fulminant presentation of Wilson's disease is not reversible with chelation therapy.

5 **Liver transplantation should be considered in any patient with severe progressive liver injury from FHF who meets criteria for a fatal outcome** (Table 2.4). The most comprehensive study of prognostic factors was performed by O'Grady and colleagues in London at the King's College Hospital Acute Liver Failure Unit.[9] These studies demonstrated a gradual improvement in survival over a 15-year period as a result of better intensive care rather than specific therapy. Overall survival improved from 20% in 1973 to >50% in 1988. The cause of liver failure was the most important variable in predicting survival; patients with acetaminophen overdose and fulminant hepatitis A had much better survival than patients with non-A, non-B hepatitis

FHF secondary to acetaminophen overdose	pH <7.30, or Prothrombin time 6.5 (INR) and serum creatinine >300 µmol/L (3.4 mg/dL)
FHF secondary to viral hepatitis or drug reaction	Prothrombin time 6.5 (INR), or Any 3 of the following: Etiology non-A, non-B hepatitis or drug reaction Age <10 and >40 years Duration of jaundice before encephalopathy >7 days Serum bilirubin >300 µmol/L (17.6 mg/dL) Prothrombin time 3.5 (INR)

Adapted from O'Grady et al. (1989).[9]
FHF, fulminant hepatic failure; INR, international normalized ratio

(Table 2.4: Prognostic indicators associated with adverse outcome and need for liver transplantation FHF)

Other predictors of prognosis in patients with FHF include stage of encephalopathy and factor V levels. Bernuau and colleagues[3] have shown that factor V levels of <20% in patients under age 30 years or <30% in patients > age 30 years predicts that survival is unlikely

6 Extracorporeal liver assist devices, using hepatocytes or whole organs, and hepatocyte transplantation are promising experimental techniques that may play a role in the management of patients with FHF in the future. Hepatocytes can be attached to various microcarriers and injected into the peritoneal cavity. Other techniques that have occasionally been employed include auxiliary partial heterotopic liver transplantation or transplantation of partial liver grafts from living related donors. These procedures provide hepatic support while allowing a period of time for the native liver to recover

Contraindications to liver transplantation in the setting of FHF

a Irreversible disease

- severe irreversible brain damage
  - cerebral perfusion pressure <40 mmHg for >2 hours
  - sustained elevation of ICP to >50 mmHg
- inability to oxygenate during anesthesia due to ARDS or severe cardiopulmonary disease
- evidence of multiorgan failure syndrome
- septic shock
- widespread mesenteric vein thrombosis
- active alcohol or drug abuse
- any other major complicating or lethal disorder (e.g., AIDS, severe depression)

b Improving liver function

Full recovery is expected if patient survives the acute hepatic insult

References

1   Lee WM. *Acute liver failure.* (N Engl J Med 1993) 329: 1862–72

2   Hoofnagle JH, Carithers RL Jr, Shapiro C, Ascher N. *Fulminant hepatic failure: summary of a workshop.* (Hepatology 1995) 21: 240–52

3   Bernuau J, Rueff B, Benhamou J-P. *Fulminant and subfulminant liver failure: definitions and causes.* (Semin Liv Dis 1986) 6: 97–106.

4   O'Grady JG, Schalm SW, Williams R. *Acute liver failure: redefining the syndromes.* (Lancet 1993) 342: 273–5

5   Lidofsky SD. *Fulminant hepatic failure.* (Crit Care Clin 1995) 11: 415–30

6   Keeffe EB. *Acute liver failure.* In: Grendell JH, McQuaid KR, Friedman SL, (eds). *Current Diagnosis and Treatment in Gastroenterology.* (Stanford, CT: Appleton & Lange, 1996) 475–83

7   Bismuth H, Samuel D, Castaing D, Adam R, Saliba F, Johann M, Azoulay D, Ducot B, Chiche L. *Orthotopic liver transplantation in fulminant and subfulminant hepatitis. The Paul Brousse experience.* (Annals of Surgery 1995) 222: 109–19

8   *Consensus conference on indications for liver transplantation.* (Hepatology 1994) 20: 1S–68S

9   O'Grady JG, Alexander GJM, Hayllar KM, Williams R. *Early indicators of prognosis in fulminant hepatic failure.* (Gastroenterology 1989) 97: 439–45

CHAPTER 3

Acute viral hepatitis

RAYMOND S. KOFF, M.D.

Key Points

1 Acute viral hepatitis is the most common cause of liver disease in the world; it is responsible for 1–2 million deaths annually

2 The nonenveloped and enterically transmitted hepatitis viruses (HAV and HEV), in general, are self-limited infections, but severe hepatitis may develop in some cases; the bloodborne hepatitis viruses (HBV, HDV, HCV, and HGV) are enveloped agents associated with persistent infection, prolonged viremia, and the development of chronic liver disease (?HGV) and its sequelae

3 A wide spectrum of clinical illness is well documented, ranging from asymptomatic, anicteric infection to fulminant hepatitis; no specific treatment of acute viral hepatitis is available; liver transplantation is indicated in fulminant hepatitis when recovery seems unlikely

4 Highly effective and safe vaccines are available for pre-exposure immunoprophylaxis of HAV and HBV infection; for post-exposure immunoprophylaxis of HAV, immune globulin is used, while for post-exposure immunoprophylaxis of HBV both HBIG and HBV vaccine are used

5 Neither immune globulin preparations nor vaccines are available for the prevention of HEV, HCV, or HGV. HBV vaccination prevents HDV infection, but for persons with established HBV infection HDV vaccines to prevent HDV superinfection are not available

---

1   Acute Viral Hepatitis: Importance

Worldwide, hepatitis virus infections are the most common cause of liver disease
Many hepatitis episodes are anicteric, inapparent, or subclinical
Globally, viral hepatitis is the major cause of persistent viremia
With its sequelae, viral hepatitis is responsible for 1–2 million deaths annually

2   The Agents of Viral Hepatitis

The agents of acute viral hepatitis can be broadly classified into two groups: the enterically transmitted and the bloodborne agents

A   Enterically transmitted agents

These agents, namely hepatitis A virus (HAV), hepatitis E virus (HEV), and possibly a third agent (?HFV):

Are nonenveloped viruses
Survive intact when exposed to bile
Are shed in feces
Are not linked to chronic liver disease
Do not result in a viremic or intestinal carrier state

1 HAV
- classified as a picornavirus, subclassified as a "hepatovirus"
- 27–28 nm in diameter with cubic symmetry
- single-stranded, linear RNA molecule, 7.5 kb
- one serotype in human beings; three or more genotypes
- contains a single immunodominant neutralization site
- contains three or four virion polypeptides in capsomere
- replication in cytoplasm of infected hepatocyte; no evidence of replication in intestine
- propagated in nonhuman primate and human cell lines

2 HEV
- tentatively classified as a member of the alpha-like supergroup of positive-strand RNA viruses
- 27–34 nm in diameter
- linear RNA molecule, 7.5 kb
- RNA genome with three overlapping open reading frames encoding structural proteins and nonstructural proteins involved in HEV replication:
  - RNA-dependent RNA polymerase
  - helicase

- – cysteine protease
- – ?methyltransferase
- only one serotype identified in human beings; minor genetic diversity
- immunodominant neutralization site on structural protein encoded by second open reading frame
- propagation in human embryo lung diploid cells
- replication in vivo limited to hepatocytes

3 Other enterically transmitted agents (?HFV)

- occasional outbreaks of enterically transmitted hepatitis, without serologic markers of HAV or HEV
- HFV reported to be a 27–37 nm DNA-containing virus – requires confirmation

B   Bloodborne agents

These agents, namely hepatitis B virus (HBV), hepatitis D virus (HDV), hepatitis C virus (HCV), and hepatitis G virus (HGV) are:

Enveloped viruses
Disrupted by exposure to bile/detergents
Not shed in feces
Linked to chronic liver disease (?HGV)
Associated with persistent viremia

1 HBV

- human-infecting member of hepatotropic DNA-containing viruses, the "Hepadnaviridae"
- 42 nm spherical particle with:
  - – a 27 nm diameter, electron-dense, nucleocapsid core
  - – a 7 nm thickness outer lipoprotein envelope
- HBV core contains circular, partially double-stranded DNA and:
  - – DNA polymerase protein with reverse transcriptase activity
  - – hepatitis B core antigen (HBcAg), a structural protein
  - – hepatitis B e antigen (HBeAg), a nonstructural protein that correlates with active HBV replication
- HBV outer lipoprotein envelope contains:
  - – hepatitis B surface antigen (HBsAg), with three envelope proteins: major, large, and middle proteins
  - – minor lipid and carbohydrate components
  - – HBsAg present in 22 nm spherical or tubular noninfectious particles, in excess of intact HBV particles
- one major serotype; many subtypes based on HBsAg protein diversity
- HBV mutant viruses are a consequence of poor proof-reading ability of reverse transcriptase; these include:

- – HBeAg-negative precore/core mutant (uncommon in USA)
- – HBV vaccine-induced escape mutant (rare)
- liver is major but not only site of HBV replication

2 HDV

- a defective RNA virus, requiring helper function of HBV for its expression and pathogenicity but not for its replication
- only one serotype recognized, three genotypes
- 35–37 nm spherical particle, enveloped by HBV lipoprotein coat
  - – ?19 nm core-like structure
- contains an antigenic nuclear phosphoprotein (HDV antigen)
  - – binds RNA
  - – exists in two isoforms: smaller 195 amino acid and larger 214 amino acid proteins
  - – smaller HDV antigen transports RNA into the nucleus and is essential for HDV replication
  - – larger HDV antigen is prenylated and inhibits HDV RNA replication and participates in HDV assembly
- HDV RNA is single stranded, covalently closed, and circular
- HDV antigenome is a genome complementary, circular RNA found in the infected hepatocyte and, to a lesser extent, in purified HDV particles
- with slightly less than 1680 nucleotides, HDV RNA is the smallest RNA genome among the animal viruses; HDV resembles plant satellite viruses
- RNA genome can form an unbranched rod-like structure by folding on itself through intramolecular base pairing
- replication limited to hepatocyte
- cell lines transfected with HDV cDNA constructs express HDV RNA and HDV antigens

3 HCV

- an enveloped, single-stranded RNA virus
- 55 nm spherical particle; 33 nm nucleocapsid core
- classified among the Flaviviridae, but distinct from the known flaviviruses and pestiviruses
- HCV genome comprises about 9400 nucleotides encoding a large polyprotein of about 3000 amino acids
  - – one third of the polyprotein comprises a series of structural proteins (an internal nucleocapsid or core (C) protein and two glycosylated envelope proteins, termed E1 and E2/NS1, present in the lipid-containing envelope of the virus)
  - – envelope proteins may generate neutralizing antibodies
  - – remaining two thirds of the polyprotein consists of nonstructural proteins (termed NS2, NS3, NS4A, NS4B, NS5A, and NS5B) involved in HCV replication
- only one HCV serotype identified; multiple HCV genotypes exist; genotypes are variably distributed throughout the world

4 HGV

- positive-strand RNA virus, with 9392 nucleotides encoding a polyprotein with 2873 amino acids
- classified as a member of the Flaviviridae, closely related to, if not identical with, an agent known as GB virus type C (GBV-C), but distinct from HCV
- nonstructural regions of the genome encode a helicase, two protease, and an RNA-dependent RNA polymerase motifs

3 Epidemiology and Risk Factors

A HAV

1 Incubation period: 15–50 days (mean of about 30 days)
2 Worldwide distribution; highly endemic in developing countries
3 HAV is excreted in the stools of infected persons for 1–2 weeks before and for at least 1 week after onset of illness
4 Viremia is short lived (no viremic carriers)
5 Prolonged fecal excretion (months) reported in infected neonates; frequency, level of virus in stool, and epidemiological importance uncertain
6 Enteric (fecal–oral) transmission predominant via person-to-person household spread; occasional outbreaks linked to common-source vehicles:
- Contaminated food, bivalve mollusks, water

7 Other risk factors include exposure:
- in day care centers for infants, diapered children
- in institutions for developmentally disadvantaged
- via international travel to developing countries
- oral–anal homosexual behavior

8 No evidence for maternal–neonatal transmission
9 Prevalence correlates with sanitary standards and large household size
10 Percutaneous transmission rare
11 Overall seroprevalence in USA: 33%

B HEV

1 Incubation period averages about 40 days
2 Widely distributed; epidemic and endemic forms but rare in USA
3 HEV RNA in serum and stool during acute phase
4 The most common form of sporadic hepatitis in young adults in the developing world
5 A largely waterborne epidemic disease
6 Intrafamilial, secondary cases are uncommon
7 Maternal–neonatal transmission has been documented
8 In the USA imported cases in returning travelers and in recent immigrants from endemic regions
9 Prolonged viremia or fecal shedding unusual

C HBV

1 Incubation period ranges from 15 to 180 days (average 60–90 days)

2 HBV viremia lasts for weeks to months after acute infection

3 1–5% of adults, 90% of infected neonates, and 50% of infants develop chronic infection and persistent viremia

4 Persistent infection linked with chronic hepatitis, cirrhosis, hepatocellular carcinoma

5 Worldwide distribution: HBV carrier prevalence <1% in USA, >15% in Asia

6 HBV present in blood, semen, cervicovaginal secretions, saliva, other body fluids

7 Modes of transmission

   a Bloodborne

- recipients of multiple blood products
- injecting drug users
- hemodialysis patients
- health care and other workers exposed to blood

   b Sexual transmission

   c Tissue penetrations (percutaneous) or permucosal transfer

- needlestick accidents
- shared razorblades
- tattoo
- acupuncture
- shared toothbrushes

   d Maternal–neonatal, maternal–infant transmission

   e No evidence for fecal–oral spread

D HDV

1 Incubation period estimated to be 4–7 weeks

2 Endemic in Mediterranean basin, Balkan peninsula, European parts of former Soviet Union, parts of Africa, Middle East, and Amazon basin

3 Viremia short lived (acute infection) or prolonged (chronic infection)

4 HDV infections occur solely in individuals at risk for HBV infection (coinfections or superinfections)

- injecting drug abusers
- homosexual men
- recipients of high-risk blood products
- sexual partners

5 Modes of transmission

   a Bloodborne

   b Sexual transmission

   c Maternal–neonatal spread

E HCV

1 Incubation period ranges from 15 to 160 days (major peak at about 50 days)

2 Prolonged viremia and persistent infection common; wide geographic distribution

3 Persistent infection linked with chronic hepatitis, cirrhosis, hepatocellular carcinoma

4 Seroprevalence of past/present infection 1.9% in USA

5 Modes of transmission

   a Bloodborne (the predominant mode)

     • injecting drug use

     • recipients of blood/blood products

   b Sexual transmission: low efficiency, low frequency

   c Maternal–neonatal: low efficiency, low frequency

   d No evidence of fecal–oral transmission

F HGV

1 Incubation period uncertain

2 Prolonged viremia and persistent infection common

3 HGV RNA in 1.5–1.7% of US blood donors

4 HGV RNA in 10–20% of patients with

   • chronic hepatitis

   • chronic hepatitis B

   • chronic hepatitis C

   • cryptogenic cirrhosis

5 Modes of transmission

   a Bloodborne

     • injecting drug users

     • recipients of blood/blood products

4 Pathophysiology

1 Cell-mediated immune mechanisms of hepatocyte injury – responsible in HAV and HBV, uncertain for HCV

   • membrane attack complex of complement demonstrated in both fulminant and acute hepatitis

   • activation of the complement terminal pathway, leading to deposition of the membrane attack complex on hepatocytes, may be involved in pathogenesis of necrosis

2 Direct viral cytopathic effect

   • postulated for HCV and HDV, but no direct evidence

3 Limited information: HEV, HGV

5 Clinical Features

A Self-limited disease

1 Spectrum of severity ranging from asymptomatic, inapparent infection to fulminant, fatal disease

2 Similar clinical syndromes for all agents beginning with nonspecific prodromal constitutional and gastrointestinal symptoms:

- malaise, anorexia, nausea, and vomiting
- flu-like symptoms of pharyngitis, cough, coryza, photophobia, headache, and myalgias

3 Onset of symptoms tends to be abrupt for HAV and HEV; in the others onset is usually insidious

4 Fever is uncommon except in HAV infection

5 Immune-complex-mediated, serum-sickness-like syndrome in less than 10% of patients with HBV infection; rarely in others

6 Prodromal symptoms abate or disappear with onset of jaundice, although anorexia, malaise, and weakness may persist

7 Jaundice heralded by the appearance of dark urine; pruritus (usually mild and transient) may occur as the jaundice increases

8 Physical examination reveals mild enlargement and slight tenderness of the liver

9 Mild splenomegaly and posterior cervical lymphadenopathy in 15–20%

B Fulminant disease (acute liver failure) (see Ch. 2)

1 Changes in mental status (encephalopathy)

- lethargy, drowsiness, coma
- reversal of sleep patterns
- personality changes

2 Cerebral edema (usually without papilledema)

3 Coagulopathy

4 Multiple organ failure

- adult respiratory distress syndrome
- cardiac arrhythmias
- hepatorenal syndrome
- sepsis
- gastrointestinal bleeding
- hypotension

5 Development of ascites, anasarca

6 Case fatality rate: 60%

7 Serial physical examinations: shrinking liver

8 Extraordinarily high rates, approaching 10–20%, in pregnant women with hepatitis E, particularly during the third trimester

C   Cholestatic hepatitis

1   Jaundice may be striking and persist for several months prior to complete resolution

2   Pruritus may be prominent

3   Persistent anorexia and diarrhea in a few patients

4   Excellent prognosis for complete resolution

5   Most commonly seen in HAV infection

D   Relapsing hepatitis

1   Symptoms and liver test abnormalities recur weeks to months after improvement or apparent recovery.

2   Most commonly seen in HAV infection – IgM anti-HAV may remain positive, and HAV may once again be shed in stool

3   Arthritis, vasculitis, and cryoglobulinemia may be seen

4   Prognosis is excellent for complete recovery even after multiple relapses (particularly common in children)

6   Laboratory Features

A   Self-limited disease

1   Most prominent biochemical feature: marked elevation of serum aminotransferase levels

2   Peak aminotransferases (ALT and AST): vary from 500 to 5000 U/L

3   Serum bilirubin level uncommonly above 10 mg/dL, except in cholestatic hepatitis (see below)

4   Serum alkaline phosphatase normal or mildly elevated

5   Prothrombin time normal or increased by 1–3 seconds

6   Serum albumin normal or minimally depressed

7   Peripheral blood counts: normal or mild leukopenia with or without a relative lymphocytosis

B   Fulminant disease (see Ch. 2)

1   Striking coagulopathy

2   Leukocytosis, hyponatremia, and hypokalemia common

3   Hypoglycemia

4   Marked elevations of serum bilirubin and aminotransferases, but the latter may decline towards normal despite disease progression

C   Cholestatic disease

1   Serum bilirubin levels may exceed 20 mg/dL

2   Serum aminotransferase levels may decline toward normal despite cholestasis

3   Variable elevation of serum alkaline phosphatase

D Relapsing hepatitis

1 After apparent normalization or near-normalization of serum aminotransferase and bilirubin levels during convalescence, both may rise again

2 Peak levels may or may not exceed those of initial bout

7 Histology (liver biopsy rarely performed in acute self-limited viral hepatitis)

A Self-limited disease

1 Major hepatocyte injury
- focal hepatocyte necrosis
- loss of hepatocytes (cell dropout)
- ballooning degeneration
- Councilman-like bodies (mummified, hyalinized, necrotic hepatocytes, extruded into a hepatic sinusoid)

2 Endophlebitis, affecting the central vein

3 Diffuse mononuclear cell (CD+8 and natural killer cell) infiltrate
- within widened portal tracts
- segmental erosion of the limiting plate
- within hepatic parenchyma
- Kupffer's cells enlarged, hyperplastic, with lipofuscin pigment and debris, remnants of injured hepatocytes

B Fulminant disease

1 Liver biopsy usually precluded by coagulopathy

2 Extensive confluent hepatocyte dropout (disappearance)

3 Collapse of reticulin framework

4 Lobular inflammation

5 Variable cholestasis

C Cholestatic disease

1 Hepatocyte degeneration, inflammation as in self-limited hepatitis

2 Prominence of bile plugs in dilated hepatocyte canaliculi and bilirubin staining of hepatocytes

3 Hepatocytes form multiple, scattered, duct-like structures (pseudoglandular transformation)

D Relapsing hepatitis

Changes similar to self-limited disease

8   Diagnosis

A   Differential diagnosis

1 Drug- and toxin-induced liver disease (see Ch. 8)
2 Ischemic hepatitis (see Ch. 20)
3 Autoimmune hepatitis (see Ch. 5)
4 Alcoholic hepatitis (see Ch. 6)
5 Acute biliary tract obstruction (see Ch. 33)

B   Serologic diagnosis (see Table 3.1)

Agent	Acute phase	Convalescence
HAV	Total anti-HAV positive IgM anti-HAV positive	Development of IgG anti-HAV Disappearance of IgM anti-HAV
HEV	IgM anti-HEV positive and/or HEV RNA (in stool) IgG anti-HEV may be present	Loss of HEV RNA; development of IgG anti-HEV Loss of IgM anti-HEV
HBV	HBsAg positive and IgM anti-HBc positive	Loss of HBsAg; later loss of IgM anti- HBc; development of IgG anti-HBc; late development of anti-HBs
HDV	HDV RNA positive or HDV antigen positive or IgM anti-HDV positive in HBsAg-positive patient	Loss of HDV RNA or antigen; development of IgG anti-HDV or loss of anti-HDV
HDV/HBV	Coinfection: IgM anti-HBc positive	Above plus usual loss of HBsAg
HDV/HBV	Superinfection:IgG anti-HBc positive	Above usually without loss of HBsAg
HCV	Early presence of HCV RNA; presence of or development of anti-HCV	Loss of HCV RNA (in a minor proportion of patients); anti-HCV persistence
HGV	HGV RNA positive	?

(Table 3.1: Serologic patterns in the diagnosis of acute viral hepatitis)

1 Enterically transmitted infections
   a HAV (see Fig. 3.1)
   - IgM antibody to HAV (IgM anti-HAV) detected during acute phase and for 3–6 months thereafter
   - presence of positive anti-HAV without IgM anti-HAV indicative of past infection
   b HEV
   - no Food and Drug Administration (FDA)-approved commercial serologic assays available
   - IgM and IgG antibodies to HEV (anti-HEV) detected early by research assays

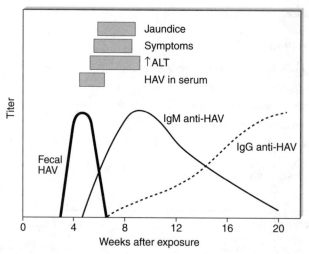

Fig. 3.1 Serologic course of HAV

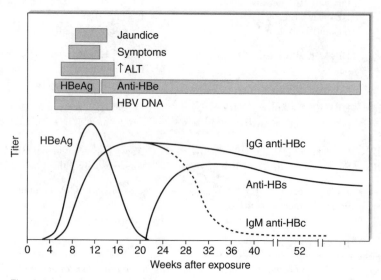

Fig. 3.2 Serologic course of HBV

- IgM anti-HEV may persist for at least 6 weeks after peak of illness
- IgG anti-HEV may remain detectable for as long as 20 months

2 Bloodborne infections

  a HBV (see Fig. 3.2)

  - serologic diagnosis established by detection of presence of IgM antibody to hepatitis B core antigen (IgM anti-HBc) and HBsAg:
    - both usually present at onset of symptoms
    - IgM anti-HBc usually preceded by HBsAg
    - HBsAg is first serologic marker of HBV infection to appear

- HBsAg may disappear, usually within several weeks to months after appearance, before loss of IgM anti-HBc
- HBeAg and HBV DNA:
    - detectable after appearance of HBsAg
    - both markers disappear after weeks to months in self-limited infection
    - not necessary for routine diagnosis
- IgG anti-HBc:
    - replaces IgM anti-HBc in resolving infection
    - indicative of past or continuing infection
    - not induced by HBV vaccine
- antibody to HBsAg (anti-HBs):
    - last antibody to appear
    - a neutralizing antibody
    - generally indicative of recovery and immunity to reinfection
    - elicited by HBV vaccine

b HDV
- HBsAg-positive individual with:
    - antibody to HDV (anti-HDV) and/or circulating HDV RNA (assays for latter currently unapproved in USA)
    - IgM anti-HDV may be present transiently
- HBV/HDV coinfection:
    - HBsAg positivity
    - IgM anti-HBc-positive
    - anti-HDV and/or HDV RNA
- HDV superinfection of HBV carrier:
    - HBsAg positivity
    - IgG anti-HBc positive
    - anti-HDV and/or HDV RNA
- anti-HDV titers decline to undetectable levels with resolution of infection

c HCV (see Fig. 3.3)
- serologic diagnosis:
    - detection of antibodies to recombinant HCV antigens (anti-HCV)
    - second- and third-generation assays include antigens from structural and nonstructural regions
    - anti-HCV detected in about 60% of patients during acute phase of illness; anti-HCV appears weeks to months later in about 35%
    - <5% of infected patients do not develop anti-HCV
    - assays for IgM anti-HCV under development
    - anti-HCV generally persists for prolonged periods following acute infection, both in the relatively few self-limited infections and in the more common chronic HCV infections

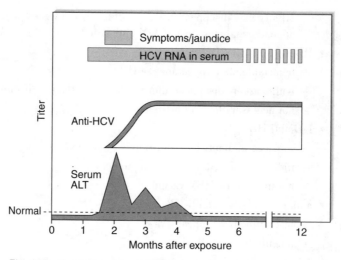

Fig. 3.3   Serologic course of HCV

- HCV RNA:
  - the earliest marker of acute HCV infection
  - appears within a few weeks of exposure
  - expensive, investigational, not routinely used for diagnosis
  - present in chronic HCV infection
- d HGV
  - detection of HGV RNA (not commercially available)
  - no serologic test available

9   Natural History and Outcome

A   Enterically transmitted infections (HAV and HEV)

1 Complete clinical, histologic, and biochemical recovery within 3–6 months
2 Occasional instances of fulminant hepatitis
   - age-dependent fatalities in HAV infection (increased risk after age 40 years)
   - increased risk in pregnant women with HEV infection
3 No chronic liver disease or prolonged carriage of virus

B   Bloodborne infections (HBV, HDV, HCV and HGV)

1 HBV

a Risk of persistent infection is age dependent and declines progressively with increasing age:
   - 90% of infected neonates become carriers
   - 1–5% of adult patients develop chronic HBV infection

    b Fulminant hepatitis in <1% of acute infections

    c Persistent infection (HBsAg positive with or without active HBV replication)

- asymptomatic carrier with normal or nonspecific liver histologic changes
- chronic hepatitis, cirrhosis, hepatocellular carcinoma
- associated with membranous glomerulonephritis, polyarteritis nodosa, and, less certainly, with mixed cryoglobulinemia

2 HDV

    a HDV/HBV coinfections usually self-limited and resolve without sequelae

    b Fulminant HDV hepatitis more often in superinfection than in coinfection

    c HDV superinfection of HBV-infected individuals may lead to chronic HDV infection superimposed on chronic HBV infection with development of severe chronic hepatitis and cirrhosis

3 HCV

    a Relatively few self-limited infections

    b Rarely associated with fulminant hepatitis uncertain

    c Persistent HCV infections with prolonged viremia and elevated serum aminotransferase levels are common

    d Histology in persistent HCV infection

- chronic hepatitis
- cirrhosis

    e Risk of hepatocellular carcinoma in HCV-related cirrhosis

    f Associated with:

- mixed cryoglobulinemia
- cutaneous vasculitis
- membranoproliferative glomerulonephritis
- porphyria cutanea tarda

4 HGV

    a Frequency of self-limited infections uncertain

    b Association with fulminant hepatitis uncertain

    c Persistent HGV infection with viremia documented

    d Histology in persistent HGV infection

- ?chronic hepatitis
- ?cirrhosis
- ?hepatocellular carcinoma

    e ?Linkage with extrahepatic disorders

10 Treatment

A Self-limited infection

1 Outpatient care unless persistent vomiting or severe anorexia leads to dehydration

2 Maintenance of adequate caloric and fluid intake

- no specific dietary recommendations
- a large breakfast may be best-tolerated meal
- prohibition of alcohol during acute phase

3 Vigorous or prolonged physical activity should be avoided

4 Limitation of daily activities and rest periods determined by the severity of fatigue and malaise

5 No specific drug treatment; corticosteroids of no value

6 All nonessential drugs discontinued

B   Fulminant hepatitis (see Ch. 2)

1 Hospitalization required
- as soon as diagnosis made
- management best undertaken in a center with a liver transplantation program

2 No specific therapy available

3 Goals
- continuous monitoring and supportive measures while awaiting spontaneous resolution of infection and restoration of hepatic function
- early recognition and treatment of life-threatening complications
- maintenance of vital functions
- preparation for liver transplantation if recovery appears unlikely

4 Survival rates of about 65% or greater achieved by early referral for liver transplantation

C   Cholestatic hepatitis

1 Course may be shortened by short-term treatment with prednisone or ursodeoxycholic acid, but no clinical trials available

2 Pruritus may be controlled with cholestyramine

D   Relapsing hepatitis

1 Management identical to that of self-limited infection

11   Prevention of Enterically Transmitted Infections

A   HAV: immunoprophylaxis is the cornerstone of preventive efforts

1 Pre-exposure immunoprophylaxis
- inactivated HAV vaccine
  - highly effective (protective efficacy rate 95–100%)
  - highly immunogenic (nearly 100% in healthy subjects)
  - protective antibodies induced in 15 days in 85%
  - safe, well tolerated
  - injection site soreness major adverse event
- inactivated HAV vaccine dose and schedule

Adults 19 years of age or older: two dose regimen (1440 Elisa Units), with second dose at 6–12 months after first

Children over 2 years of age: three-dose regimen (360 Elisa Units), 0, 1, and 6–12 months or two-dose regimen (720 Elisa Units), 0 and 6–12 months

- inactivated HAV vaccine indications
  - travelers to high-risk areas (for those leaving immediately, immune globulin may be given simultaneously, at a different site)
  - homosexual and bisexual men
  - injecting drug users
  - native peoples of the Americas and Alaska
  - children and young adults in communities experiencing community-wide outbreaks
  - susceptible patients with chronic liver disease
  - laboratory workers handling HAV
  - ?food-handlers
  - ?staff in day care centers
2 Post-exposure immunoprophylaxis
  - efficacy of HAV vaccine in the postexposure setting not established
  - efficacy of immune globulin well established but imperfect

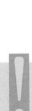

Immune globulin schedule and dose
  - 0.02 mL/kg body weight, deltoid injection, as early as possible after exposure

  - well tolerated, injection site soreness
  - indications: household and intimate contacts of individuals with acute HAV infection

B **HEV: presence of IgG anti-HEV in contacts of patients with hepatitis E may be protective, but efficacy of immune globulin containing anti-HEV uncertain**

- ?development of high-titer, hyperimmune globulin
- ?development of HEV vaccine

12 Prevention of Bloodborne Infections

A **HBV: the cornerstone of immunoprophylaxis is the pre-exposure administration of HBV vaccine**

1 Pre-exposure immunoprophylaxis with HBV vaccine
  a Recombinant yeast-derived vaccines
    - contain HBsAg as the immunogen

- highly immunogenic, inducing protective levels of anti-HBs in >95% of healthy young (under 40 years of age) recipients after all three doses
- 85–95% effective in preventing HBV infection or clinical hepatitis B
- major side effects
  - transient pain at injection site in 10–25%
  - short-lived, mild fever in fewer than 3%
- boosters not recommended even as long as a decade after initial immunization. Boosters only for immunocompromised individuals if anti-HBs titer below 10 mU/mL
- immunotherapeutic value in the individual with established HBV infection under study

b HBV vaccine dose and schedules

Intramuscular (deltoid) injection in a dose of 10 or 20 µg of HBsAg protein for adults; infants receive 2.5, 5, or 10 µg doses
Initial injection, repeated 1 and 6 months later

c Indications
- universal infant immunization recommended
- catch-up vaccination of all pre-teenagers (11–12 year olds) not previously vaccinated
- targeted high-risk groups
  - household and spouse contacts of HBV carriers
  - Alaskan natives, Pacific Islanders
  - health care and other workers exposed to blood
  - injecting drug users
  - homosexual and bisexual men
  - individuals with multiple sexual partners
  - workers in institutions for the developmentally disadvantaged
  - recipients of high-risk blood products
  - maintenance hemodialysis patients
  - inmates of prisons (in which injecting drug use and homosexual behavior may occur)

2 Post-exposure immunoprophylaxis with HBV vaccine and hepatitis B immune globulin (a preparation of immune globulin containing high titers of anti-HBs)

a Indications
- susceptible sexual contacts of acutely HBV-infected individuals

0.04–0.07 mL/kg HBIG as early as possible after exposure
First of three HBV vaccine doses given at another site (deltoid) at the same time or within days
Second and third vaccine doses given 1 and 6 months later

- neonates of HBsAg-positive mothers identified during pregnancy

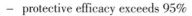

A dose of 0.5 mL of HBIG given within 12 hours of birth into the anterolateral muscle of the thigh

HBV vaccine, in doses of 5–10 µg, given within 12 hours of birth (at another site in the anterolateral muscle), repeated at 1 and 6 months

- – protective efficacy exceeds 95%
- b HDV
  - neither specific high-titer anti-HDV containing immune globulin nor HDV vaccine is available
  - immunoprophylaxis is dependent on the prevention of HBV by use of HBV vaccine
- c HCV: immunoprophylaxis of HCV infection not available, although neutralizing antibodies identified; work on HCV vaccine in progress
  - anti-HCV screening of blood and donor selection has reduced risk of transfusion-associated hepatitis C
  - safe sexual practice for contacts of HCV-infected individuals may be appropriate
- d HGV: no information on immunoprophylaxis available

References

1 Andre FE, Zuckerman AJ. *Review: protective efficacy of hepatitis B vaccines in neonates.* (J Med Virol 1994) 44: 144–51

2 Choo QL, Kuo G, Ralston R, et al. *Vaccination of chimpanzees against infection by the hepatitis C virus.* (Proc Natl Acad Sci USA 1994) 91: 1294–8

3 Hyams KC. *Risks of chronicity following acute hepatitis B virus infection: a review.* (Clin Infect Dis 1995) 20: 992–1000

4 Innis BL, Snitbhan R, Kunasol P, et al. *Protection against hepatitis A by an inactivated vaccine.* (JAMA 1994) 271: 1328–34

5 Koff RS. *Viral hepatitis.* In: Schiff L, Schiff ER, (eds). *Diseases of the Liver,* 7th ed Philadelphia: Lippincott, 1993) 492–577

6 Linnen J, Wages J Jr, Zhen-Yong ZK, et al. *Molecular cloning and disease association of hepatitis G virus: a transfusion-transmissible agent.* (Science 1996) 271: 505–8

7 Margolis HS, Coleman PJ, Brown RE, Mast EE, Sheingold SH, Arevalo JA. *Prevention of hepatitis B virus transmission by immunization: an economic analysis of current recommendations.* (JAMA 1995) 274: 1201–1208

8 McQuillan G, Alter MJ, Everhart JE. *Viral hepatitis.* In: Everhart JE, (ed.). *Digestive Diseases in the United States.* (Washington, DC: NIH, Publication No. 94–1447, 1994) 127–56

9 Polish LB, Gallagher M, Fields HA, Hadler SC. *Delta hepatitis: molecular biology and clinical and epidemiological features.* (Clin Microbiol Rev 1993) 6: 211–29

10 Thomas DL, Zenilman JM, Alter HJ, et al. *Sexual transmission of hepatitis C virus among patients attending sexually transmitted diseases clinics in Baltimore: an analysis of 309 sex partnerships.* (J Infect Dis 1995) 171: 768–75

11   West DJ, Watson B, Lichtman J, et al. *Persistence of immunologic memory for twelve years in children given hepatitis B vaccine in infancy.* (Pediatr Infect Dis J 1994) 13: 745–7

12   Yoshiba M, Okamoto H, Mishiro S. *Detection of the GBV-C hepatitis virus genome in serum from patients with fulminant hepatitis of unknown aetiology.* (Lancet 1995) 346: 1131–2

Chronic viral hepatitis

LORNA M. DOVE, M.D.   TERESA L. WRIGHT, M.D.

▼

Key Points

1 Hepatitis B, C and D represent the major viral agents currently shown to cause chronic hepatitis

2 Chronic hepatitis implies persistence of viral infection and secondary inflammation for greater than 6 months after initial exposure

3 The long-term complications of chronic hepatitis are cirrhosis, with attendant problems resulting from hepatic synthetic failure and portal hypertension, and hepatocellular carcinoma

4 Interferon, the only FDA approved drug for the treatment of chronic hepatitis, has a sustained effect in approximately 15–25% of HCV-infected patients and 35% of HBV-infected patients treated Promising antiviral agents are in clinical development for the treatment of chronic HBV infection. Effective therapies for treatment of HCV infection lag behind

5 Interferon has been demonstrated to improve long-term prognosis in patients with chronic hepatitis B; the long-term benefits of this drug in the treatment of chronic HCV infection are more controversial

6 Chronic viral hepatitis is a major indication for liver transplantation in both the USA and around the world. The availability of effective antiviral agents is reducing the incidence of post-transplantation recurrence, particularly in patients with HBV infection, and improving long-term prognosis

▲

1   Overview

1 Chronic hepatitis describes persistent inflammation of the liver for 6 months or more after initial exposure and/or initial detection of liver disease

2 The primary cause of chronic hepatitis is viral infection. Chronic hepatitis is caused by hepatitis B, C, and D. Whether there is a causative association between hepatitis G virus and chronic liver disease is under investigation

3 Complications of chronic hepatitis are cirrhosis, with attendant problems resulting from hepatic synthetic failure and portal hypertension, and hepatocellular carcinoma (HCC)

4 There are substantial differences in the virology, epidemiology, methods of diagnosis, and pathology/pathogenesis of disease among these viruses (see also Ch. 3)

2   Hepatitis B

A   Virology

1 Partially double-stranded DNA virus which replicates via an RNA intermediate that is used both for production of viral DNA and for translation of four major viral proteins

2 4.2 kb in length

3 Four open reading frames in the viral genome encode these major proteins:
- surface gene for hepatitis B surface antigen (HBsAg), pre-S proteins
- core gene for hepatitis B core antigen, hepatitis B e antigen (HBeAg)
- polymerase gene for the DNA polymerase (P protein) which catalyzes several steps in viral replication and assembly
- X gene for the X protein, the function of which is unknown but which may control the replication of HBV, as well as the replication of other viruses such as human immunodeficiency virus (HIV)

B   Epidemiology

1 Approximately 5% of the world's population are carriers of HBV

2 There are wide ranges world wide in the prevalence of this virus. Highest prevalences (8–15%) are in the Far East, Middle East, and Africa; lowest prevalences are in the USA and Western Europe (0.2–1.0%)

3 Overall prevalence in the USA is 1%. Within the USA, prevalence is greatest in Alaskan natives, Pacific Islanders, first-generation immigrants from South East Asia, injection drug users, and homosexual men. Prevalence in healthy blood donors is less than 0.5%

4 Risk factors for transmission include:
- high-risk sexual activity (multiple sexual partners, homosexual sexual activity)
- injection drug use
- hemodialysis
- living in or being born in areas of high endemnicity

- working in the health care profession (note: HBV has been documented to be transmitted on occasion from health care worker to patient)
5 There are four antigenic subtypes of HBV (adw, ayw, adr, ayr), with geographic variation in the distribution of these subtypes, but little clinical significance associated with infection by different subtypes

C   Clinical manifestations/natural history

1 Acute illness is usually mild; the risk of chronicity is dependent on the age and immune function of the patient (see Table 4.1)

Age at acquisition	Risk of HBV chronicity
Immunocompetent adult	<5%
Immunocompromised adult[a]	>50%
Early childhood	50%
Newborn	90%

[a]Immunocompromised adults include those with reduced ability to recognize and/or clear viral infections (patients who are on chronic hemodialysis, receive chemotherapy or exogenous immunosuppression, or are coinfected with HIV)

(Table 4.1: Risk of HBV chronicity varies with age)

2 Symptoms of chronic hepatitis range from asymptomatic infection to nonspecific complaints (fatigue, right upper quadrant pain, arthralgias), and, in advanced disease, to complications of cirrhosis (variceal bleeding, encephalopathy, ascites, infection, and hepatocellular carcinoma)
3 Extrahepatic manifestations include
- arthralgias (common)
- glomerulonephritis (rare)
- polyarteritis nodosa (rare)
- HBV-associated vasculitis (rare)
- mixed essential cryoglobulinemia (rare)
- pericariditis (rare)
- pancreatitis (rare)
4 50% of all carriers have evidence of viral replication (HBeAg and/or HBV DNA positivity)
5 In longitudinal follow-up, spontaneous loss of HBeAg is 7–20% per year; thus, the prevalence of HBeAg declines with age
6 Spontaneous loss of HBsAg occurs less frequently (1–2% per year)
7 15–20% of carriers develop cirrhosis within 5 years of disease onset, and in those with cirrhosis medium-term survival is significantly impaired
- Weissberg (1984)[1] published mortality data based on a prospective study of 379 patients

- 5-year survival was dependent on histologic staging found on liver biopsy; early histologic changes 97%; chronic active hepatitis 86%; cirrhosis 55%

8 Those with evidence of active viral replication are at increased risk for development of progressive disease

9 Hepatocellular carcinoma
- risk is increased >10-fold in patients with chronic HBV infection
- mechanism of oncogenesis is unknown
- cirrhosis of the liver is present in the majority

10 In regions where HBV is endemic, HCC is the leading cause of cancer-related deaths (see Ch. 27)

D   Serological and virological tests (see Table 4.2; see also Ch. 3)

HBV serologic and virologic markers	Stage of disease/interpretation
HBsAg	Ongoing infection
IgM anti-HBc	Recent infection or reactivation of chronic infection
IgG anti-HBc with anti-HBs	Prior infection
IgG anti-HBc alone	Prior infection, low-level infection or false-positive test
anti-HBs alone	Vaccine-induced immunity
HBeAg	Active viral replication
anti-HBe	Low replication and infectivity
HBV DNA (various methods of detection)	Active disease with active viral replication; when present in inactive disease, sensitive molecular methods needed for detection
HBV DNA in the absence of HBeAg	Mutations in the precore gene results in failure of HBeAg production; associated with fulminant acute infection and aggressive chronic disease

(Table 4.2: Interpretation of serologic and virologic test results)

1 Diagnosis of HBV infection relies largely on detection of HBsAg

2 Early events in acute infection which progresses to chronicity are similar to those in acute infection which resolves (seropositivity for HBsAg, anti-HBc, and HBeAg and detectable HBV DNA)

3 In persistent or chronic infection, these markers remain positive for 6 months or longer, and ALT levels remain elevated (from 50 to 200 U/L) in many

4 Acute and chronic infections are distinguished by the presence of IgM and IgG antibodies to hepatitis B core antigen (anti-HBc). Typically IgM anti-HBc is seen with acute infection, although it is also present on occasion with reactivation of chronic HBV infection

5 Active viral replication is defined by the presence of HBeAg and/or HBV DNA

E Pathology/pathogenesis

1 HBV is strongly hepatotropic, but viral sequences are also present in extrahepatic tissues (lymph nodes and peripheral blood mononuclear cells)

2 Most damage from HBV is caused by the host immune response to the virus rather than by the virus directly

3 Cell-mediated response directed against cellular HBcAg causes immune lysis of infected hepatocytes and resulting hepatitis and/or viral clearance

4 Cytotoxic T lymphocytes are the effector cells that have traditionally been believed to mediate cell damage

5 Recent evidence supports a central role of cytokines in mediating viral clearance

6 A hyperactive host response may lead to fulminant hepatitis, whereas a reduced host response increases the risk of chronic infection

7 Findings on liver histology include a predominantly portal-based lymphocytic infiltrate. Characteristic of chronic HBV infection is the appearance of ground-glass hepatocytes in which the cytoplasm is stained pink with hematoxylin and eosin, reflecting the massive overproduction of HBsAg. HBcAg can be demonstrated in the hepatocyte nuclei, within the cytoplasm, and on the cell membrane.

A standardized scale for the interpretation of histology in chronic hepatitis was developed by Batts & Ludwig (1995)[2]. The grading scale measures the necro-inflammatory process; the staging scale measures the degree of fibrosis (see Tables 4.3 and 4.4)

Grade (Semi-quantitative)	Descriptive	Lymphocytic piecemeal necrosis	Lobular inflammation and necrosis
0	Portal inflammation	None	None
1	Minimal	Minimal, patchy	Minimal; occasional spotty necrosis
2	Mild	Mild; involving some or all portal tracts	Mild; little hepatocellular damage
3	Moderate	Moderate	Moderate; with noticeable hepatocellular change
4	Severe	Severe	Severe; with prominent diffuse hepatocellular damage

(Table 4.3: Grading of disease activity in chronic hepatitis)

F Therapy

1 Goals of therapy include:
  - prevention of long-term complications
  - reduction in mortality
  - symptomatic improvement
  - loss of HBV DNA

Stage (Semi-quantitative)	Descriptive	Criteria
0	No fibrosis	Normal connective tissue
1	Portal fibrosis	Fibrous portal expansion
2	Periportal fibrosis	Periportal or rare portal – portal septa
3	Septal fibrosis	Fibrous septa with architectural distortion; no obvious cirrhosis
4	Cirrhosis	Cirrhosis

(Table 4.4: Staging of chronic hepatitis)

- seroconversion from HBeAg positivity to anti-HBe positivity
- normalization of serum alanine aminotransferase (ALT)
- reduction in hepatic inflammation (determined histologically)
- prevention of secondary spread of infection

Proof of long-term benefit is difficult since complications of chronic hepatitis occur over years

2 Drugs

- approaches to therapy have included modification of the host defenses against infection and inhibition of viral replication
- intermediate markers have been used to assess therapeutic efficacy
- interferon is the only drug approved by the FDA in the USA
- other drugs are in development (see Table 4.5); the nucleoside analogs appear to have the greatest promise
- future therapies may include combinations of antivirals and immune modulators

3 Specific drugs

a **Interferon** – Loss of HBeAg and HBV DNA is seen in approximately one third of treated patients. Loss of HBeAg (usually induced with therapy) results in increased survival overall and reduced HBV complication rate

- recommended dosage: interferon alpha 5 MU per day or 10 MU three times per week for 16 weeks

- cost–efficacy analysis suggests that interferon increases life expectancy and decreases projected lifetime cost
- patient characteristics associated with response to therapy include:

High aspartate aminotransferase (AST) and ALT levels
Low HBV DNA levels (<200 pg/ml)
Short duration of infection
Histologic picture of active hepatitis

	Status of development	Efficacy/side effects
Immunomodulators		
Interferon alpha-2b	FDA approved	Moderate efficacy and safety
Interferon beta, gamma	On hold	Limited US data
Corticosteroids	On hold	Significant toxicity
Thymosin alpha-1	Phase III trial complete	Limited efficacy safe
Interleukin 2	On hold	Limited data on efficacy/significant toxicity
Therapeutic vaccine (Theradigm)	Phase I trial complete Phase II trial underway	Safety and efficacy under evaluation
Antivirals		
Lamivudine (3TC, Epivir)	Phase III trial of 100 mg/day orally under way	Good safety profile, promising efficacy
Famciclovir (Famvir)	Phase III trial of 750 mg/day orally under way	Good safety profile, promising efficacy
Lobucovir	Phase I trial under way	Efficacious in vitro
Acyclovir	On hold	Limited efficacy; nephrotoxic at high doses
Ganciclovir	On hold	Poor oral bioavailability; limited efficacy
AZT/ddI	On hold	Limited efficacy in those with HBV/HIV coinfection
Ara-A	On hold	Significant neurotoxicity
FIAU (Fialuridine)	On hold	Significant hepatotoxicity

(Table 4.5: Options for the treatment of chronic HBV)

b **Lamivudine**
- (–) enantiomer of 3′-thiacytidine
- orally available
- inhibitor of viral reverse transcriptase (P protein)
- initial randomized placebo-controlled study demonstrated a 98% reduction in circulating HBV DNA with doses of 100 mg/day or higher; rebound after discontinuation of drug was observed in the majority
- phase II study of 25 mg, 100 mg and 300 mg demonstrated fall in HBV DNA levels in all patients, becoming undetectable at 4 weeks in those receiving 100 and 300 mg/day. Post-treatment rebound in 84%

c **Famciclovir**
- orally available guanosine analog
- converted in the liver to penciclovir, the active compound
- mechanism of action unknown
- 83% reduction in HBV DNA levels on therapy shown in uncontrolled studies
- phase III trial under way

4 **Liver transplantation** (see Ch. 31)
- treatment of choice in patients with end-stage chronic liver disease
- without specific precautions, HBV recurrence is universal and post-transplantation survival reduced
- peri- and postoperative hepatitis B immune globulin (HBIg) reduces recurrence and improves survival

- HBIg is expensive and must be given indefinitely
- nucleoside analogs (lamivudine and famciclovir) have been given pre-emptively (prior to and following transplantation) as well as for post-transplantation recurrence
- potential advantages of nucleoside analogs include low cost, oral availability, and good safety profile
- preliminary results of nucleoside analogs are encouraging, but their use is still experimental

3   Hepatitis C

A   Virology

1 Single-stranded, enveloped RNA virus which belongs to the Flaviviridae family
2 Approximately 9.4 kb in length
3 Genome has a single open reading frame which encodes a polypeptide of approximately 3010 amino acids in length
4 The long polypeptide is cleaved after translation by at least two viral proteases into structural (core and two envelope) proteins and nonstructural (helicase and RNA polymerase) proteins
5 Preferential replication in hepatocytes; extrahepatic virus has been demonstrated
6 Inherently high mutation rate which results in considerable heterogeneity throughout the genome
7 Classified into genotypes
   - genetically distinct groups of viral isolates that have arisen during the evolution of the virus
   - epidemiological differences in geographical distribution and mode of acquisition
   - major types and, within these types, 40 different *subtypes* (designated by a lower-case letter)
   - in the USA, genotype 1 is most prevalent (approximately 70% of all infections), with equal distribution between *subtypes* 1a and 1b
   - genotype 1 has been associated with lower response to interferon than has other genotypes
8 Classified into quasispecies
   - closely related, yet heterogeneous, sequences of virus within an infected individual which result from mutations occurring during viral replication
   - postulated to be important for escape from the host immune response
   - may play a role in pathogenesis of disease

B   Epidemiology

1 Worldwide prevalence of HCV is estimated to be 1%
2 Marked geographical variation in prevalence exists from 0.4–1.1% in North America to 9.6–13.0% in North Africa
3 Infects 3.9 million people in the USA

Prior to screening of blood, HCV was the etiologic agent in >85% of cases of post-transfusion hepatitis (see Table 4.6)

Risk factors for acquisition	Proportion in the USA
Percutaneous	
Transfusion associated	<5%
Injection drug use	40%
Needlestick exposure	1%
Non percutaneous	
Sexual contact	Unknown (probably low)
Perinatal exposure	Unknown (probably low)
Sporadic	40%

(Table 4.6: Risk factors for acquisition of HCV)

4 Risk of transmission/acquisition with exposure depends on mode of acquisition
- sexual (<5%)
- injection drug use (90%)
- needlestick exposure (5–10%)
- perinatal exposure (0–50% depending on titer of virus in the mother)

C   Clinical manifestations/natural history

1 Clinical findings
- with acute infection, the majority are asymptomatic, although jaundice can occur
- with chronic infection, fatigue is the most frequent complaint, the degree of which is unrelated to the severity of liver disease
- other complaints include depression, nausea, anorexia, abdominal discomfort, and difficulty with concentration
- with advancing liver disease, ascites, encephalopathy, and gastrointestinal bleeding may occur as complications of portal hypertension
- jaundice is rare until hepatic decompensation is profound

2 **Natural history**
- infection, once established, persists in the vast majority (>80%)
- progression of disease is largely silent, with infection/disease often identified only on routine biochemical screening or during the course of blood donation
- death from end-stage liver disease is uncommon, but clearly liver failure and HCC can occur
- HCC occurs in approximately 15% of those with cirrhosis
- while limited in their duration of follow-up, available prospective studies indicate that at least 20–30 years of infection are required to develop clinically significant disease
- in a large observational study by Seeff and colleagues (1992)[3], outcome of 568 patients with post-transfusion non-A, non-B hepatitis was compared to 984

matched controls who received transfusions but did not develop hepatitis. After an average of 18 years of follow-up, mortality from all causes was similar in cases and controls

- death rate attributable to liver disease was low but was higher in cases than in controls (3.3% versus 1.5%)
- however, morbidity was significant; after 20 years, liver biopsies were obtained in patients with biochemical abnormalities and serologic evidence of HCV infection, and almost 90% had evidence of chronic hepatitis or cirrhosis

- findings have been confirmed in a large study by Clarke et al. (1996)[4], which evaluated natural history in 438 young women who were exposed to HCV. Prolonged follow-up (more than 18 years) revealed few patients with cirrhosis and none who had developed complications of liver disease

3 Extrahepatic manifestations may be secondary to immune complex deposition in association with intact virus or viral proteins

- membranoproliferative glomerulonephritis (rare)
- mixed cryoglobulinemia (common)
- porphyria cutanea tarda (common)
- leukocytoclasitc vasculitis (rare)
- focal lymphocytic sialadenitis (rare)
- idiopathic pulmonary fibrosis (rare)

D   Serologic and virologic tests (see also Ch. 3)

1 Diagnosis largely depends on detection of antibodies to the virus. Currently three generations of serological assays exist which use recombinant antigens derived from cloned HCV transcripts (see Table 4.7)

Serologic test	Antigens	Sensitivity (%)	Specificity (%)
EIA-1	c-100–3	89	92
EIA-2	c-100–3, c22–3, c33c	100	68
RIBA-2[a]	c100–3, c22–3, c33c, c1–1, SOD	98	97
RIBA-3	c100–3, c22, c33c, NS5		99.35

[a](+) result: two or more bands are detectable representing at least two gene products
(–) result: no bands reacts
EIA, ezyme immuoassay; RIBA, recombinant immunoblot assay

(Table 4.7: Indeterminate: one band from one region, superoxide dismutase, and two or more antigen bands)

- sensitivities and specificities above are based on a small study of 54 patients with clinical chronic non-A, non-B hepatitis, compared with patients with nonviral liver disease (Silva et al. 1994)[5]
- sensitivity and specificity of these tests depend on the prevalence of disease in the population under study

2 viral RNA detected by amplification methods such as polymerase chain reaction (PCR) or hybridization methods such as the branched DNA (bDNA)

3 HCV RNA (quantitative or qualitative) may also be used prior to the initiation of therapy and for monitoring during therapy

4 Figure 4.1 shows an algorithm for testing for HCV infection

E Pathology/pathogenesis

1 Pathology ranges from minimal periportal lymphocytic inflammation to active

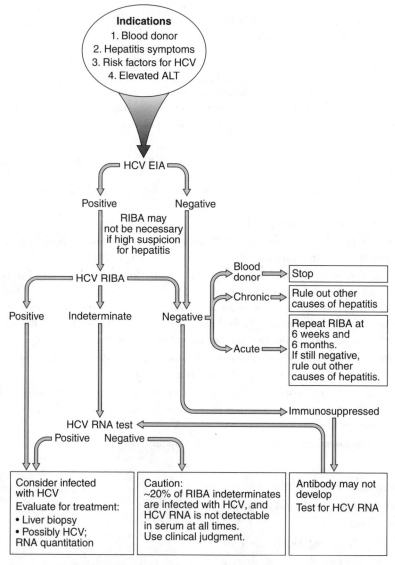

Fig. 4.1: Algorithm for the diagnosis of HCV infection (Reproduced from Wilber and Polito 1995[6])

hepatitis with bridging fibrosis, hepatocyte necrosis, and frank cirrhosis. Steatosis, lymphoid aggregates, and bile duct damage are frequently found in the liver biopsies of patients with HCV infection, but there is considerable overlap with the histologic findings in patients with chronic HBV infection and autoimmune hepatitis

2   Grading and staging of liver histology are the same as for HBV infection

3   Three mechanisms of pathogenesis of HCV-related liver injury have been proposed:
   * direct cytopathic damage
   * immune-directed hepatocyte inflammation and destruction
   * viral-induced autoimmunity

The weight of evidence suggests that immune-mediated mechanisms predominate, with destruction of hepatocytes by sensitized T cells

F   Therapy

Knowledge of the natural history of untreated infection and factors contributing to disease progression are essential when assessing the need for therapeutic intervention. HCV clearly can cause progressive liver disease; thus, treatment is justified

1   Drugs

a   Interferon

* interferon alpha-2b is currently the only approved treatment for chronic HCV infection in the USA

* early results revealed an initial response rate of only 40–50% and a sustained biochemical response rate of only 25%. In most studies biochemical response is defined by normalization of serum aminotransferase activity

* **standard dose of interferon alpha is 3 mU three times weekly for 6 months**. Increasing the duration of therapy (to 12–18 months) increases the sustained response rates by about 10%, but it increases the cost of treatment. Increasing the dose to 5–10 mU three times weekly increases rate of sustained response by 5–10% but this substantially increases side effects

* current standards define a response to therapy as normal serum ALT and absent HCV RNA 6 months or more after treatment cessation

* duration of post-treatment follow-up in most trials has been short; thus, interferon has not been proven to influence progression to decompensated disease or development of HCC

* features associated with an improved therapeutic response:

Low pre-treatment HCV RNA level
Infection with non-type 1 viral genotype
Absence of cirrhosis
Treatment for 12–18 months
Low hepatic iron content
Mutations in NS5b

- combination of interferon with other agents including ribavirin, thymosin, or ursodeoxycholic acid may improve response rates

b **Ribavirin**
- ribavirin is an antiviral agent with activity against DNA and RNA viruses
- monotherapy results in transient decreases in ALT levels, minor improvements in liver histology, but no changes in HCV RNA levels
- ribavirin in combination with interferon has shown promise in improving sustained response rates, and a phase III trial is under way

2 **Liver transplantation** (see also Ch. 31)
- chronic HCV is the most common indication for liver transplantation
- post-transplantation recurrence (determined by presence of virus) is universal
- histologic evidence of liver injury is present in approximately 50% at 1 year, a proportion which increases with follow-up
- serological assays underestimate post-transplantation HCV infection and virological tests may be required for diagnosis
- histologic findings typical of post-transplantation HCV infection include fatty infiltration, portal and parenchymal mononuclear infiltrates, and hepatocyte swelling and necrosis
- short-term survival is similar to that in patients who undergo liver transplantation for non-viral liver disease
- interferon therapy has been used to treat post-transplantation recurrence. Transient reductions in HCV RNA levels have been observed, but sustained biochemical and virologic responses are rare
- interferon should be used in transplant recipients with caution, since treatment may increase the risk of allograft rejection

4 Hepatitis D (HDV)

A Virology

1 Single-stranded positive-sense RNA molecule
2 HBsAg is used as the envelope protein. Thus, HDV assembly occurs only in the presence of HBV infection
3 Unlike HBV, HDV infects only hepatocytes, with no extrahepatic sites of viral replication
4 In coinfection, HDV frequently appears to inhibit or suppress replication of HBV
5 Two highly conserved regions of the genoune exist, each approximately 265 nucleotides in length, which are believed to be important for viral replication as well as autocleavage and ligation
6 Comparison of full-length RNA sequences reveals significant heterogeneity. Currently, three genotypes have been proposed:
  - type 1 – predominant type in most areas of the world
  - type 2 – more common in Taiwan/less severe disease
  - type 3 – South America/associated with severe hepatitis

B   Epidemiology

1 HDV infection occurs only in the presence of HBV infection
   - coinfection – when both viruses are acquired simultaneously
   - superinfection – when HDV infection occurs in a patient with chronic HBV infection

2 Approximately 15 million individuals are infected worldwide

3 Areas of high prevalence include southern Italy, the Amazon Basin, Columbia, Venezuela, Western Asia, Eastern Europe, and some Pacific Islands

4 Injection drug use is the single most important risk factor

C   Clinical manifestations/natural history

1 Symptoms of HDV are nonspecific; therefore, diagnosis is rarely made based on clinical presentation

2 HDV infection should be suspected in
   - fulminant HBV infection
   - acute HBV infection that improves but subsequently relapses
   - progressive chronic HBV in the absence of active HBV replication

3 Coinfection with HBV and HDV produces more severe acute illness than HBV infection alone and is associated with an increased risk of fulminant hepatic failure

4 Rate of chronicity following coinfection with HBV and HDV is similar to that for HBV infection alone (<5%)

5 Superinfection with HDV in a patient with chronic HBV accelerates the natural history of chronic HBV

D   Serological and virologic tests

1 Currently available tests are enzyme-linked immunosorbent assay (ELISA) for IgG and IgM anti-HDV

2 Using only anti-HDV, differentiation between chronic HDV infection with active replication and resolved HDV infection in the absence of HDV replication is difficult

3 Persistence of IgM anti-HDV and/or very high titers of IgG anti-HDV is suggestive of ongoing HDV infection

4 Detection of HDV RNA in serum is suggestive of persistent infection, but this test is only available on a research basis

E   Pathology/pathogenesis

1 Necroinflammatory activity is often severe, but histologic features are not specific for chronic HDV

2 Hepatitis D antigen (HDAg) is readily demonstrated in nuclei and to a lesser extent in the cytoplasm of infected cells

3 HDV appears to be directly cytopathic, but the mechanism of cell death is unknown

F Therapy

1 Drugs
- interferon alpha therapy results in an initial response in 50%, but biochemical and virological response is rarely sustained
- typical interferon dose is 9 MU three times per week

2 Transplantation
- patients with chronic HDV infection are at lower risk for HBV recurrence than are those with chronic HBV alone
- HDV recurrence can be detected prior to signs of HBV reactivation
- decreased recurrence rates and improved survival in HDV cirrhosis may be due to the inhibitory effects of HDV on HBV replication
- post-transplantation there are two distinct pathological findings:
  - inflammatory changes and active HBV replication
  - hepatocyte necrosis in the absence of inflammation and in the absence of HBV active replication
- there are no convincing data on the treatment of post-transplantation recurrent hepatitis with interferon

5 Hepatitis G

- recently identified RNA virus which is transfusion transmitted
- causes persistent infection for many years
- present in patients with various other liver diseases, including cryptogenic cirrhosis, chronic HBV, chronic HCV
- viremia present in approximately 1.5% of healthy US blood donors, irrespective of the presence or absence of elevated serum ALT levels
- causative association with liver disease has not been demonstated
- clinical manifestations, natural history and pathogenesis are under investigation
- diagnosis is currently dependent on virologic assays avialable only in research setting

References

1   Weissberg JL, Andres LL, Smith CI, et al. *Survival in chronic hepatitis B: an analysis of 379 patients*. (Ann Intern Med 1984) 101: 613–16

2   Batts KP, Ludwig J. *Chronic hepatitis. An update on terminology and reporting*. (Am J Pathol 1995) 19: 1409–17

3   Seeff LB, Buskell-Bales Z, Wright EC. Long-term mortality after transfusion-associated non-A, non-B hepatitis. (N Engl J Med 1992) 327: 1906–11

4   Clarke G, Pathmakanthan S, Sullivan A, et al. *Interferon–Ribavirin combination therapy for chronic hepatitis C, type 1B in a unique Irish cohort 18 years post inoculation*. (Gastroenterology 1996) 110: A1173

5   Silva AE, Hosein B, Boyle R. *Diagnosis of chronic hepatitis C: comparison of immunoassays and the polymerase chain reaction*. (Am J Gastroenterol 1994) 89: 493–6

6   Wilber JC, Polito A. *Serological and virological diagnostic tests for hepatitis C virus infection.* (Semin Gastrointest Dis 1995) 6: 13–19

7   Dienstag J, Perrillo RP, Schiff ER, Bartholomew M, et al. *A preliminary trial of lamivudine for chronic hepatitis B infection.* (N Engl J Med 1995) 333: 1657–61

8   Niederau C, Heintges T, Lange, S et al. *Long-term follow-up of HBeAg-positive patients treated with interferon alpha for chronic hepatitis B.* (N Engl J Med 1996) 334: 1422–7

9   Perrillo RB, Schiff ER, Davis EL, et al. *A randomized controlled trial of interferon alpha-2b alone and after prednisone withdrawal.* (N Engl J Med 1990) 323: 295–301

10 Terrault NA, Wright TL. *Therapy for chronic hepatitis B.* (Adv Exp Med Biol 1996) 394: 189–205

11 Wong DKH, Cheung AM, O'Rourke K, et al. *Effect of alpha-interferon treatment in patients with hepatitis Be antigen-positive chronic hepatitis: a meta-analysis.* (Ann Intern Med 1993) 1194: 312–23

CHAPTER 5

Autoimmune hepatitis

ALBERT J. CZAJA, M.D.

Key Points

1 Criteria for diagnosis have been codified and a quantitative scoring system exists

2 Definite diagnosis requires absence of viral infection and includes clinical disease of any duration

3 Prognosis relates to severity of inflammatory activity and HLA risk factors. Patients with HLA DR3 are younger, respond less well to corticosteroids, and require liver transplantation more commonly than patients with HLA DR4

4 Two subtypes are valid based on distinctive immunoserologic findings, clinical differences, and treatment outcomes

5 Variant forms are present, and empiric therapies are appropriate

6 Two treatment regimens are equally effective and each is superior to no therapy or nonsteroidal regimens. Prednisone in combination with azathioprine is preferred over prednisone alone because of fewer side effects

7 Indefinite therapy with low-dose prednisone (≤10 mg daily) or azathioprine (2 mg/kg/day) controls disease after multiple relapses

8 Higher than conventional doses of medication improve clinical and laboratory features of treatment failure but liver transplantation may be necessary

▶

9 Liver transplantation is effective for patients who have decompensated on corticosteroid therapy but recurrence after transplantation is possible

10 Multiple immunosuppressive and cytoprotective agents have theoretical or anecdotal bases for efficacy but are unproven

1 Diagnosis

A Clinical definition

1 Self-perpetuating hepatocellular inflammation of unknown cause characterized by periportal hepatitis (also referred to as piecemeal necrosis or interface hepatitis) on histologic examination, hypergammaglobulinemia, and liver-associated autoantibodies in serum

2 Requires exclusion of other chronic liver diseases that have similar features, including Wilson's disease, chronic viral hepatitis, alpha-1 antitrypsin deficiency, hemochromatosis, drug-induced liver disease, nonalcoholic steatohepatitis, and the immune cholangiopathies of primary biliary cirrhosis (PBC), primary sclerosing cholangitis (PSC), and autoimmune cholangitis

3 Minimum diagnostic studies at presentation are shown in Table 5.1

B Nomenclature

1 Designation, *autoimmune hepatitis*, replaces terms such as autoimmune liver disease and autoimmune chronic active hepatitis

2 No subtypes formally recognized, but types 1, 2, and 3 autoimmune hepatitis (defined by principal autoantibody reactivity) used in clinical practice

C Diagnostic criteria

1 Criteria for the *definite* and *probable* diagnosis established by consensus of an international panel are shown in Table 5.2

2 Requirement for 6 months of disease activity to establish chronicity is not necessary, reflecting tendency for acute presentation

3 Lobular hepatitis is in the histologic spectrum, but periportal hepatitis remains the sine qua non for diagnosis

4 Cholestatic histologic changes, including bile duct injury and ductopenia, or features suggestive of another disease (fat, copper, or iron overload, portal tract lymphoid aggregates) argue against the diagnosis

5 Evidence of an infection with a hepatitis virus (hepatitis A, hepatitis B, hepatitis C, Epstein–Barr virus, cytomegalovirus) precludes *definite* diagnosis

6 Patients who lack conventional autoantibodies but who satisfy other criteria and are seropositive for antibodies to asialoglycoprotein receptor (anti-ASGPR),

Diagnostic studies	Purpose
Serum aspartate (AST) and alanine aminotransferase (ALT), bilirubin, alkaline phosphatase, and gamma globulin levels	Estimate severity of inflammatory activity Confirm predominant hepatocellular pattern of injury
Serum albumin level and prothrombin time	Estimate impairment of hepatic synthetic function
Antinuclear antibodies (ANA), smooth muscle antibodies (SMA), antibodies to liver/kidney microsome 1 (anti-LKM1), antimitochondrial antibodies (AMA)	Document presence and nature of immunologic activity
Serum immunoglobulin levels	Confirm mainly IgG elevation
Liver tissue examination	Document histologic changes compatible with the diagnosis Exclude findings suggestive of other diagnoses
HBsAg, anti-HBc, IgM anti-HAV, and anti-HCV (second-generation assays)	Document absence of concurrent viral infection
Recombinant immunoblot assay (second generation) for anti-HCV and/or HCV RNA in serum by polymerase chain reaction if anti-HCV positive by enzyme immunoassay (ELISA)	Exclude false-positive ELISA for anti-HCV Confirm absence of concurrent infection with hepatitis C virus
Ceruloplasmin level	Exclude Wilson's disease (< age 40)
Alpha-1 antitrypsin phenotype	Exclude alpha-1 antitrypsin deficiency
Serum iron, transferrin and ferritin levels	Exclude hemochromatosis

(Table 5.1: Minimum diagnostic tests at presentation)

soluble liver antigen (anti-SLA), liver–pancreas (anti-LP), or liver cytosol type 1 (anti-LC1) warrant a *probable* diagnosis

7 Scoring system accommodates diverse manifestations of the disease and renders an aggregate score that reflects net strength of diagnosis before and after corticosteroid treatment. It is useful in evaluating patients with mixed features (see Table 5.3)

2 Pathogenesis

A Hypotheses: two prevailing theories:

- autoantigen-driven cell-mediated cytotoxicity
- antibody-dependent cell-mediated cytotoxicity

Diagnostic features	Definite diagnosis	Probable diagnosis
Epidemiologic factors	No exposure to drugs or hepatotoxic chemicals No blood transfusions Limited average daily alcohol use (<35 g in men and <25 g in women)	Exposure to drug, chemicals or excess alcohol but continued liver injury despite withdrawal Moderate average daily alcohol use (35–50 g in men and 25–40 g in women)
Viral markers	No HBsAg, IgM anti-HBc, anti-HCV, IgM anti-HAV by current assays Negative Epstein–Barr virus and cytomegalovirus assays	False-positive anti-HCV Past HBV infection (HBsAg negative, anti-HBc and anti-HBs positive)
Inflammatory indices	Predominant serum aspartate (AST) or alanine aminotransferase (ALT) abnormality Hypergammaglobulinemia Normal alpha-1 antitrypsin phenotype (or level) Normal serum copper level Normal serum ceruloplasmin	Abnormal serum copper or ceruloplasmin if Wilson's disease excluded Partial alpha-1 antitrypsin deficiency
Autoantibodies	ANA, SMA or anti-LKM1 titers $\geq 1:80$ in adults and $\geq 1:20$ in children	ANA, SMA, or anti-LKM1 titers $\geq 1:40$ in adults or $\geq 1:10$ in children Other liver-related antibodies
Immunoglobulins	Total globulin, gamma globulin, or IgG level ≥1.5 times normal limit	Globulin abnormality of any degree
Histologic findings	Moderate to severe piecemeal necrosis with or without lobular hepatitis or central – portal bridging necrosis No biliary or other lesions	Same changes as for definite diagnosis

(Table 5.2: Consensus criteria for the definite or probable diagnosis)

1 **Autoantigen-driven cell-mediated hypothesis** (preferred theory) requires:
   - aberrant display of HLA class II antigens on hepatocyte surface because of viral, drug, toxic, environmental, or idopathic factors
   - enhanced presentation of normal liver cell constituents as autoantigens
   - activation of antigen processing cells that stimulate clonal expansion of autoantigen-sensitized cytotoxic T lymphocytes
   - liver cell destruction by tissue-infiltrating cytotoxic T lymphocytes which release noxious cytokines
   - modulation of disease susceptibility and severity by human leukocyte antigens (HLA) DR3 and DR4

2 **Antibody-dependent cell-mediated cytotoxicity** hypothesis requires:
   - intrinsic defect in suppressor T lymphocyte function that facilitates

	Score		Score
Gender		*Blood transfusion*	
Female	+2	Yes	–2
		No	+1
Alkaline phosphatase : asparatate			
aminotransferase levels		*Alcohol consumption*	
≥3	–2	<25 g/day	+2
<3	+2	<60 g/day	–2
Gamma globulin or IgG levels		*Immune disease*	
above normal		Patient or relative	+1
>2.0	+3		
1.5–2.0	+2	*Histologic findings*	
1.0–1.5	+1	Lobular hepatitis + bridging	+3
<1.0	0	Piecemeal necrosis only	+2
		Rosettes	+1
		Marked plasma cells	+1
ANA, SMA, or Anti-LKM1		Biliary changes	–1
>1 : 80	+3	Other etiologic features	–3
1 : 80	+2		
1 : 40	+1	*HLA*	
<1 : 40	0	B8-DR3 or DR4	+1
Antimitochondrial antibodies		*Treatment responses*	
Positive	–2	Complete	+2
		Partial	0
Viral markers		Treatment failure	0
HBsAg or IgM anti-HAV	–3	No response	–2
HCV RNA or other viruses	–3	Relapse	–3
Anti-HCV/RIBA reactive	–2		
All negative	+3	**Diagnostic scores**	
		Pretreatment: definite	**>15**
Drugs		**probable**	**10–15**
Yes	–2	**Post-treatment: definite**	**>17**
No	+1	**probable**	**12–17**

(Table 5.3: Scoring system for quantitative diagnosis)

unmodulated B cell production of IgG against normal hepatocytic membrane proteins

- antigen–antibody complex on hepatocyte surface targeted by natural killer cells with Fc receptors
- Linkage of natural killer cell to antigen–antibody complex and subsequent cytolysis
- HLA A1-B8-DR3 predisposition for suppressor T cell defect

B   Shortcomings

1 None of the autoantibodies associated with autoimmune hepatitis is pathogenic
2 Reasons for aberrant HLA display on hepatocyte surface uncertain

3 Only one autoantigen (P-450 IID6) incriminated in pathogenesis, and it relates to a rare form of disease (type 2 autoimmune hepatitis)

4 No reproducible animal model that fully reflects human disease

5 Only *non-antigen-specific* suppressor T cell defect demonstrated, which may not be disease specific

6 Multiple viruses proposed as etiologic agents but none established

3 Subclassifications

A Types

1 Type 1 autoimmune hepatitis (see Table 5.4)

- characterized by the presence of smooth muscle antibodies (SMA) and/or antinuclear antibodies (ANA) in serum

- antibodies to actin (anti-actin) specific for the diagnosis but low sensitivity (38–74%) and best assay for detection unestablished
- occurs at any age but typically has bimodal age distribution
- majority (78%) are women (female : male ratio, 3.6 : 1).
- concurrent extrahepatic immunologic diseases in 41%, including:

  - autoimmune thyroiditis (12%)
  - Graves' disease (6%)
  - chronic ulcerative colitis (CUC) (6%)
  - rheumatoid arthritis (1%)
  - pernicious anemia (1%)
  - systemic sclerosis (1%)
  - Coomb's positive hemolytic anemia (1%)
  - idiopathic thrombocytopenic purpura (1%)
  - leukocytoclastic vasculitis (1%)
  - nephritis (1%)
  - erythema nodosum (1%)
  - fibrosing alveolitis (1%)

- concurrent CUC compels cholangiography to exclude PSC
- acute onset in 40%; may resemble fulminant hepatitis. Typically, clinical (ascites, esophageal varices, and/or spider telangiectases), laboratory (thrombocytopenia, hypoalbuminemia, and/or hypergammaglobulinemia), and histologic changes (cirrhosis) suggest pre-existing chronic disease
- target autoantigen unknown but ASGPR promising candidate because of

membrane surface location, antigen trafficking function, association with high-titer autoantibodies in serum, and presence of ASGPR-sensitized liver-infiltrating lymphocytes in patients

- antibodies to ASGPR, especially those directed against human-derived antigen, have diagnostic and prognostic value, since they are specific for diagnosis; titers correlate with degree of inflammatory activity; and their persistence during therapy is associated with relapse after drug withdrawal
- HLA DR3 and DR4 are independent risk factors for susceptibility and suggest a polygenic disorder. DRB1*0301 allele associated most closely with the disease in white patients of northern European extraction in the USA, whereas DRB1*0401 has secondary association

2 Type 2 autoimmune hepatitis (see Table 5.4)

- characterized by antibodies to liver/kidney microsome type 1 (anti-LKM1) in serum

- afflicts mainly children (age range 2–14 years)
- 20% of European patients are adults whereas only 4% of American patients are adults
- genetic polymorphisms affect expression of cytochrome monooxygenase P-450 IID6 and influence regional prevalence
- acute or fulminant presentation possible
- commonly associated with concurrent immune diseases, including vitiligo, insulin-dependent diabetes mellitus, or autoimmune thyroiditis
- frequent concurrence of organ-specific autoantibodies, including antibodies to parietal cells, thyroid, or islets of Langerhans
- lower serum concentrations of immunoglobulins, especially IgA, than type 1 autoimmune hepatitis
- progresses to cirrhosis more frequently during therapy than type 1 disease (82% versus 43% within 3 years) and probably has poorer prognosis
- cytochrome monooxygenase, P-450 IID6 (CYP2D6), is putative target autoantigen
  - epitopes of anti-LKM1 included in linear 33 amino acid sequence of recombinant P-450 IID6 and some within even shorter eight amino acid sequence
  - 254–271 peptide sequence of recombinant P-450 IID6 designated as "core motif" for anti-LKM1 reactivity in type 2 disease
  - antibodies to LKM1 present in chronic hepatitis C but reactive to epitopes usually outside core motif
- HLA B14, DR3 and C4A–Q0 are possible susceptibility factors

3 Type 3 autoimmune hepatitis

- unestablished as distinct subgroup
- characterized by antibodies to soluble liver antigen (anti-SLA), which are directed against cytokeratins 8 and 18

Clinical features	Type 1	Type 2
Diagnostic autoantibodies	Smooth muscle antibodies Antinuclear antibodies Antibodies to actin	Antibodies to liver/kidney microsome type 1 Antibodies to P-450 IID6 Antibodies to synthetic peptides 254–271
Age (years)	Bimodal (10–20 and 45–70)	Pediatric (2–14) Rare adults (4%)
Women (%)	78	89
Concurrent immune diseases (%)	41	34
Concurrent organ-specific antibodies (%)	4	30
Gamma-globulin elevation	+++	+
Low IgA	No	Occasional
Human leukocyte antigen (HLA) associations	B8, DR3, DR4	B14, DR3, C4A-Q0
Allelic risk factors	DRB1*0301 DRB1*0401 DRB3*0101 DRB4*0103	Uncertain
Steroid response	+++	++
Progression to cirrhosis (%)	45	82

(Table 5.4: Features of type 1 and type 2 autoimmune hepatitis)

- ANA and anti-LKM1 absent but SMA (35%), antibodies to mitochondria (AMA) (22%), rheumatoid factor (22%), and antibodies to liver–membrane antigen (26%) commonly present
- antibodies to SLA absent in chronic viral hepatitis but present in 11% of type 1 autoimmune hepatitis, suggesting type 3 is a variant rather than separate condition. Seropositivity for anti-SLA not associated with distinctive clinical or prognostic features
- antibodies to liver–pancreas (anti-LP) are better markers for type 3 autoimmune hepatitis but also lack exclusivity. Sixty-three percent with anti-LP are anti-actin positive; 12% have ANA; and 30% have antibodies to cytokeratins 8 and 18

B Variants (see Table 5.5)

1 Overlap syndrome with PBC

- defined by features of autoimmune hepatitis in conjunction with AMA seropositivity and/or histologic findings of bile duct injury or loss
- majority (88%) have AMA titers ≤ 1 : 160 and rare seropositivity for antibodies to M2 autoantigens (8%) (see Ch. 14)

- AMA reactivity may be false because of confusion with anti-LKM1 by indirect immunofluorescence
- hepatic copper accumulation in 19% suggests PBC component
- empiric corticosteroid treatment (3–6 months) improves autoimmune-predominant disease and argues against diagnosis of PBC

2 Overlap syndrome with PSC

- defined by features of autoimmune hepatitis in conjunction with inflammatory bowel disease, cholestatic biochemical changes, histologic evidence of bile duct injury, and/or recalcitrance to corticosteroid therapy
- cholangiography required for diagnosis and warranted in those with chronic liver disease and inflammatory bowel disease, regardless of other diagnostic features
- radiologic changes of intra- and/or extrahepatic bile duct damage diagnostic of overlap in clinical context of autoimmune hepatitis
- histologic features of fibrous cholangitis or fibrous obliterative cholangitis and normal cholangiogram indicate small duct variant
- clues to diagnosis are inflammatory bowel disease, suboptimal response to corticosteroid therapy, and/or rising serum alkaline phosphatase level
- histologic findings range from periportal hepatitis only to periportal hepatitis and background bile duct injury or obstruction
- resistance to corticosteroids is typical; drug withdrawal justified as soon as lack of efficacy shown

3 Overlap syndrome with viral hepatitis

- concurrence of viral infection and autoantibodies constitutes overlap between autoimmune hepatitis and chronic viral hepatitis
- true positive reactions for antibodies to hepatitis C virus (anti-HCV) and serologic evidence of hepatitis B virus infection (antibodies to hepatitis B core antibody and/or hepatitis B surface antigen) in only 4% of autoimmune hepatitis
- HCV RNA in serum by polymerase chain reaction in 11% of autoimmune hepatitis that does not respond to corticosteroids or that relapses after corticosteroid withdrawal
- SMA in 11%, ANA in 28%, diverse autoantibodies (SMA, ANA, thyroid antibodies, rheumatoid factor, and/or IgG antibodies to double-stranded DNA) in 62%, and concurrent immune disease in 23% of chronic viral hepatitis
  - SMA and ANA titers are typically low in chronic viral hepatitis ($\leq 1 : 80$ in 89%). Only 11% with serum titers $\geq 1 : 160$ and rarely titers $\geq 1 : 320$
  - concurrent seropositivity for SMA and ANA rare (4%)
- median serum titers of SMA and ANA $1 : 160$ and $1 : 320$, respectively, in autoimmune hepatitis. Only 6% with isolated titers $\leq 1 : 80$ and 60% have concurrent SMA and ANA
- Treatment directed against predominant disease:
  - **autoimmune-predominant disease** defined by SMA or ANA titers $\geq 1 : 320$ or concurrent SMA and ANA seropositivity regardless of titer
  - **viral-predominant disease** defined by true viral infection and anti-LKM1 or true viral infection and low-titer ($<1 : 320$) SMA or ANA seropositivity

- histologic changes can define autoimmune or viral predominance but with uncertain sensitivity:
  - moderate to severe portal plasma cell infiltration (66% versus 21%), lobular inflammation (47% versus 16%), and piecemeal necrosis (23% versus 0%) more commonly in autoimmune-predominant disease
  - portal lymphoid aggregates (49% versus 10%), steatosis (72% versus 19%), and bile duct damage or loss (91% versus 20%) more frequently in viral-predominant disease (chronic hepatitis C)
- treatment is appropriate to the prevailing condition: corticosteroids for autoimmune-predominant disease and interferon for viral-predominant disease. Results must be assessed at 3 months and alternative therapies considered if response is poor

- corticosteroids in viral-predominant disease are ineffective and increase virus burden. Interferon in autoimmune-predominant disease enhances immunoreactivity and may exacerbate inflammatory activity

4 Autoimmune cholangitis
- has composite features of autoimmune hepatitis and AMA-negative PBC
- ANA and/or SMA typically present in conjunction with cholestatic biochemical changes, normal cholangiogram, and/or histologic findings of bile duct injury
- antibodies to carbonic anhydrase commonly present; occurrence greater than in autoimmune hepatitis or PBC
- variable responsiveness to corticosteroids or ursodeoxycholic acid. Therapies improve clinical and laboratory findings but not histologic changes

5 Cryptogenic chronic hepatitis
- satisfies consensus criteria for diagnosis of autoimmune hepatitis but lacks characteristic autoantibodies
- similar in age, female predominance, frequency of concurrent immunologic diseases, histologic features, occurrence of HLA B8, DR3 and A1-B8-DR3, and laboratory findings to autoimmune hepatitis
- respond as well to corticosteroid treatment as autoantibody-positive counterparts
- represent form of autoimmune hepatitis that has escaped detection by conventional immunoserologic assays
- reclassification to autoimmune hepatitis possible by testing for anti-SLA (18%) and anti-LP (33%) and successive testing for conventional autoantibodies that may have late or variable appearance.

4 Prevalence

1 0.69 cases per 100 000 persons per year in Western Europe (or in other ethnically similar populations)
2 Frequency of 11–23% among chronic liver diseases of North America

Variant	Features	Treatment
Overlap with primary biliary cirrhosis (PBC)	Low-titer antimitochondrial antibodies Absent antibodies to M2 antigens Antibodies to liver/kidney microsome 1 confused with mitochondrial antibodies Histologic features of cholangitis Hepatic iron accumulation possible	Empiric therapy with prednisone (20 mg daily maintenance) × 3–6 months
Overlap with primary sclerosing cholangitis (PSC)	Inflammatory bowel disease Cholestatic biochemical changes Histologic evidence of cholangitis Abnormal cholangiogram (except in "small duct" variant) Resistance to corticosteroids	Discontinuation of corticosteroids Empiric therapy with ursodeoxycholic acid (15–20 mg/kg/day) Investigational protocols
Overlap with viral hepatitis	True positive antibodies to hepatitis C HCV RNA in serum Smooth muscle or antinuclear antibodies Autoimmune or viral predominance determined by autoantibody titer, concurrent immunoserologic markers, and histologic changes	Autoimmune predominant: prednisone trial (20 mg daily) × 3–6 months Viral predominant: interferon trial (3 million units s.c. thrice weekly) × 6 months
Autoimmune cholangitis	Antinuclear antibodies and/or smooth muscle antibodies present Cholestatic biochemical changes No antimitochondrial antibodies Histologic features of cholangitis Normal cholangiogram Antibodies to carbonic anhydrase	Prednisone (20 mg daily maintenance) × 3–6 months Ursodeoxycholic acid (15 mg/kg daily) × 3–6 months
Cryptogenic chronic hepatitis	Autoimmune hepatitis but no conventional autoantibodies	Prednisone (20 mg daily) or prednisone and azathioprine combination

(Table 5.5: Variants forms of autoimmune hepatitis)

3 Prevalence greatest among white groups of northern Europe, North America, and Australia with a high frequency of HLA DR3 and DR4

4 Japanese patients have HLA DR4 association

5   Prognostic Indices

A   Severity of inflammation

1 Biochemical indices

- serum aspartate aminotransferase (AST) and gamma globulin levels most useful
- 3-year mortality of 50% and 10-year mortaility of 90% in patients with sustained serum AST level of at least 10-fold normal or at least 5-fold normal in

conjunction with serum gamma globulin level of at least twice normal

- 10-year mortality of 10% and low frequency of cirrhosis (49% after 15 years) in patients with less severe laboratory abnormalities
- spontaneous resolution in 13–20% regardless of disease activity
- untreated patients with initially severe disease who survive the first 2 years of illness survive long term. Such survivors commonly (41%) develop inactive cirrhosis

2 Histologic indices

- periportal hepatitis (piecemeal necrosis or interface hepatitis) associated with normal 5-year survival and 17% frequency of cirrhosis
- bridging necrosis or multilobular necrosis associated with 5-year mortality of 45% and frequency of cirrhosis at 5 years of 82%
- cirrhosis at presentation associated with 5-year mortality of 58%. Esophageal varices develop in 54% with cirrhosis, and death from hemorrhage occurs in 20% of those with varices

B HLA status

1 HLA B8 and DR3 identify younger patients with more severe inflammatory activity, less responsiveness to corticosteroid therapy, and greater frequency of liver transplantation

2 HLA DR4 identifies patients with different clinical features and better outcomes than those with HLA DR3. Patients with HLA DR4 are older and more commonly women than counterparts with HLA DR3. They have concurrent immunologic diseases more frequently, and they enter remission more often and fail corticosteroid therapy less commonly than patients with HLA DR3

3 DQA1*0101 and DQA1*0102 alleles associated with a lower frequency of autoimmune hepatitis in men and may have protective effect

4 DRB1*0301 (86% versus 45%, $p = 0.008$) and DRB1*0301-DRB3*0101 (79% versus 42%, $p = 0.02$) occur more commonly in patients who fail corticosteroid treatment. In contrast, DRB1*0401 and DRB1*0401-DRB4*0103 are associated with a lower frequency of death from liver failure or need for transplantation than other alleles (0% versus 37%, $p = 0.03$)

5 Patients with DRB1*0301 differ from those with DRB1*0401 in that they are younger and fail treatment more commonly (27% versus 5%, $p = 0.04$)

6 Null allotypes at the complement C4A and C4B locus occur in 90% of patients with early-onset disease

7 21-Hydroxylase A pseudogene in adults associated with increased mortality and frequent relapses

6 Clinical Features

1 Most common symptom is easy fatigability (85%). Weight loss unusual, and intense pruritus against diagnosis

2 Most common physical findings are hepatomegaly (78%) and jaundice (69%).

Splenomegaly may occur in patients with and without cirrhosis (56% and 32%, respectively) as may spider telangiectases

3 Hyperbilirubinemia in 83%, but serum level infrequently higher than threefold normal (46%). Serum alkaline phosphatase level commonly increased (81%) but not more than twofold (33%) or fourfold (10%) normal

4 Polyclonal hypergammaglobulinemia is required for diagnosis; IgG fraction predominates

5 Diverse, nonspecific immunoserologic findings are common: antibodies to bacteria (*Escherichia coli*, *Bacteroides* and *Salmonella*) and viruses (measles, rubella and cytomegalovirus). Cryoglobulinemia possible, but symptomatic disease rare

6 Concurrent immunologic diseases frequent (41%) and involve diverse organ systems, most frequently the thyroid

7 SMA, ANA and anti-LKM1 required for the diagnosis but other autoantibodies possible, including antibodies to ASGPR, actin, SLA, LP, and LC1. These latter autoantibodies do not have routine clinical applications and are investigational in nature

7   Treatment

A   Indications (see Table 5.6)

	Indications	
Absolute	**Relative**	**None**
Incapacitating symptoms	Mild or no symptoms	Asymptomatic with mild laboratory changes
Relentless clinical progression		Previous intolerance of prednisone and/or azathioprine
AST ≥ 10-fold normal	AST 3–9-fold normal	AST < 3-fold normal
AST ≥ 5-fold normal and gammaglobulin ≥ 2-fold normal	AST ≥ 5-fold normal and gamma globulin < 2-fold normal	Severe cytopenia
Bridging necrosis	Periportal hepatitis	Inactive cirrhosis
Multilobular necrosis		Portal hepatitis Decompensated cirrhosis with variceal bleeding

(Table 5.6: Treatment indications)

Treatment is indicated by the severity of hepatic inflammation rather than the degree of hepatic dysfunction. Hypoprothrombinemia and/or hyperbilirubinemia in the absence of severe inflammation does not compel therapy nor does histologic cirrhosis contraindicate treatment if inflammatory activity is severe

B Treatment regimens (see Table 5.7)

Combination regimen			Single drug regimen	
Prednisone (mg/day)	Azathioprine (mg/day)	Treatment candidates	Prednisone (mg/day)	Treatment candidates
30 mg × 1 week	50 mg until endpoint	Postmenopausal women and/or osteoporosis	60 mg × 1 week	Pregnancy or considering pregnancy
20 mg × 1 week		Cushingoid features/ obesity	40 mg × 1 week	Severe cytopenia
15 mg × 2 weeks		Brittle diabetes	30 mg × 2 weeks	Azathioprine intolerance
10 mg until endpoint		Labile hypertension	20 mg until endpoint	Short empiric trial (≤6 months)
		Emotional lability		Concurrent malignancy

(Table 5.7: Treatment regimens)

1 Prednisone alone or a lower dose of prednisone in combination with azathioprine is effective. The combination regimen is preferred because of a lower risk of corticosteroid-related side effects !

2 Combination regimen with azathioprine requires determinations of leukocyte and platelet counts at 3–6-week intervals throughout treatment period to monitor for bone marrow toxicity

3 Follow-up assessments should be every 6 months during treatment, or sooner if symptoms of liver failure or drug intolerance

4 **No findings at presentation preclude a satisfactory response to treatment.** Ascites and hepatic encephalopathy identify patients with a poor prognosis, but they do not contraindicate therapy

5 Patients with multilobular necrosis on histologic examination who fail to normalize at least one laboratory parameter or improve pretreatment hyperbilirubinemia during a 2-week treatment period have high immediate mortality. They should be evaluated for liver transplantation if there are features of decompensation !

6 Patients who improve by the above parameters have an excellent immediate survival; their drug treatment should be continued until satisfactory endpoint is reached (see below)

C Drug-related side effects

1 Cosmetic changes (facial rounding, dorsal hump formation, obesity, acne, or hirsutism) in 80% after 2 years regardless of regimen

2 Severe side effects (osteopenia with vertebral compression, diabetes, cataracts, severe emotional lability, and hypertension) usually after protracted therapy (>18 months) with prednisone only

3 Prednisone and azathoprine regimen preferred because of fewer corticosteroid-related side effects during comparable periods of treatment (10% versus 44%)

4 Premature discontinuation of treatment necessary in 13%, mainly because of intolerable obesity, cosmetic changes, or osteoporosis

5 Postmenopausal women at risk for vertebral compression, especially during retreatment after relapse

6 Regular program of exercise, calcium (1–1.5 g/day) intake, vitamin D (50 000 units/week) supplementation, and hormonal replacement appropriate for skeletal integrity

7 Azathioprine therapy complicated by cholestatic hepatotoxicity, nausea, emesis, rash, and cytopenia in ≤10% treated with 50 mg daily. Side effects reversible with dose reduction or termination of therapy

8 Teratogenicity and oncogenicity are theoretical complications of azathioprine therapy. Risk of nonhepatic malignancy ≥1.4-fold that in age- and sex-matched normal population

D   Treatment endpoints (see Table 5.8)

Features	Remission	Treatment failure	Incomplete response	Drug toxicity
Definition	No symptoms AST ≤ 2-fold normal Normal other tests Inactive or minimally active biopsy	Progressive symptoms AST ≥ 67% previous level Bilirubin ≥ 67% previous level Worsening inflammation on liver biopsy	No remission after 3 years of continuous treatment	Intolerable obesity Vertebral compression Severe cytopenia Psychosis Rash Nausea/emesis
Occurrence	65% within 2 years	9%	13%	13%
Action after endpoint	Tapered discontinuation of medication over 6-week period	Prednisone 60 mg daily or prednisone 30 mg daily and azathioprine 150 mg daily	Long-term maintenance with low-dose prednisone (≤10 mg daily)	Dose reduction or drug withdrawal
Consequence	Relapse (50% in 6 months) or sustained remission	Indefinite treatment or liver transplantation	Indefinite treatment with balanced benefit – risk ratio	Indefinite low-dose therapy Investigational therapy

(Table 5.8: Treatment endpoints)

1 Continue therapy until remission, treatment failure, incomplete response, or drug toxicity

2 Histologic resolution lags behind clinical and laboratory resolution by 3–6 months, and therapy must be extended for this duration

3 **Liver biopsy examination prior to drug withdrawal is necessary to establish remission**. Significant residual inflammatory activity on liver tissue examination in 55% with normal laboratory studies during therapy

4 Degree of histologic improvement during therapy influences frequency of relapse after drug withdrawal:
   - reversion to normal liver architecture associated with 20% frequency of relapse
   - improvement to portal hepatitis associated with 50% frequency of relapse
   - progression to cirrhosis during therapy or persistence of periportal hepatitis associated with 100% frequency of relapse

5 Many side effects are reversible. Consequences such as cataracts and osteopenia with vertebral compression have effective therapies. Weight gain, acne, edema, and diabetes may be consequences of the disease rather than the drugs

6 Gradual corticosteroid withdrawal over 6-week period after treatment endpoint (see Table 5.9). In patients entering remission, laboratory tests (serum AST, bilirubin, and gamma globulin levels) should be performed every 3 weeks during treatment withdrawal and then every 3 weeks for 3 months. Thereafter, tests should be performed every 6 months for 1 year and then at annual intervals if remission is sustained

Withdrawal intervals	Prednisone and azathioprine regimen		Prednisone regimen
Weeks after remission	Prednisone dose (mg/day)	Azathioprine dose (mg/day)	Prednisone dose (mg/day)
1	7.5	50	15
2	7.5	50	10
3	5	50	5
4	5	25	5
5	2.5	25	2.5
6	2.5	25	2.5
Thereafter	None	None	None

(Table 5.9: Withdrawal schedule after remission)

E   Treatment results

1 **Remission**
   - accomplished in 65% within 3 years
   - average treatment interval until remission, 22 months

2 **Relapse after drug withdrawal**
   - occurs in 50% within 6 months and majority (70–86%) within 3 years
   - defined by recrudescence of symptoms, increase serum AST level ≥ threefold normal, and/or reappearance of periportal hepatitis on histologic examination

- reinstitution of original treatment induces another remission, but relapse commonly recurs after termination of therapy
- major consequence of relapse and retreatment is development of drug-related complications. These occur in 70% of those who relapse multiply. Requirement for more than two treatments diminishes net benefit–risk ratio of conventional therapy
- patients who have relapsed at least twice require indefinite therapy with either prednisone or azathioprine (see Table 5.10)

Features	Prednisone alone		Azathioprine alone	
Schedule	Induce clinical and biochemical remission with standard regimen Discontinue azathioprine Reduce prednisone dose by 2.5 mg per month until lowest dose to prevent symptoms and maintain serum AST level $\leq$ 5-fold normal Periodic attempts to reduced dose further		Induce clinical and biochemical remission with standard regimen Discontinue prednisone in tapered fashion and increase azathioprine to daily dose of 2 mg/kg Nonsteroidal medications as needed for withdrawal arthralgias Continuous therapy thereafter	
Outcomes	Remission	8%	Remission[a] (10 years)	83%
	Continuous therapy	73%	Weight loss	43%
	Improvement side effects	85%	Hypertension improved	13%
	Hepatic mortality	9%	Hepatic mortality	1%
Side effects	New side effects	0%	Withdrawal arthralgias	53%
			Required dose reduction	32%
			Withdrawal myalgias	14%
			Lethargy	10%
			Malignancy	7%
			Myelosuppression	6%
Contra-indications	None		Pregnancy or contemplation of pregnancy Severe cytopenia	
Duration of follow-up	170 ± 12 months		67 months (median) Range, 12–128 months	

[a]Different from Mayo definition

(Table 5.10: Long-term treatment regimens after multiple relapses)

- long-term regimens have not been compared directly and reasons for preference have not been established. Risks of teratogenicity and oncogenicity uncertain

3 Treatment failure (9%)

- deterioration despite compliance with conventional therapy
- high-dose prednisone alone (60 mg daily) or prednisone (30 mg daily) in conjunction with azathioprine (150 mg daily) induces clinical and biochemical improvement in 70% within 2 years
- histologic resolution in only 20%; long-term therapy frequently necessary

- liver transplantation at the first sign of decompensation (usually ascites formation)
- re-establish legitimacy of original diagnosis by excluding viral infection, primary sclerosing cholangitis, primary biliary cirrhosis, autoimmune cholangitis, and drug-induced chronic liver disease

4 Incomplete response (13%)

- improvement during therapy but not enough to satisfy remission criteria after 3 years
- diminishing benefit–risk ratio of protracted therapy justifies empiric trial with low-dose prednisone schedule similar to that used after multiple relapses
- goal is to control disease activity on the lowest dose of medication possible

5 Survival

- 10-year life expectancies for treated patients with and without cirrhosis at presentation are 89% and 90%, respectively. Overall 10-year survival is 93%
- survival comparable to that of an age- and sex-matched cohort from the population at large (94% over 10 years)
- patients with histologic cirrhosis respond as well as noncirrhotic patients and should be treated similarly with the same expectations of success

F Liver transplantation

1 Effective in decompensated patient who has failed corticosteroid therapy

2 Autoantibodies and hypergammaglobulinemia disappear within 2 years

3 5-year survival is 96%

4 Recurrent disease after transplantation possible but uncommon

5 Recurrence mainly in patients inadequately immunosuppressed or in HLA DR3-positive recipients of HLA DR3-negative donors

6 Adjustments in immunosuppressive regimen usually sufficient to suppress manifestations of recurrent disease

G Drugs of unproven efficacy (see Table 5.11)

1 Cyclosporine

- anecdotal use (5–6 mg/kg daily) in patients unresponsive to or intolerant of corticosteroids
- improvement in all instances within 1 year (small numbers)
- relapse usual after drug withdrawal; indefinite cyclosporine maintenance required
- consequences of long-term treatment, including renal insufficiency, hypertension and malignancy, unknown

2 Tacrolimus (FK-506)

- improvement in serum ALT and AST levels and bilirubin concentration after 1 year at a dose of 4 mg twice daily in small, open-labeled trial
- abnormalities in serum creatinine and blood urea nitrogen levels mild and well tolerated
- treatment not continued long enough to determine benefit–risk ratio

3 Budesonide

- potent second-generation corticosteroid with high first-pass hepatic clearance, low systemic availability, and metabolites devoid of glucocorticoid activity
- improvement in serum ALT and immunoglobulin levels in small open-labeled treatment trial (6–8 mg daily for 6–10 weeks, then individualized doses for ≤9 months)
- low frequency of systemic side effects and only marginal reduction in plasma cortisol levels in noncirrhotic patients
- requires further study

4 Polyunsaturated phosphatidylcholine

- cytoprotective agent
- improves histologic features to greater degree than prednisone alone when given in combination with prednisone (double-blind controlled trial)
- similar results with arginine thiazolidinecarboxylate
- histologic improvement modest and of uncertain clinical significance
- not frontline agent

5 Ursodeoxycholic acid

- improves serum AST and gamma glutamyltransferase levels in patients with chronic hepatitis (diverse group) when administered in doses of 250 mg, 500 mg, or 750 mg daily for 2 months
- clinical significance of improvements unknown
- experiences too preliminary to justify routine clinical use

6 Intravenous immunoglobulin

- isolated use in patient with aseptic necrosis of the femoral head after long-term corticosteroid treatment
- symptoms diminished; liver test abnormalities resolved; circulating immune complexes disappeared; and liver biopsy findings improved
- uncertain durability of the response
- little justification for such expensive therapy except in highly selected patients in investigational settings

7 Thymic hormone extracts

- improve suppressor T cell function and inhibit immunoglobulin production
- unable to prevent relapse after corticosteroid withdrawal
- possible value in other clinical situations but additional trials needed, especially following drug toxicity or incomplete response

8 Rapamycin and brequinar

- immunosuppressive agents with theoretical actions of potential value
- no meaningful clinical evaluation in autoimmune hepatitis
- emphasize need to systematically import and effectively study promising immunomodulatory agents used in transplantation

9 6-Mercaptopurine

- purine analog inhibits nucleic acid synthesis and lymphocyte proliferation
- may be effective in patients who are unresponsive to azathioprine in combination with prednisone

Immunosuppressive agents		Cytoprotective agents	
Drug	**Putative actions**	**Drug**	**Putative actions**
Cyclosporine	Inhibits lymphokine release	Phosphatidyl choline	Modifies liver cell surface membrane
FK-506 (Tacrolimus)	Prevents expansion of cytotoxic T cells by inhibiting interleukin 2 receptor	Thiazolidine carboxylate	Modifies liver cell surface membrane
Thymic extracts	Stimulates suppressor cells Inhibits antibody production	Ursodeoxycholic acid	Alters expression class I antigens and reduces hydrophobic bile acids
Intravenous immunoglobulin	Interferes with Fc receptors Induces suppressor cells Suppresses anti-idiotypes		
Brequinar	Inhibits pyrimidine synthesis and lymphocyte proliferation		
Rapamycin	Blocks transmission signal after interleukin 2 and receptor binding and immunocyte expansion		
Budesonide	Improves suppressor function and decreases antibody production		
Mercaptopurine	Purine analog inhibits nucleic acid synthesis		

(Table 5.11: Unproven therapies)

- used as azathioprine substitute in combination regimen
- effective dose, 25 mg daily; then slow increase to 1.5 mg/kg daily as tolerated
- uncertain reasons for efficacy (azathioprine-induced hepatitis, different intestinal absorption, alternative detoxification pathway)

8 Future Research

1 Clarification of pathogenic mechanisms
2 Characterization of target autoantigens
3 Definition of host susceptibility factors
4 Identification of susceptibility gene(s)
5 Alternative treatment strategies using drugs with highly selective actions aimed at critical pathogenic pathways (immunosuppressive agents, cytoprotective drugs, or combinations of both)

References

1   Czaja AJ. *Low dose corticosteroid therapy after multiple relapses of severe HBsAg-negative chronic active hepatitis.* (Hepatology 1990) 11: 1044–9

2   Czaja AJ. *Autoimmune hepatitis: evolving concepts and treatment strategies*. (Dig Dis Sci 1995) 40: 435–56

3   Czaja AJ, Carpenter HA, Santrach PJ, Moore SB. *Significance of HLA DR4 in type 1 autoimmune hepatitis*. (Gastroenterology 1993) 105: 1502–7

4   Czaja AJ, Carpenter HA, Santrach PJ, Moore SB, Homburger HA. *The nature and prognosis of severe cryptogenic chronic active hepatitis*. (Gastroenterology 1993) 104: 1755–61

5   Doherty DG, Donaldson PT, Underhill JA, et al. *Allelic sequence variation in the HLA class II genes and proteins in patients with autoimmune hepatitis*. (Hepatology 1994) 19: 609–15

6   Johnson PJ, McFarlane IG, Alvarez F, et al. *Meeting Report. International Autoimmune Hepatitis Group*. (Hepatology 1993) 18: 998–1005

7   Johnson PJ, McFarlane IG, Williams R. *Azathioprine for long-term maintenance of remission in autoimmune hepatitis*. (N Engl J Med 1995) 333: 958–63

8   Poralla T, Treichel U, Lohr H, Fleischer B. *The asialoglycoprotein receptor as target structure in autoimmune liver diseases*. (Semin Liver Dis 1991) 11: 215–22

9   Roberts SK, Therneau T, Czaja AJ. *Prognosis of histologic cirrhosis in type 1 autoimmune hepatitis*. (Gastroenterology 1996) 110: 848–57

10   Yamamoto AM, Cresteil D, Homberg JC, Alvarez F. *Characterization of the anti-liver–kidney microsome antibody (anti-LKM1) from hepatitis C virus-positive and -negative sera*. (Gastroenterology 1993) 104: 1762–7

Alcoholic liver disease

GILLIAN ANN ZELDIN, M.D.   ANNA MAE DIEHL, M.D.

Key Points

1 Alcoholic liver disease is the most prevalent form of liver disease in the USA; worldwide, numerous epidemiologic studies have documented the correlation between per capita alcohol consumption and deaths from cirrhosis

2 The risk of hepatotoxicity increases if a threshold level of alcohol consumption is exceeded, but even consistently high consumption rarely causes cirrhosis. Variables affecting the development of cirrhosis include genetic polymorphisms of alcohol-metabolizing enzymes, gender differences, nutritional status, concomitant viral hepatitis, exposure to drugs or toxins, and immunologic factors

3 Alcoholic liver disease is believed to progress through histologic stages: from normal to steatosis (fatty liver) then steatohepatitis (alcoholic hepatitis), and finally to cirrhosis (when fibrogenesis predominates)

4 Treatment of alcoholic liver disease includes discontinuation of alcohol consumption, treatment of extrahepatic complications of alcoholism (electrolyte abnormalities, withdrawal syndromes, cardiac dysfunction, poor nutrition, pancreatitis, gastritis, infection), and management of the sequelae of cirrhosis (ascites, portal hypertensive bleeding, and encephalopathy). Liver transplantation should be considered in the abstinent patient with cirrhosis

1 Epidemiology

A Overview

1 Alcohol is used by three quarters of Americans; alcohol abuse and dependence are common, with approximately 10% of Americans who drink experiencing alcohol-related problems

2 Alcoholic liver disease is one of the most serious medical consequences of long-term alcohol abuse and is the most common cause of cirrhosis in the Western world. In 1988 approximately 44% of deaths from cirrhosis in the USA were the result of alcoholic liver disease

3 Alcohol abuse and dependence rates are higher for men (11%) than for women (4%) and higher for non-blacks than for blacks (non-black males 11%, females 4%; black males 8%, females 3%). Despite these differences, progression to cirrhosis occurs at a higher rate in blacks than non-blacks

B Criteria for the diagnosis of alcohol dependence or abuse

1 Alcohol dependence (three items required)

- alcoholic beverages often taken in larger amounts or over a longer period than intended
- persistent desire for alcohol or one or more unsuccessful attempts to cut down or control use
- a great deal of time spent in obtaining alcohol, drinking it, or recovering from its effects
- (a) recurrent use at times when alcohol use is physically hazardous (e.g. driving while intoxicated) or (b) frequent intoxication or withdrawal symptoms despite major obligations at work, school, or home
- social, occupational, or recreational activities discontinued or reduced because of alcohol use
- continued alcohol use despite knowledge of having persistent or recurrent social, psychological or physical problems that are caused or exacerbated by alcohol use
- marked tolerance: need for markedly increased amounts of alcohol (at least 50% increase) to achieve intoxication or desired effect, or markedly diminished effect with continued use of the same amount
- characteristic withdrawal symptoms
- alcohol taken to relieve or avoid withdrawal symptoms

2 **Alcohol abuse** (one item required)

- continued use despite knowledge of having persistent or recurrent social, occupational, psychological, physical problem that is caused or exacerbated by the use of the substance
- recurrent use in situations in which its use is physically hazardous

C Screening for alcohol problems

CAGE questionnaire

a Have you ever felt you ought to **cut down** on your drinking?

b Have people **annoyed** you by criticizing your drinking?

c Have you ever felt bad or **guilty** about your drinking?

d Have you ever had a drink first thing in the morning (**eye opener**) to steady your nerves or get rid of a hang over?

Two or more positive responses is a positive test.

2   Risk Factors for Alcoholic Liver Disease

A   Overview

1 In all societies studied, a positive correlation exists between average per capita consumption of alcohol and frequency of cirrhosis

2 Amount ingested and duration of intake correlate with incidence of alcohol-related liver disease

3 Once a threshold level of consumption is exceeded (estimated to be 80 g/day for men and 20 g/day for women), the risk of hepatotoxicity increases dramatically

4 Consistently high intake of alcohol uncommonly induces cirrhosis. Less than 20% of men consuming more than two six-packs of beer per day for 10 years become cirrhotic

5 Recently, several advisory committees have recommended that alcohol consumption be limited to moderate levels, defined as not more than two drinks per day for healthy males and not more than one drink per day for healthy non-pregnant females

B   Factors that influence the development of alcoholic liver disease

1 **Gender**: women experience more toxicity per dose than men, but this cannot be explained solely by differences in body composition or alcohol distribution. Gastric mucosal alcohol dehydrogenase activity is lower in women; this may allow for greater hepatic metabolism of ingested alcohol

2 **Genetic variability in alcohol-metabolizing enzymes**: polymorphisms of the alcohol dehydrogenase and aldehyde dehydrogenase enzymes seem to protect certain individuals from ethanol toxicity. For example, Asians frequently inherit a "slow" aldehyde dehydrogenase isoenzyme, thereby increasing serum levels of acetaldehyde. This causes flushing, nausea, and dysphoria (disulfiram-like reaction). This may explain why habitual alcohol use and alcoholic liver disease are rare in this group

3 **Nutrition**: ethanol interferes with intestinal absorption and storage of nutrients and reduces appetite for nonalcoholic sources of calories. This may result in deficiencies of protein, vitamins, and minerals

4 **Infections with hepatotropic viruses**: acute and chronic hepatitis B or C accelerate the progression of alcoholic liver disease

5 **Co-exposure to drugs or toxins**: chronic consumption of alcohol induces the activity of microsomal enzymes, potentiating the metabolism of drugs, solvents, and xenobiotics. For example, therapeutic doses of acetaminophen can cause severe hepatic damage in alcoholic individuals; similarly, tolbutamine, isoniazid, and industrial solvents accelerate alcoholic liver disease

6 Immunologic derangements: alcoholic liver disease is modulated by alterations in the cellular immune system and include increased reactivity of T and B cells and increased expression of MHC class I and class II DR antigens. Increased levels of immune modulatory cytokines tumor necrosis factor, interleukin 1 and interleukin 6 are also seen. Alterations of the humoral immune system that include increased levels of circulating immunoglobulins, the presence of autoantibodies (against nuclear, smooth muscle, liver cell membrane, liver-specific proteins, and alcoholic hyaline antigens), and the development of antibodies against neo-antigens, proteins altered by reaction to acetaldehyde, malondialdehyde, and various radicals

3   Clinical Features

A   History

1 A history of habitual alcohol consumption is useful in suggesting alcohol as the cause of liver disease, but given the dearth of pathognomonic symptoms and signs of alcoholic liver disease, the elimination of other potential causes of injury is mandatory
2 The type of alcoholic beverage consumed does not influence the likelihood of developing hepatotoxicity. The amount of ethanol (grams) consumed in spirits, wine, or beer can be estimated by multiplying the volume of the beverage in milliliters by the percentage of that beverage that is pure ethanol (spirits = 40%, wine = 12%, beer = 5%) times the specific gravity (0.8) of ethanol
3 The CAGE questionnaire is sensitive for detecting alcohol abuse
4 Accelerated disease progression is likely when alcohol abuse is accompanied by one or more of the following: viral hepatitis, acetaminophen intake, exposure to solvents, a family history of alcoholic liver disease, hemochromatosis, Wilson's disease, or alpha-1 antitrypsin deficiency

B   Signs and symptoms of alcoholic liver disease

1 The clinical features of alcoholic liver disease are variable, ranging from a complete absence of symptoms to the florid features of advanced parenchymal cell failure and portal hypertension
2 Patients can have one or more of the following: fever, weakness, anorexia, nausea and vomiting, malaise, confusion, sleep–wake cycle alterations, hepatomegaly, splenomegaly, cachexia, jaundice, spider telangiectases, Dupuytren's contractures, gynecomastia, testicular atrophy, parotid/lacrimal gland enlargement, asterixis, Muehrcke's lines, white nails, decreased libido. None is specific or pathognomonic for alcoholic liver disease

C   Laboratory abnormalities: variable and often (see Table 6.1)

Parameter	Result
Aspartate aminotransferase (AST)/ alanine aminotransferase (ACT) ratio	greater than 2 and both generally under 300 U/L
Alkaline phosphatase	Increased to much increased
Bilirubin	Normal to very high
Prothrombin time	Normal to very high
Albumin	Normal to decreased
Ammonia	Normal to high
Hematocrit	Typically mild macrocytic anemia, may be normal
White blood cell count	Leukemoid reactions can be associated with steatohepatitis
Platelets	Normal to decreased
Triglycerides	Typically increased, esp. in active drinkers
Potassium, phosphate, magnesium	Deficiency is common in active drinkers
Glucose	Hyperglycemia common

(Table 6.1: Laboratory abnormalities in alcoholic liver disease)

4   Histology

A   Fatty liver (steatosis)

- a consequence of alcohol oxidation. Results when the intracellular-redox potential and redox-sensitive nutrient metabolisms are disturbed. An excessive accumulation of reducing equivalents favors metabolic pathways that lead to the accumulation of intracellular lipid. The excess lipid is stored in large droplets within individual hepatocytes. With abstinence, the normal redox potential is restored, the lipid is mobilized and fatty liver resolves completely. Although there have been reports of fatal outcomes, this is generally considered a benign, reversible condition. See Figure 6.1, plate section

B   Alcoholic hepatitis

- characterized by steatosis, hepatocellular necrosis, and acute inflammation. As for steatosis, most pronounced in zone three of the hepatic acinus. Characteristic eosinophilic fibrillar material (Mallory's hyaline bodies) may be seen in ballooned hepatocytes. These condensations of cytoskeletal intermediary filaments result from the formation of acetaldehyde–tubulin adducts. Although characteristic of alcoholic hepatitis, they are not specific and are also seen in other forms of hepatitis. Focally

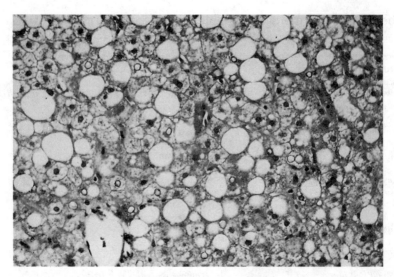

Fig. 6.1   Fatty liver (steatosis) in alcoholic liver disease. See page xv.

intense lobular infiltration of polymorphonuclear leukocytes distinguishes alcoholic hepatitis from other types of liver disease. In most other types of hepatitis, the inflammatory infiltrate is composed of monocytes predominately localized around the portal triads

- until recently, alcoholic hepatitis was felt to be the prerequisite for alcoholic cirrhosis. However, it is now known that acetaldehyde may initiate fibrogenesis in the absence of demonstrable necro-inflammation. Nonetheless, the severity of the clinical syndrome which occurs in some patients with alcoholic steatonecrosis and the lesion's potential to progress to cirrhosis have made it the target of many therapeutic trials. See Figure 6.2, in the plate section

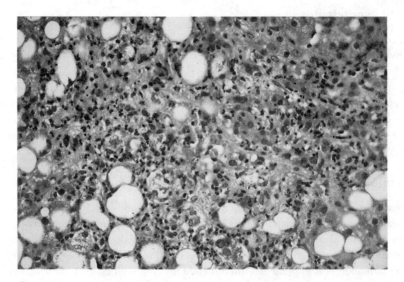

Fig. 6.2   Alcoholic hepatitis. See page xv.

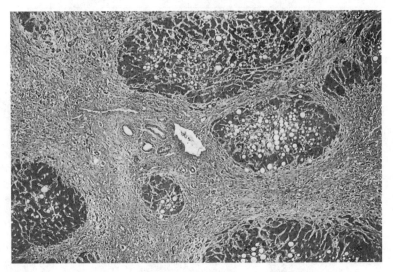

Fig. 6.3   Fibrogenic damage as a consequence of cirrhosis. See page xvi.

C   Cirrhosis

- considered the end stage of alcoholic liver disease However, most patients with alcoholic fatty liver never progress to cirrhosis despite continued and prolonged consumption of alcohol. In others, fibrogenic damage ensues. See Figure 6.3, in the plate section. In some of these individuals, features of all three histologic "stages" coexist

- alcoholic liver damage is typically associated with the deposition of collagen around the terminal hepatic vein (i.e., perivenular fibrosis) and along the sinusoids. This results in a "chicken wire" pattern of scarring that is rarely seen in other types of cirrhosis

- chronic consumption of alcohol also impairs the regenerative response that is normally triggered by liver cell death. This results in nodules of regenerating parenchyma that are small. For this reason, **micronodular cirrhosis** is seen in actively drinking patients

- abstinence releases the liver from the anti-proliferative actions of alcohol and is associated with the development of **macronodular cirrhosis**

5   Indices of Liver Dysfunction

Formulae for estimating the short term prognosis of patients with alcoholic liver disease.

1   **Composite Clinical Laboratory Index (CCLI):** Orrego and co-workers (1978)[1] defined a group of parameters that correlate with mortality in hospitalized patients with alcoholic hepatitis. Calculation of the CCLI permits a linear estimate of acute mortality (see Table 6.2).

Sign/symptoms	Score
Hepatomegaly	1
Splenomegaly	1
Ascites	
1+	1
2+	2
3+	3
Encephalopathy	
grade 1	1
grade 2	2
grade 3	3
Clinical bleeding	1
Spider nevi	1
Palmar erythema	1
Collateral circulation	1
Peripheral edema	1
Anorexia	1
Weakness	1
AST > 200	1
ALT	
> 100	1
> 200	2
Alk. Phos. > 80 U	1
Albumin < 2.59%	1
Prothrombin time (seconds prolonged)	
< 3	1
3–5	2
> 5	3
Bilirubin (mg/100 mL)	
1.2–2	1
2–5	2
> 5	3

(Table 6.2: Composite Clinical Laboratory Index)

2   **Maddrey's discriminant function (DF)**: Maddrey and co-workers (1978)[2] simplified the assessment of outcome of alcoholic liver disease by developing a discriminant function.

DF = 4.6 × (the difference between the patient's and control prothrombin time) + serum bilirubin

- Patients with a DF greater than 32 have a 50% chance of dying during current hospitalization. This index offers the advantage of few variables and easy computation (and therefore recall), but it is relatively imprecise. Fifty percent of patients with a DF greater than 32 will survive the hospitalization

6   Therapy

A   General measures to treat acute and chronic alcoholic liver disease

1   Discontinuation of alcohol use and resumption of a nutritious diet remain the cornerstones of therapy for alcoholic patients even after cirrhosis has developed

2   Vigorous efforts to enroll patients in a detoxification program are justified

3   Hospitalization benefits those patients with significant extrahepatic complications of alcoholism, notably electrolyte abnormalities, cardiac dysfunction, pancreatitis, hemorrhagic gastritis, major alcohol withdrawal syndromes, and infection

4   The risk of hepatocellular cancer is increased in any patient with cirrhosis, but is especially high in alcoholics. Although it is assumed that periodic ultrasound examinations and measurement of alpha fetoprotein levels may be helpful in detecting hepatocellular cancer at an early stage, there is little evidence that this improves survival in alcoholic liver disease. Chronic infection with hepatitis B or C virus also has a significant role in predisposition to liver cancer. The effect of interferon therapy on the evolution of hepatocellular cancer in alcoholic patients with chronic viral infection is unknown

B   Specific therapies for acutely decompensated alcoholic liver disease

1   **Corticosteroids**: meta-analysis of multiple studies and two prospectively randomized, placebo-controlled trials has demonstrated that patients with clinically severe alcoholic hepatitis benefit from treatment with corticosteroids once serious infection and/or gastrointestinal bleeding have been controlled. **A 4-week course of prednisone (32 mg methylprednisolone or the equivalent daily) halves the 1-month mortality rate of patients with a Maddrey discriminant function of more than 32**. It is important to note that these results were obtained in carefully selected patients who did not have clinically significant diabetes, pancreatitis, cancer, or viral hepatitis. The efficacy of corticosteroids in patients with these comorbid conditions and alcoholic hepatitis is not established

2   **Diet**: ethanol interferes with intestinal absorption and storage of nutrients and reduces appetite for nonalcoholic sources of calories. This may result in deficiencies of protein, vitamins and minerals. Such malnutrition correlates with mortality in patients with alcoholic liver disease. Trials of supplemental amino acid therapy have yielded conflicting results. Parenteral amino acids have been reported to improve nutritional status, serum bilirubin levels, and aminopyrine breath test results but not to increase the rates of short- or long-term survival

3   **Other supplements**: patients who are actively drinking are generally severely depleted of magnesium, potassium, and phosphate. This can precipitate multi-organ system dysfunction. Therefore, these elements should be repleted promptly

4   **Thiamine**: to prevent Wernicke's encephalopathy, thiamine must be administered

5   **Other treatments**: these include therapies aimed at reducing oxidative stress (propylthiouracil and cyanidanol), improving hepatic regeneration (anabolic steroids), and preventing fibrosis (d-penicillamine and colchicine). Since none reproducibly improves short-term survival, these agents are not recommended for general clinical use

C Specific therapies for decompensated chronic alcoholic liver disease

1 **Drug therapy**: few long-term treatment trials of patients with alcoholic liver disease have been conducted, and these are confounded by noncompliance and large dropout rates. However, two prospective randomized controlled trials have reported improvements in 5–10-year survival. A Mexican trial showed a survival advantage when **colchicine** was taken daily. A Canadian study also evaluated **propylthiouracil** (PTU) and demonstrated improved long-term survival. Both studies, however, included a small number of patients and may have been too small to detect uncommon adverse reactions. At the present time these are not standard treatments for chronic alcoholic liver disease

2 **Liver transplantation**: clearly improves survival in patients with decompensated alcoholic cirrhosis when compared with medically treated controls. Patients with a history of alcohol dependence or alcohol abuse and end-stage liver disease should be considered for liver transplantation (see Ch. 31). Abstinent patients (for greater than 6 months) who are evaluated by a multidisciplinary committee, and determined to be at low risk for recidivism and noncompliance, are good candidates for liver transplantation. A signed "contract" stipulating abstinence is occasionally helpful in maintaining commitment. Screening programs now in place have reduced recidivism rates to less than 10% post-liver transplantation. Emerging evidence suggests an accelerated form of alcoholic liver disease may develop in patients who resume alcohol abuse after transplantation

References

1 Orrego H, Kalant H, Israel Y, et al. *Effect of short-term therapy with propylthiouracil in patients with alcoholic liver disease.* (Gastroenterology 1978) 75: 105

2 Maddrey W, Boitnott J, Bedine M, et al. *Corticosteroid therapy in alcoholic hepatitis.* (Gastroenterology 1978) 75: 193

3 Carithers RL, Herlong HF, Diehl AM, et al. *Methylprednisolone therapy in patients with severe alcoholic hepatitis: a randomized multicenter trial.* (Ann Intern Med 1989) 110: 685

4 Isreal Y, Orrego H, Niemela O. *Immune responses to alcohol metabolites: pathogenic and diagnostic implications.* (Semin Liver Dis 1988) 8: 81

5 Leiber CS. *Biochemical factors in alcoholic liver disease.* (Semin Liver Dis 1993) 13: 134

6 Lucey MR, Merion RM, Henley KD, et al. *Selection for and outcome of liver transplantation in alcoholic liver disease.* (Gastroenterology 1992) 102: 1736

7 Lumeng L, Crabb DW. *Genetic aspects and risk factors in alcoholism and alcoholic liver disease.* (Gastroenterology 1994) 107: 572

8 Mezey E. *Interaction between alcohol and nutrition in the pathogenesis of alcoholic liver disease.* (Semin Liver Dis 1991) 11: 340

9 Morse R, Hurt R. *Screening for alcoholism.* (JAMA 1979) 242: 2688

Fatty liver and nonalcoholic steatohepatitis

BRENT A. NEUSCHWANDER-TETRI, M.D.
BRUCE R. BACON, M.D.

▼

Key Points

1 Hepatic steatosis, both benign and inflammatory (i.e., NASH), is a common cause of minor serum aminotransferase elevations (<4 × upper limit of normal), especially in the patient with obesity, type II diabetes mellitus, and corticosteroid therapy

2 Hepatic steatosis is reliably identified by imaging techniques when the degree of fatty infiltration is substantial. Ultrasonography reveals increased liver echogenicity, whereas noncontrast CT imaging reveals decreased liver density compared to the spleen

3 Focal steatosis is a variant that is typically detected incidentally during sonographic or CT imaging of the abdomen. The appearance is usually characteristic, although biopsy confirmation is occasionally required to exclude malignancy when the imaging appearance is atypical

4 Steatosis without accompanying inflammation is a benign condition. However, NASH can be associated with progressive fibrosis, cirrhosis, and liver failure. A liver biopsy is warranted to diagnose NASH or other causes of occult liver disease when the aminotransferases are persistently elevated

5 The pathogenetic mechanisms of hepatic steatosis are generally related to either increased delivery of fatty acids to the liver or defects in the complex process of VLDL synthesis and export of triglycerides from the liver

▲

95

1   Clinical Manifestations of Hepatic Steatosis and NASH

A   Symptoms

1 Patients with benign steatosis and nonalcoholic steatohepatitis (NASH) are typically asymptomatic, whereas patients with alcoholic hepatitis are nearly always symptomatic

2 The most common symptoms are constitutional and nonspecific: fatigue, weakness, and malaise

3 Right upper quadrant pain or fullness is a less frequent complaint. Liver capsule distention probably underlies the pain. Occasionally, patients present with right upper quadrant abdominal pain as a chief complaint; hepatic steatosis as the cause is diagnosed only after imaging excludes other intrahepatic or biliary causes

B   Physical findings

1 Hepatomegaly is common but can be difficult to detect on physical examination of the obese patient

2 Signs of chronic liver disease such as spider telangiectasias, muscle wasting, jaundice, and ascites point to cirrhosis

C   Risk factors

1 **Obesity** (see Table 7.1)

Body habitus	Prevalence of hepatic steatosis
Normal	21%
>10% over ideal body weight	75%
Morbidly obese	100%

(Table 7.1: Relationship between obesity and prevalence of hepatic steatosis)

- hepatic steatosis occurs in all morbidly obese children and adults
- an increased ratio of abdominal fat to hip fat predicts hepatic steatosis
- hepatic inflammation is found in 8–20% of obese individuals with hepatic steatosis

2 **Diabetes mellitus**
- hepatic steatosis is present in one third of type II diabetics
- steatosis is unusual in type I diabetics unless glycemic control is poor
- the evidence linking diabetes (in the absence of obesity) to progressive liver disease is weak

3 **Lipid abnormalities**
- hypertriglyceridemia may be a risk factor for hepatic steatosis; factors known to contribute to both hypertriglyceridemia and hepatic steatosis include: 1 obesity; 2 excessive fat intake; 3 lipodystrophies
- hypercholesterolemia is not a risk factor for hepatic steatosis

4 **Gender**
- female gender is *not* a risk factor for benign steatosis or NASH: 1 steatosis is

equally prevalent among males and females on computed tomography (CT); 2 NASH is equally prevalent in both sexes at autopsy; 3 a greater prevalence of NASH in women has not been confirmed by recent clinical studies

2 Diagnosis

A Terminology

1 Benign steatosis is a descriptive term for the accumulation of droplets of lipid (triglyceride) within hepatocytes of an otherwise normal liver

2 NASH is a clinical syndrome of steatosis and hepatic inflammation that is diagnosed by liver biopsy after other causes of liver disease have been excluded

B History

1 The diagnosis of NASH can be established only when alcohol abuse (>20 g daily) is convincingly excluded as a contributing factor

2 In the absence of alcohol abuse, other causative factors should be considered (see Table 7.2)

Nutritional abnormalities	Obesity Total parenteral nutrition Choline deficiency Rapid weight loss Kwashiorkor
Drugs	Estrogens Corticosteroids Chloroquine
Metabolic diseases	Abetalipoproteinemia Hypobetalipoproteinemia Wilson's disease Weber–Christian disease Limb lipodystrophy
Surgical alterations of gastrointestinal anatomy	Jejunoileal bypass Jejunocolic bypass Extensive small bowel loss Gastroplasty
Occupational exposure	Hydrocarbons

(Table 7.2: Causes of NASH)

C Laboratory findings

1 There are no blood tests that point unequivocally to steatosis or NASH

2 Aminotransferase (AST, ALT) elevations are commonly the only biochemical indicator of steatosis and NASH

3 The aminotransferases can be normal in both benign steatosis and NASH. Screening liver biopsies of morbidly obese individuals have shown that progressive liver disease can occur despite normal biochemical indices

4 The AST/ALT ratio can be helpful in distinguishing alcoholic hepatitis from nonalcoholic steatosis or NASH (see Table 7.3). Whereas an AST/ALT ratio greater than 2 points to alcohol as an etiology, patients with NASH typically have ALT levels that exceed the AST in the absence of cirrhosis

Alcoholic hepatitis	AST > ALT, typically > 2 : 1 ratio
Nonalcoholic steatohepatitis	ALT > AST, sometimes > 2 : 1 ratio

(Table 7.3: Steatohepatitis and serum aminotransferase patterns)

5 Serum triglycerides are not typically elevated in adults with benign steatosis or steatohepatitis whereas children often have elevated triglycerides
6 Serum levels of aminotransferases or other liver enzymes do not help to identify the presence of liver fibrosis or cirrhosis
7 Serum alkaline phosphatase can be elevated up to 2× normal
8 Viral, autoimmune, and metabolic causes of liver disease must be excluded as causes of aminotransferase elevations

D Imaging

- imaging techniques cannot distinguish benign steatosis and NASH, although NASH is usually diffuse, whereas benign steatosis can be either focal or diffuse
- focal or diffuse steatosis is often an incidental imaging finding

1 **Ultrasonography**
- liver is echogenic or "bright"
- ultrasonography detects steatosis only when there is substantial fat accumulation and thus has suboptimal sensitivity for detecting mild degrees of steatosis
- cirrhosis can also cause an echogenic appearance of the liver but the texture is typically coarser

2 **Computed tomography (CT)**
- steatotic liver is low in density compared with the spleen on noncontrast images

3 **Magnetic resonance imaging (MRI)**
- generally contributes little to CT findings
- phase shifting can be useful for identifying focal fat based on its loss of intensity on T1-weighted images

4 **Radionuclide scanning**
- focal fat appears as filling defects with technetium-99m sulfur colloid scanning
- areas of "focal sparing" in an otherwise fatty liver demonstrate tracer uptake, a finding helpful for identifying these unusual lesions noninvasively
- ^{133}Xe retention is a highly sensitive, rarely used method for detecting hepatic steatosis

5 **Focal fat**
- found in up to one third of patients with CT evidence of hepatic steatosis
- can be peripheral (especially in the diabetic receiving insulin by peritoneal dialysis), central, or periportal

- typically aspherical or geometric in shape
- does not exert a mass effect on adjacent structures
- fine-needle biopsy occasionally needed to establish the diagnosis when doubt persists

6 Focal sparing

- regions of normal liver in an otherwise steatotic liver
- appears relatively hypoechoic by sonography (compared with surrounding liver)
- appears relatively hyperdense by CT
- shape is typically geometric
- location is commonly in the caudate lobe
- may be caused by isolation of spared regions from mesenteric blood flow
- location and appearance usually make tissue diagnosis unnecessary

7 Problems identifying other lesions in the steatotic liver

- hemangiomas, which are usually characteristically hyperechoic by ultrasonography, can appear relatively hypoechoic in a steatotic liver
- identifying dilation of intrahepatic bile ducts can be difficult due to loss of contrast between the usually hyperechoic bile duct wall and the liver parenchyma

E   Liver biopsy

1 A liver biopsy is often needed to evaluate unexplained aminotransferase elevations. Unless a therapeutic trial of discontinuing specific medications or avoiding occupational exposures is planned, evaluation of liver enzyme elevations by liver biopsy should not be delayed. Arbitrarily established waiting periods of observation cause unnecessary delays in reaching a diagnosis

2 Liver biopsy is not indicated when the aminotransferases are normal yet imaging suggests steatosis. Although progressive and severe liver injury can occur with normal aminotransferases, such progression does not occur with sufficient frequency to warrant biopsy of all fatty livers

3 Specific histological findings of NASH	
Steatosis	fat droplets (triglyceride) within hepatocytes can be large, displacing cellular contents to the periphery
Inflammation	mixed neutrophilic and mononuclear cell infiltrate within the lobule; portal infiltrates are not a feature of NASH and suggest an alternative cause (e.g., hepatitis C)
Mallory bodies	eosinophilic cytoplasmic aggregates of cytoskeletal proteins which are typically smaller than those seen in alcoholic hepatitis
Glycogen nuclei	clear intranuclear vacuoles which nearly fill the nucleus; also seen in diabetes, Wilson's disease, and many other diseases

| Fibrosis | similar to alcoholic liver disease with perivenular deposition around the central vein and a "chicken wire" pattern of sinusoidal fibrosis; fortunately, an infrequent finding as it signifies a risk for progression to end-stage liver disease |

3 Pathogenetic Factors

The causes of steatosis-induced inflammation (steatohepatitis) are unknown. One possibility is that fatty acids serve as substrates for lipid peroxidation, a process capable of initiating an inflammatory response

The causes of hepatic steatosis are attributable to one or more of the following defects in the trafficking of fatty acids through the liver

A Increased peripheral mobilization of fatty acids

The ability of the liver to metabolize or secrete fat is easily overwhelmed by the capacity of peripheral stores to deliver fatty acids via the circulation. When hepatic steatosis results, impaired secretion of fat by the liver may also be present, although this second defect is not necessary

1 Adipose tissue releases fatty acids in response to cAMP-mediated signaling from glucagon, epinephrine, and ACTH. Released fatty acids are transported to the liver bound to albumin in the circulation

2 Starvation is associated with the release of fat from peripheral stores and development of hepatic steatosis

B Increased hepatic synthesis of fatty acids

1 The liver disposes excess carbohydrates by converting carbohydrate to fatty acids; excess carbohydrates from dietary sources (overindulgence) or provided parenterally (e.g., TPN) cause hepatic steatosis

C Impaired hepatic catabolism of fatty acids

1 Impaired mitochondrial beta oxidation of fatty acids is probably one of the major contributing factors in alcoholic steatosis, whereas it is not a major factor in NASH

2 Mitochondrial beta oxidation requires carnitine; carnitine deficiency causes hepatic steatosis

3 Factors which cause microvesicular steatosis may do so through impaired mitochondrial function, e.g., 1 valproic acid; 2 alcohol; 3 acute fatty liver of pregnancy

D Impaired synthesis and excretion of very-low-density lipoproteins (VLDL) from the liver

1 Fatty acids delivered to the liver but not metabolized are re-esterified to form triglycerides. (Human metabolic pathways do not allow synthesis of glucose from fatty acids)

2 Fatty acid esterification ensures that the level of fatty acids within hepatocytes remains low, thus avoiding fatty acid-induced cellular injury

3 Once triglyceride is formed, a variety of components are needed to form and secrete intact VLDL. These include: 1 choline to form lecithin; 2 necessary amino acids and unimpaired transcription, translation, and synthesis of protein to form apolipoproteins; 3 unimpaired cholesterol esterification; 4 intact cytoskeleton for exocytosis.

4 Any deficiency or metabolic aberration which interferes with any one of these steps can cause accumulation of hepatic triglyceride and hepatic steatosis. The complexity of the secretory pathway for VLDL, with its myriad potential defects, explains the multiple and seemingly disparate causes of hepatic steatosis

4   Prognosis (see Fig. 7.1)

A   Steatosis

- steatosis alone is a benign condition, although it may be associated with clinically significant symptoms

B   NASH

- steatohepatitis develops in 8–20% of obese individuals with hepatic steatosis
- the presence of fibrosis on liver biopsy identifies patients at risk for developing cirrhosis
- risk of developing fibrosis and cirrhosis is 10–50% in patients with NASH
- risk of developing cirrhosis when fibrosis is absent on initial biopsy is low

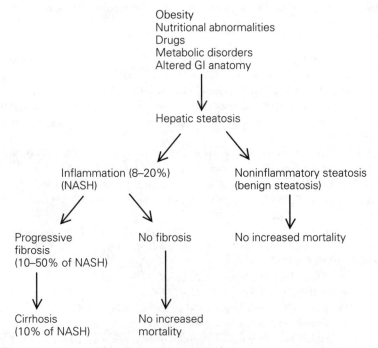

Fig. 7.1   Prognosis for patients with hepatic steatosis

- cirrhosis developing from NASH is the underlying liver disease in up to 1% of patients requiring liver transplantation

5 Therapeutic Considerations

A Weight loss

1 For the obese individual with hepatic steatosis or NASH, gradual and sustained weight loss will result in: 1 resolution of steatosis; 2 normalization of aminotransferases

2 Weight loss achieved with protein malnutrition will not improve hepatic steatosis

3 Hepatic steatosis in obese diabetics will improve with weight loss; improved glycemic control in type II diabetics will not help

B Identifying and treating nutritional deficiencies

Many of the causes of hepatic triglyceride accumulation may be related to treatable nutritional abnormalities such as:

- protein deficiency
- carbohydrate excess
- choline deficiency during prolonged parenteral nutrition; the resulting hepatic steatosis responds to choline supplementation
- coenzyme A deficiency caused by pantothenic acid deficiency has been suggested as a reversible cause of hepatic steatosis mediated by impaired mitochondrial function

References

1 Bacon BR, Farahvash MJ, Janney CG, Neuschwander-Tetri BA. *Nonalcoholic steatohepatitis: an expanded clinical entity.* (Gastroenterology 1994) 107: 1103–9

2 Baldridge AD, Perez-Atayde AR, Graeme-Cook F, Higgins L, Lavine JE. *Idiopathic steatohepatitis in childhood: a multicenter retrospective study.* (J Pediatr 1995) 127: 700–4

3 Diehl AM, Goodman Z, Ishak KG. *Alcohol-like liver disease in nonalcoholics.* (Gastroenterology 1988) 95: 1056–62

4 Galambos JT, Wills CE. *Relationship between 505 paired liver tests and biopsies in 242 obese patients.* (Gastroenterology 1978) 74: 1191–5

5 Lee RG. *Nonalcoholic steatohepatitis: a study of 49 patients.* (Hum Pathol 1989) 20: 594–8

6 Ludwig J, Viggiano TR, McGill DB, Ott BJ. *Nonalcoholic steatohepatitis.* (Mayo Clin Proc 1980) 55: 434–8

7 Powell EE, Cooksley WGE, Hanson R, Searle J, Halliday JW, Powell LW. *The natural history of nonalcoholic steatohepatitis: a follow-up study of forty-two patients for up to 21 years.* (Hepatology 1990) 11: 74–80

8 Teli MR, James OFW, Burt AD, Bennett MK, Day CP. *The natural history of nonalcoholic fatty liver: a follow-up study.* (Hepatology 1995) 22: 1714–19

9 Van Ness MM, Diehl AM. *Is liver biopsy useful in the evaluation of patients with chronically elevated liver enzymes?* (Ann Intern Med 1989) 111: 473–8

10 Wanless IR, Lentz JS. *Fatty liver hepatitis (steatohepatitis) and obesity: an autopsy study with analysis of risk factors.* (Hepatology 1990) 12: 1106–10

CHAPTER 8

Drug-induced and toxic liver disease

THOMAS D. SCHIANO, M.D.   MARTIN BLACK, M.D.

▼

Key Points

1 It is estimated that adverse reactions to drugs account for 2–5% of all cases of jaundice in hospitalized patients, 40% of cases of hepatitis in patients over age 50, and up to 25% of cases of fulminant hepatic failure

2 The spectrum of drug-related hepatotoxicity can range from subclinical liver disease with mildly abnormal liver function tests to subfulminant and fulminant hepatic failure requiring liver transplantation. Drug-induced liver disease can mimic clinically and histologically almost every type of liver disease

3 Many different medications and toxins have been implicated in causing fulminant hepatic failure; the likelihood of spontaneous recovery is low and the

overall prognosis poor without liver transplantation

4 Over-the-counter preparations and herbal medications may have significant hepatotoxicity, and their use should be searched for in cases of unexplained acute or chronic liver disease

5 Early suspicion of drug-induced liver injury is essential since morbidity is greatly increased if the medication is continued after symptoms develop or liver function test abnormalities appear.

6 The main treatment for drug hepatotoxicity is withdrawal of the agent. Physicians should caution their patients to be cognizant of signs of drug-induced liver injury, especially in the case of agents with well-recognized hepatotoxic potential

▲

1 Overview of Drug-Induced Hepatotoxicity

- may occur as an unexpected idiosyncratic reaction to a medication's therapeutic dose or as an expected consequence of the agent's intrinsic toxicity
- hepatotoxicity may be the only manifestation of the adverse drug effect, or it may be accompanied by injury to other organ systems or by systemic manifestations
- **acute liver injury** may develop within days of ingestion of a known hepatotoxin or after several weeks of taking a drug which provokes an immunoallergic reaction. It may be *necroinflammatory* (characterized by hepatocellular damage), *cholestatic* (manifested by arrested bile flow with little parenchymal injury), or a *mixed* type with features of both parenchymal and cholestatic injury
  - aminotransferases (AST, ALT) and lactate dehydrogenase may be elevated 10–100 times the normal range in acute hepatocellular injury, while alkaline phosphatase levels are usually less than three times the upper limit of normal. The serum bilirubin may be elevated or within the normal range
  - cholestatic drug injury resembles obstructive jaundice in its clinical manifestations and biochemical parameters. Serum alkaline phosphatase, gamma glutamyl transpeptidase (GGTP), and direct bilirubin are variably elevated with or without aminotransferase elevation (usually no higher than five to eight times the normal range)
- **subclinical hepatic injury** reflected only by minor liver enzyme elevation (e.g., AST, ALT in the 100–250 U/L range) is a common phenomenon and may not worsen and may even subside despite continued administration of a medication
- **acute (microvesicular) steatosis**, as is seen in Reye's syndrome, may present with modest aminotransferase elevations and only mild jaundice
  Table 8.1 shows the disorders associated with particular hepatotoxic agents.

2 Characterization of Drug-induced Liver Injury

A Intrinsic hepatotoxicity

- Causes include acetaminophen, carbon tetrachloride, alcohol. May occur secondary to metabolite-mediated hepatocellular necrosis or interference with specific hepatocellular metabolic pathways, leading to structural injury. In some cases there may be disruption of hepatic excretory pathways resulting in cholestasis. This form of injury is almost always dose dependent and reproducible in laboratory animals

B Idiosyncratic hepatotoxicity

- causes include isoniazid, sulfonamides, valproate, phenytoin. Occurs unpredictably in a small number of recipients of a medication as an expression of some unidentified reaction by the patient. There is no dose dependency, and toxicity is not reliably reproduced in laboratory animals nor is it revealed in preclinical animal testing
- immunologically mediated injury can be accompanied by a mononucleosis-like illness and extrahepatic hallmarks of generalized hypersensitivity like fever, rash, and eosinophilia. Usually develops after a sensitization period of several weeks.

Disorder	Hepatotoxic agents
Acute disorders	
Hepatitis-like syndromes (acute necroinflammatory liver disease)	Dapsone, disulfiram, isoniazid, indomethacin, phenytoin, sulfonamides
Fulminant hepatic failure	Acetaminophen, fialuridine (FIAU), fluconazole, ketoconazole, halothane, isoniazid, methyldopa, niacin, nitrofurantoin, propylthiouracil, valproic acid, flutamide
Cholestatic syndromes	Amitriptyline, ampicillin, carbamazepine, chlorpromazine, prochlorperazine, cimetidine, ranitidine, captopril, estrogens, trimethoprim-sulfamethoxazole, thiabendazole, tolbutamide
Mixed necroinflammatory	Carbimazole, chlorpropamide, dicloxacillin, methimazole, naproxen, phenylbutazone, sulindac, phenytoin, thioridazine, clinoril
Granulomatous hepatitis	Allopurinol, dapsone, diazepam, diltiazem, hydralazine, penicillin, phenylbutazone, phenytoin, quinidine, procainamide, sulfonamides
Macrovesicular steatosis	Alcohol, glucocorticoids, L-asparaginase, methotrexate, minocycline, nifedipine, total parenteral nutrition
Microvesicular steatosis	Alcohol, amiodarone, aspirin, zidovudine (AZT), didanosine (DDI), FIAU, piroxicam, tetracyclines, tolmetin, valproic acid
Budd–Chiari syndrome	Oral estrogens
Ischemic necrosis	Cocaine, sustained-release niacin, methylenedioxyamphetamine
Chronic disorders	
Chronic active hepatitis	Alpha-methyldopa, isoniazid, nitrofurantoin, oxyphenisatin
Fibrosis/cirrhosis	Alcohol, alpha-methyldopa, isoniazid, methotrexate
Peliosis hepatis	Anabolic/androgenic steroids, azathioprine, hydroxyurea, oral contraceptives, tamoxifen
Phospholipidosis	Amiodarone, perhexilene, diltiazem, nifedipine
Primary biliary cirrhosis	Chlorpromazine, haloperidol, prochlorperazine
Sclerosing cholangitis	Floxuridine FUDR via hepatic artery infusion
Steatohepatitis	Amiodarone, diethylstilbesterol, total parenteral nutrition
Veno-occlusive disease	Azathioprine, busulfan, cyclophosphamide, daunorubicin, pyrrolizidine alkaloids, thioguanine, x-irradiation
Oncogenic effects	
i. Cholangiocarcinoma	Thorotrast
ii. Focal nodular hyperplasia	Estrogens, oral contraceptives
iii. Hepatic adenoma	Estrogens, oral contraceptives
iv. Hepatoma	Alcohol, anabolic/androgenic steroids
v. Hepatoblastoma	Estrogens
vi. Angiosarcoma	Arsenic, vinyl chloride, thorotrast

(Table 8.1: Clinicopathologic patterns of drug injury to the liver)

Symptoms recur if the agent is used again. Lack of clinical hallmarks of hypersensitivity and of symptomatic recurrence with rechallenge suggest the production of hepatotoxic metabolites or a metabolic defect in detoxifying them. This form of liver injury may become manifest after latent periods of varying duration

3 Pathophysiology

- the liver is exposed to high concentrations of ingested drugs, particularly those with a high first-pass metabolism. Because the liver is extremely efficient in filtering substances from the bloodstream, it is exposed to high concentrations of compounds toxic in their native form or following metabolism in hepatocytes
- hepatic uptake of drugs may occur via specific transport mechanisms; the majority of drugs are lipophilic, however, and diffuse across the hepatocellular sinusoids. Back-diffusion may be deterred via binding to specific intracellular proteins that in turn facilitate transfer to the endoplasmic reticulum, where drug metabolism occurs, and to the bile canaliculi, where other transport proteins secrete substances into the bile
- many of the mechanisms involved in the pathophysiology of drug-induced liver injury at the molecular level are shown in Table 8.2.

Peroxidation of lipids
Denaturation of protein
ATP depletion
Mitochondrial dysfunction
Free radical generation
Electrophilic radical generation and hapten formation
Biotransformation via cytochrome P-450
Binding of active metabolites to nuclear or cytoplasmic molecules
Binding or blockage of transfer RNA
Attachment to membrane receptors
Disruption of calcium homeostasis
Disruption of the hepatocellular cytoskeleton

(Table 8.2: Mechanisms of drug-induced liver injury at the molecular level)

- normally the liver metabolizes drugs to more polar forms, thus facilitating their excretion in aqueous fluids. Sometimes these metabolites may be toxic (e.g., in acetaminophen overdose) but are generally converted to less toxic compounds by native detoxification enzymes. The net accumulation of toxic metabolites depends on both metabolism and detoxification.
- individual susceptibility to drug hepatotoxicity is influenced by multiple variables which affect the biotransformation of drugs (Table 8.3). Usually more than one of these is involved in any one patient. The most important of these factors is liver enzyme induction involving biotransformation of drugs and the cytochrome P-450 system of microsomal enzymes

4 Biotransformation

- this is a process by which therapeutic agents are rendered more hydrophilic, thus facilitating their excretion from the body. Biotransformation takes place in several steps, classified as phase 1 and phase 2 reactions, often involving microsomal enzyme systems

Age
Drug–drug interactions
Duration and total dose of drug
Enzyme induction
Enzyme polymorphism
Ethnic and racial factors
Gender
Nutritional status
Pregnancy
Renal function
Systemic disease
Underlying liver disease

(Table 8.3: Factors influencing patient susceptibility to drug hepatotoxicity)

A   Phase 1 reactions

- cytochrome P-450-mediated, primarily oxidative in nature, yielding active intermediate metabolites that may be responsible for liver injury. A family of isoenzymes found primarily in the liver within the endoplasmic reticulum, P-450 enzymes utilize molecular oxygen and electrons donated via a linked electron transfer chain involving NADPH and result in aliphatic and aromatic hydroxylation, dealkylation, or dehydrogenation. Products of these reactions may sometimes undergo further metabolism via a phase 2 reaction.
- Many medications may alter P-450 activity and thus promote drug toxicity (Table 8.4). Cytochrome P-450 enzymes catalyze the rate-limiting steps in the elimination of many drugs

B   Phase 2 reactions:

- mainly conjugative, converting the active metabolite to nontoxic more hydrophilic products via linkage with glutathione, sulfate, or glucuronide. This is all that is required for the hepatic metabolism of some compounds, most drugs first undergo cytochrome P-450 metabolism
- phase 1 reactions may thus be regarded as potential *"toxification"* and phase 2 as *"detoxification."* Drug injury may result from toxification (increased active metabolites) or inadequate detoxification

5   Diagnosis of Drug-induced Liver Injury

- a detailed drug history, including dosage, duration of therapy and other concomitantly administered drugs is essential
- exclude other causes of liver disease by careful assessment of clinical, radiologic, histologic, biochemical, and serologic findings
- the possibility of drug injury superimposed on pre-existing liver disease must always be considered
- elevation of serum lactate dehydrogenase levels is more indicative of toxic liver injury than viral-related disease, though this finding is nonspecific

Inhibitors	Inducers
Chloramphenicol	Carbamazepine
Cimetidine	Dexamethasone
Disulfiram	Ethanol
Erythromycin	Isoniazid
Fluoxetine	Omeprazole
Isoniazid	Phenobarbital
Ketoconazole	Phenytoin
Propoxyphene	Rifampin
Quinidine	

Substrates affected	
Benzodiazepines	Oral contraceptives
Carbamazepine	Phenytoin
Cyclosporine	Propranolol
Imipramine	Quinidine
Lidocaine	Theophylline
Metoprolol	Warfarin

(Table 8.4:   Drugs that affect cytochrome P-450 metabolism)

- nonspecific histologic lesions suggestive of drug injury include granulomas, eosinophils within an inflammatory infiltrate, a sharp zone of demarcation between necrosis and unaffected parenchyma, and a disproportionately severe degree of damage in relation to the patient's condition and the extent of liver function test abnormalities. **If histologic changes are not reconcilable with a single disease, drug-induced liver injury should be considered**

6   Hepatotoxicity of Specific Medications

Over 1000 drugs have been implicated in causing acute or chronic liver injury, ranging from subclinical elevation of liver function tests to fulminant hepatic failure. Following is a summary of some of the more frequently used medications with hepatotoxic potential and with the best-characterized mechanisms of injury

A   Acetaminophen (Paracetamol, Tylenol[R])

- typically well tolerated without many side effects. **Overdose is the most common cause of drug-induced liver injury and fulminant hepatic failure**[1]
- amount ingested as a single dose required to produce hepatic injury is quite variable. A toxic dose may be 10–20 g, while in alcoholics it can be as low as 5–10 g. In overdoses, intake exceedes 15 g in 80% of serious or fatal cases
- acetaminophen is present in dozens of other over-the-counter (e.g., Nyquil) and prescription preparations. Thus, concurrent acetaminophen toxicity should be considered in every multiple drug ingestion
- greatest risks for hepatotoxicity are influenced by the dose ingested and the interval between drug ingestion and antidote administration

- **alcoholism is a significant risk factor for toxicity, with appreciable liver injury occurring with therapeutic intent ("therapeutic misadventure") even with therapeutic doses**[2]. ALT levels may be greater than 10 000 U/L; the clinical presentation may be similar to alcoholic hepatitis, so the **extremely high aminotransferase levels should alert the clinician to the possibility of acetaminophen toxicity**. Alcoholics should be informed of this very real potential hepatotoxicity of acetaminophen. Malnutrition or fasting may play a role in acetaminophen hepatotoxicity by reducing glutathione stores[3]
- the use of concurrent medications that induce cytochromes P-450 (see Table 8.4) may heighten the risk and severity of liver injury associated with acetaminophen overdose. There have also been recent case reports of acetaminophen hepatotoxicity being potentiated by isoniazid

1 Clinical phases of massive ingestion

a Acute gastrointestinal symptoms (nausea, vomiting, anorexia) occur ½–24 hours post-ingestion.

b Cessation of gastrointestinal symptoms is followed by a period of well-being for about 48 hours. Right-sided abdominal pain occurs with oliguria and the appearance of abnormal liver function tests and prolonged prothrombin time

c Hepatic necrosis occurs 3–5 days after ingestion. Aminotransferase levels may peak at greater than 20,000 U/L. By comparison, peak aminotransferase levels with acute viral hepatitis are usually much lower. Renal failure from proximal and distal renal tubular damage occurs in up to 20% of patients, with fulminant hepatic failure developing in up to 30%. There may also be myocardial toxicity

d Recovery phase occurs 5–10 days after ingestion without residual histologic damage

2 Prognosis

a **Risk of liver injury** can be assessed based on the serum acetaminophen level obtained more than 4 hours after ingestion (Fig. 8.1)

b **Criteria for predicting death or the need for liver transplantation**[4]
  - pH < 7.3 irrespective of stage of encephalopathy or
  - prothrombin time > 6.5 (INR) and serum creatinine > 3.4 mg/dL in patients with stage 3 or 4 encephalopathy
  - factor V level of 10% or less may be a sensitive predictor of adverse outcome

3 Mechanism of hepatotoxicity

acetaminophen is normally metabolized by conjugation to glucuronide and sulfate, with a relatively small amount being metabolized by cytochrome P-450 to form oxidative metabolites, which are further conjugated prior to elimination. When large quantities are ingested, the glucuronide and sulfate conjugation pathways become saturated and more metabolism via cytochrome P-450 occurs. Increased formation of one of the oxidative metabolites, N-acetyl-p-benzoquinoneimine (NAPQI), leads to depletion of intracellular glutathione (which normally inactivates the potent electrophile), allowing it to bind covalently to certain cell macromolecules disrupting mitochondrial function (Fig. 8.2). Depletion of glutathione by pretreatment measures, including starvation or alcohol ingestion, may further augment NAPQI toxicity

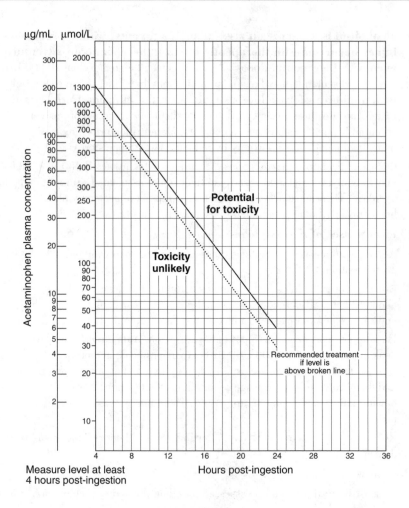

Fig. 8.1   Acetaminophen toxicity nomogram (From Rummack & Matthews 1975[5]). Note: the time coordinates refer to time post ingestion; the graph relates to plasma levels following a single acute dose of acetaminophen; levels drawn earlier than 4 hours after ingestion may not represent peak levels; the interrupted line is drawn 25% below the solid line to allow for possible errors in acetaminophen plasma assays and estimated time from ingestion of an overdose)

a   Goals are to reduce further absorption of ingested acetaminophen and to replete hepatic glutathione via acetylcysteine[6]

b   Use of **N-acetylcysteine** in a dose of 140 mg/kg orally followed by 70 mg/kg orally every 4 hours for an additional 17 doses

4 Management of overdose

- enhances glutathione synthesis
- provides a glutathione substitute to inactivate NAPQI
- may provide a substrate to enhance the nontoxic sulfation pathway

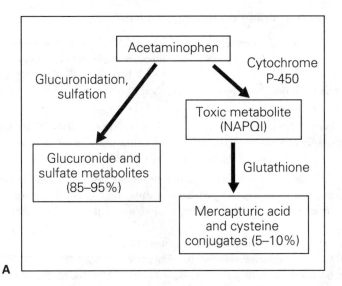

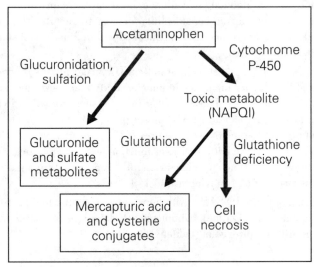

Fig. 8.2   Acetaminophen metabolism for **A**, therapeutic (non-toxic) amounts; and **B**, toxic (e.g., overdose) amounts

- may act as an antioxidant to modify secondary effects of inflammation
- may act on microcirculatory blood flow and improve tissue oxygenation

c If liver injury develops despite *N*-acetylcysteine therapy (or if the patient presents too late for the therapy to be effective), patients should be managed as for all types of acute necroinflammatory liver disease (see Ch. 2). They should be monitored for progression to fulminant hepatic failure and considered early for liver transplantation

B   Nonsteroidal anti-inflammatory agents (NSAIDs)

- despite the overall extremely low incidence of NSAID-induced hepatotoxicity, widespread use of these agents makes them an important class of potentially hepatotoxic drugs. For instance, in Denmark between 1978 and 1987, about 9% of hepatotoxic drug reactions were ascribed to NSAIDS[7]

- prevalence of isolated minor increases in liver function tests is 1–15% and is often considered a class effect of these agents. **Nearly all NSAIDs have been implicated in causing liver injury, ranging from mild to severe.** The most frequently implicated NSAIDs are discussed below

- most NSAIDs produce injury in an unpredictable fashion via an idiosyncratic mechanism and often hepatocellular in nature. Risk of clinically apparent acute liver injury is low, almost always reversible, with fatal reactions being rare

1 **Diclofenac** (Voltaren): hepatotoxicity is most likely to occur in older women with osteoarthritis. In analyzing 180 reports of hepatic injury attributable to diclofenac that had been submitted to the FDA, Banks et al (1995)[7] found that the frequency of hepatotoxicity was rivaled only by sulindac. Most cases occur within 3 months of the start of therapy, with a mixed hepatocellular/cholestatic picture. The FDA recommends that liver enzyme tests be checked within 2 months of starting treatment with diclofenac

2 **Sulindac** (Clinoril): reports submitted to the FDA suggest that sulindac is accompanied by a higher incidence of hepatotoxicity than most other NSAIDs: it was listed in 25% of the reported cases of liver injury associated with NSAIDs despite accounting for only 10% of all NSAID prescriptions. Most cases occur in older women and present frequently with features of hypersensitivity. Up to 50% of cases demonstrate a cholestatic pattern of liver function test abnormalities. Following the discontinuation of sulindac, symptoms generally improve within a few days, with biochemical dysfunction resolving within 1–3 weeks[9]

- Other commonly used NSAIDs with hepatotoxic potential include tolmetin (Tolectin), etodolac (Lodine), nabumetone (Relafen), phenylbutazone (Butazolidin), and piroxicam (Feldene).

3 **Aspirin**
- liver enzyme abnormalities are almost always mild, asymptomatic, and reversible
- in 30% of cases, serum aminotransferase levels are less than 100 U/L and in 45% between 300 and 500 U/L. Serum bilirubin and alkaline phosphatase levels are frequently normal. Liver histology demonstrates focal necrosis and mild nonspecific inflammation
- liver injury is dose dependent and related to serum salicylate levels due to intrinsic toxicity of the salicylate moiety. Ninety percent of toxic cases have a level greater than 15 mg/dL. This level is easily achieved with the large doses used in the treatment of some rheumatologic disorders

C   Antimicrobial and antiviral agents

Isoniazid, macrolide antibiotics, penicillin and its derivatives, and sulfonamides are the most frequent agents responsible for antimicrobial-related hepatotoxicity. Hepatic injury may be necroinflammatory in nature (isoniazid), cholestatic (macrolides, clavulanic acid), or a combination of the two (sulfonamides)

1 **Antibiotics**
  - hepatotoxicity is usually self-limited and idiosyncratic. The length of time for symptomatic recovery correlates with the severity of the initial toxic result
  - **penicillin** hepatotoxicity is more frequently necroinflammatory than cholestatic in nature. **Carbenicillin** and **oxacillin** are the most frequent offenders, with the latter known to cause a cholestatic hepatitis. First-generation **cephalosporins** rarely have hepatotoxic potential; ceftriaxone has been implicated in the formation of biliary sludge. **Amoxicillin–clavulanic acid** (Augmentin) can cause a predominant cholestatic injury occurring within 2 weeks of starting the drug
  - the estolate, ethylsuccinate, propionate and stearate esters of **erythromycin** have all been implicated in the production of cholestatic jaundice. Serum alkaline phosphatase levels may rise to high levels with modest elevations in aminotransferases. There is slow resolution of these abnormalities after cessation of the drug
  - **sulfonamides** (including sulfasalazine used in the treatment of inflammatory bowel disease) most frequently cause a necroinflammatory injury, but they may also provoke a cholestatic, mixed, or granulomatous hepatitis. Trimethoprim–sulfamethoxazole (Bactrim, Septra) causes a predominantly cholestatic injury that may be severe and last for many months. Patients with HIV infection are particularly susceptible to trimethoprim–sulfamethoxazole and pentamidine hepatotoxicity

2 **Antifungals**
  - **ketoconazole** can cause inconsequential biochemical abnormalities with a necroinflammatory pattern in as many as 3–10% of patients taking it. It is thought to be due to an idiosyncratic mechanism, occurring mainly in middle-aged women. Several instances of fulminant hepatic failure have been reported
  - **fluconazole** has also been associated with modest aminotransferase elevations; there have been reports of associated fatal hepatic necrosis

3 **Antituberculous agents**
  a **Isoniazid** (INH)
    - incidence of jaundice is approximately 1% in all patients. Rare in patients under age 20, with an incidence greater than 2% in patients over age 50; females and alcoholics are at greatest risk
    - up to a three-fold elevation in aminotransferases may be seen in 10–20% of patients during the first 2 months of therapy. One half of cases of symptomatic INH hepatotoxicity occur within the first 2 months
    - may resemble acute viral hepatitis with aminotransferases peaking as high as several thousand
    - continuing INH after clinical liver injury occurs may result in fulminant hepatitis with a high mortality
    - mechanism of hepatotoxicity is via cytochrome P-450 transformation of the parent compound into a toxic acetyl radical

b **Rifampin**
- injury is mainly hepatocellular but may be a mixed pattern.
- has rare hepatotoxic potential when taken alone. However, when taken with INH, there is greater hepatotoxicity than with either drug alone. This combination may result in clinical hepatitis in 5–8% of patients. Fulminant hepatitis may occur within the first week of treatment
- toxicity with concurrent INH use results from cytochrome P-450 induction by rifampin, resulting in a greater conversion of INH to toxic metabolites

Streptomycin has no reported hepatotoxic potential, while ethambutol has rarely been incriminated in causing liver injury.

4 **Antiviral agents**
  a **Zidovudine** (AZT)
  - sporadic cases of biochemical hepatitis.
  - appears to be associated with an ill-defined and potentially fatal syndrome of hepatomegaly, lactic acidosis, and hepatic steatosis in some AIDS patients
  b **Didanosine** (DDI): high incidence of causing elevated aminotransferase levels, especially when used at high doses. Several cases of fulminant hepatic failure have been reported
  c **Fialuridine** (FIAU): an investigational agent tested for the treatment of chronic hepatitis B that in 1993 induced a severe toxic reaction in 15 patients, which was characterized by fatal hepatic failure, lactic acidosis, pancreatitis, myopathy, and neuropathy. McKenzie et al (1995)[10] postulated that this toxicity was probably caused by widespread mitochondrial damage: similar, less toxic reactions can infrequently occur with other nucleoside analogues like AZT, DDI, and lamivudine (3-TC)
  d **Interferon alpha**: may provoke deterioration of hepatic enzymes when used (to treat suspected chronic hepatitis C) in patients with autoimmune hepatitis

D Hormonal agents and antihyperlipidemics

1 **Oral contraceptives**: cause frequent, reversible liver function test abnormalities; some patients may develop overt cholestatic jaundice. The molecular basis of injury is disputed but may be due to an alteration of the basolateral membrane of the hepatocyte with a resultant decrease in bile flow. Other conditions associated with use of oral contraceptives include:
  - cholestasis of pregnancy
  - hepatic adenoma (risk increases with duration of use and is higher in women over age 35)
  - hepatocellular carcinoma (possible association)
  - Budd–Chiari syndrome (may be related to thrombogenic effect of the estrogenic component)
  - focal nodular hyperplasia (relationship not firmly established)

2 **Anabolic and androgenic steroids**
  - cholestatic jaundice

- peliosis hepatis
- hepatic adenoma (possible association)
- hepatocellular carcinoma (stronger association than with oral contraceptives)

3 **Flutamide**: an oral anti-androgen used in the treatment of metastatic prostate cancer. Associated with idiosyncratically mediated modest elevation of aminotransferases and rarely massive hepatocellular necrosis. Liver function tests should be checked periodically while on flutamide and the drug immediately discontinued if significant elevations occur.

4 **Niacin** (nicotinic acid)
- widely available over the counter and one of the least expensive antihyperlipidemic agents
- hepatotoxicity is infrequent, occurring at doses that exceed 3 g/day. Its spectrum can range from asymptomatic aminotransferase elevations that resolve within a month of cessation of use to fulminant hepatic failure
- the mechanism of liver injury is unknown; liver biopsy shows both centrilobular cholestasis and hepatocellular necrosis
- sustained-release formulations appear to be better tolerated than regular niacin, and their use has been advocated to improve patient compliance. Over the past several years, there have been increasing reports of severe hepatotoxicity, including fulminant hepatic failure, associated with the use of sustained-release niacin, primarily in patients who were previously treated with conventional niacin formulations
- a Veterans Administration retrospective cohort study of Gray et al. (1994)[11] confirmed that sustained-release niacin resulted in a dose-related increase in liver enzymes over a dosage range of 1–3 g/day. There was an increased risk for hepatotoxicity in the presence of pre-existing liver disease, even when aminotransferase levels were normal. Other risk factors included excessive alcohol ingestion and diabetes mellitus

- *Niacin-prescribing guidelines*
  - liver dysfunction is an absolute contraindication to use of niacin; a history of compensated chronic liver disease is a relative contraindication
  - patients should not switch niacin formulations without consulting their physician
  - with long-term therapy, dosage increments of sustained-release niacin should not be greater than 0.5 g/day, liver enzymes should be assessed at baseline, within 6 weeks of any dosing increase, and then every 3 months
- dosages greater than 2 g/day are more likely to cause hepatotoxicity and require more frequent monitoring. If patients are switched from standard niacin to the sustained-release form, a dose reduction of 50–75% is indicated

5 **HMG CoA reductase inhibitors** (e.g., lovastatin, simvastatin): hepatotoxicity is a frequent side effect, usually asymptomatic aminotransferase elevations, typically within the first year of therapy, not accompanied by increases in serum alkaline phosphatase, and resolution with cessation of the drug

E   Halothane (see Ch. 30)

- although the incidence of hepatotoxicity is low, fear of this complication has contributed to dramatic decrease in its use
- hepatotoxicity is extremely uncommon after a first exposure (1 per 10 000 cases), typically occurring within 2 weeks of surgery. Risk is greater after repeated exposures with the clinical onset of symptoms occurring earlier. Repeated exposures over a short period of time increases risk. See Ray et al. (1991)[12]
- risk factors include female gender, obesity, increasing age and repeated exposures. There is commonly fever with or without eosinophilia after initial halothane exposure
- aminotransferases may increase 25–250 times normal with minimal elevation of serum alkaline phosphatase. Bilirubin levels may be extremely high, especially in patients with a fatal outcome. The prognosis of patients who develop jaundice is poor unless liver transplantation is performed
- the mechanism of liver injury appears to involve formation of a toxic metabolite (probably generated via cytochrome P-450 metabolism). Liver damage occurs directly or as a result of the capacity of halothane metabolites to function as neoantigens able to elicit typical hypersensitivity manifestations (e.g. fever, eosinophilia)

Other halogenated anesthetics like enflurane and isoflurane have infrequently been reported to cause a liver injury similar to that of halothane.

F   Neurologic/antipsychotic agents:

In general, phenothiazines, other neuroleptics e.g., haloperidol, and less frequently benzodiazepines and barbiturates (e.g., phenobarbital) can cause cholestatic liver injury probably secondary to delayed hypersensitivity. Hepatocellular injury can be produced by tricyclic antidepressants (e.g., amitryptiline), and anticonvulsants such as carbamazepine, phenytoin, and valproic acid

1 **Chlorpromazine** (Thorazine)
- as with many phenothiazines the incidence of drug-induced jaundice may be as high as 1–5%. Asymptomatic liver function test abnormalities have been reported in up to 25% of patients
- onset of jaundice typically occurs within 1–4 weeks of initiation of treatment. A prodrome of pruritus and constitutional and gastrointestinal symptoms occurs in most patients. Recovery usually occurs within 2–8 weeks with discontinuation of the drug, though symptoms resembling those of primary biliary cirrhosis can persist
- bilirubin levels may be as high as 5–15 mg/dL, alkaline phosphatase up to 10 times the upper limit of normal, with moderate elevations of aminotransferases

Pronounced hypercholesterolemia is often seen. Histologically, centrilobular cholestasis is seen with scattered periportal inflammation, usually comprised of eosinophils

2 Carbamazepine (Tegretol): structurally similar to tricyclic antidepressants; reported to produce mild to moderate liver function test elevations in up to 22% of patients within the first 6–8 weeks of therapy

3 Phenytoin (Dilantin)

- asymptomatic aminotransferase elevations common, with clinically significant liver injury occurring in 0.1% of patients
- the majority of patients with clinical hepatotoxicity have hypersensitivity-type symptoms, including eosinophilia, fever, leukocytosis, lymphadenopathy, and rash
- liver biopsy findings can demonstrate a lobular, cholestatic, or granulomatous hepatitis

4 Valproic acid (Depakene)

- a common cause of asymptomatic aminotransferase elevations, which are usually mild, reversible, and dose dependent
- fatal valproate hepatotoxicity is not dose-dependent, occurs in young patients who are often receiving other anticonvulsants, and appears to be idiosyncratic in nature. In a retrospective analysis of 400 000 patients treated with valproate from 1978 to 1984 by Dreifuss et al. (1989)[13] 37 fatalities were reported, of which 73% were children younger than age 10. Marked serum aminotransferase elevations are usually absent. Microvesicular steatosis accompanied by centrilobular necrosis is seen in the majority of cases

G Cardiovascular agents

1 Amiodarone

- up to five-fold aminotransferase elevations are seen in 40% of patients receiving long-term therapy. Hepatomegaly is typical, but jaundice is generally absent. There appears to be a relation between the dose of amiodarone, the plasma level of the drug, and the development of abnormal liver tests. The drug should be discontinued when aminotransferase levels are twice normal, and a liver biopsy should be considered
- acute and even fatal hepatotoxicity may occur, probably immunoallergic in nature
- chronic injury usually has an insidious onset; aminotransferases are usually mildly elevated. Liver test abnormalities resolve slowly over several weeks to months after the drug is withdrawn
- liver histology shows changes mimicking those of alcoholic hepatitis with steatosis, Mallory bodies, focal necrosis, and centrizonal fibrosis. Phospholipidosis (recognition of which requires electron microscopic examination) typically occurs due to entrapment of the drug within lysosomes, where it binds to phospholipids, protecting them from degradation by phospholipases and leading to their accumulation

2 Alpha-methyldopa (Aldomet)

- can result in a spectrum of liver disease ranging from transient aminotransferase elevations to chronic hepatitis and even fulminant hepatic failure. The frequency of symptomatic liver disease is 1% of users; 80% of these develop acute hepatocellular injury, 5% cholestatic injury, and the remainder chronic hepatitis. Acute injury may be indistinguishable clinically and histologically from viral hepatitis

- chronic hepatitis may develop in some patients and can be histologically indistinguishable from autoimmune hepatitis

3 Angiotensin-converting enzyme (ACE) inhibitors

- **captopril, enalapril and lisinopril** have each been implicated in causing hepatic injury. Hepatotoxicity is unusual and in most cases occurs in the setting of underlying medical problems and polypharmacy

- captopril typically produces cholestatic, lisinopril hepatocellular, and enalapril acute mixed hepatocellular and cholestatic injury

- liver function test abnormalities resolve with cessation of therapy in most cases, but fatal hepatic necrosis may occur. Cross-reactivity between agents has been described by Hagley et al. (1992)[14]

4 Calcium channel blockers: necroinflammatory injury has been reported with verapamil and mixed hepatocellular and cholestatic injury with nifedipine. Granulomatous hepatitis and hepatocellular injury have been reported with diltiazem usage

H   Chemotherapeutic/immunosuppressive agents

Alkylating agents like chlorambucil have low hepatotoxic potential. When used to treat vasculitis, cyclophosphamide has been associated with liver damage when administration is preceded by azathioprine. When used in conjunction with total body irradiation before allogeneic bone marrow transplantation, alkylating agents may result in veno-occlusive disease

1 Methotrexate

- hepatotoxicity has been recognized for several decades in patients being treated for psoriasis. The spectrum includes hepatic steatosis, fibrosis, and cirrhosis

- cumulative dose appears to be the greatest risk factor for the development of cirrhosis; a total dose of 1.5 g is associated with significant liver disease

- in contradistinction to psoriasis (in which there is a lack of correlation between liver test abnormalities and histopathology), elevations of aminotransferases are not uncommon in rheumatoid arthritis patients receiving methotrexate. When monitoring is performed every 4–6 weeks, the frequency of aminotransferase elevations has correlated with histologic deterioration on liver biopsy. Table 8.5 shows guidelines for monitoring the liver toxicity of methotrexate in rheumatoid arthritis

2 5-fluorouracil (5-FU): there have only been rare reports of associated hepatotoxicity with intravenous 5-FU. The combination of 5-FU and levamisole used as adjuvant therapy in Duke's stage 3 colon cancer, however, carries the potential for hepatotoxicity. Moertel et al. (1993)[15] found that 39.6% of 376 patients undergoing this treatment manifested mild and reversible elevations of aminotransferases, bilirubin, and alkaline phosphatase. They cautioned that these laboratory

Assess baseline serum aminotransferases, alkaline phosphatase, albumin, bilirubin, hepatitis B and C serologies, complete blood count, creatinine

Pretreatment liver biopsy recommended only for patients with a history of prior excessive alcohol consumption, persistently abnormal baseline aminotransferases, or chronic hepatitis B or C

Serum aminotransferase and albumin levels should be checked at 4–8-week intervals, with liver biopsy reserved for persistent liver test abnormalities, defined as an elevation in AST in 5 of 9 determinations within a 12-month period of time, or 6 of 12 determinations if monthly tests are performed, or an abnormal decrease in albumin

Routine surveillance liver biopsies are not recommended

Patients should understand about the possible risk factors for the development of significant hepatotoxicity, including alcohol consumption, cumulative dose, and increasing age

With persistent liver enzyme abnormalities, methotrexate dose should be decreased, followed by temporary discontinuation if liver enzymes remain abnormal. Liver biopsy should be considered before the drug is restarted

(Table 8.5: American College of Rheumatology guidelines for monitoring liver toxicity of methotrexate in rheumatoid arthritis)

abnormalities simulate changes that may accompany the development of liver metastases

3 Azathioprine:
- has been associated with a wide range of hepatotoxic reactions, including nodular regenerative hyperplasia, veno-occlusive disease, peliosis hepatis, and, most commonly, cholestasis and asymptomatic aminotransferase elevations
- the presumed mechanism of hepatoxicity is via damage to endothelial cells within terminal hepatic venules and sinusoids

4 Cyclosporine: infrequent cause of hepatotoxicity, usually manifested by cholestasis with prominent hyperbilirubinemia. Appears to be mediated by inhibition of canalicular bile acid transport. There seems to be a direct relationship between the hyperbilirubinemia and elevated cyclosporine levels

I   Total parenteral nutrition (TPN)

- hepatotoxicity occurs frequently and in the absence of underlying liver disease. In adults, aminotransferase elevations may occur within the first 2–3 weeks of TPN; this is usually reversible within 10–14 days of cessation of TPN. Elevations of alkaline phosphatase and bilirubin occur after more prolonged treatment. In most cases, TPN can be safely continued in these patients. In neonates and infants, liver test abnormalities are present in 90% of patients receiving TPN for more than 10 days. Elevation in direct bilirubin is seen early
- histologically, steatosis, steatohepatitis, and intrahepatic cholestasis may all be found with TPN use in adults. There is infrequent progression to clinically significant chronic liver disease. Histologic progression to cirrhosis and chronic liver disease occurs with long-term TPN use, and commonly in the pediatric population

Composition of TPN
Excess glucose (maximal rate of utilization is 4–5 g/kg, beyond which fat synthesis occurs)
Excess fat (leads to hepatic phagocytosis of lipid droplets)
Imbalance between amino acids and glucose (may increase intrahepatic lipid synthesis)
Deficiency states
Carnitine
Choline
Essential fatty acids
Glutamine
Increased bacterial translocation
Toxic amino acid metabolites and bile acids
Altered gastrointestinal hormonal milieu

(Table 8.6: Possible mechanisms of TPN-associated hepatotoxicity)

- the mechanism of TPN-induced liver dysfunction is still unknown but is probably multifactorial in nature (see Table 8.6)
- gallbladder sludge is detected in 50% of patients receiving TPN for 4–6 weeks and in almost all patients after 8–13 weeks of treatment. Bile stasis is related to prolonged fasting, associated ileal disorders, and reduced gallbladder contractility. TPN-induced gallstones are pigmented, composed primarily of calcium bilirubinate
- there is a higher incidence of both calculous and acalculous cholecystitis in patients receiving long-term TPN. Radionucleotide hepatobiliary scanning has been shown to be of limited diagnostic utility because of a high false-positive rate

J Alternative health agents/herbal medicines

- traditional and nontraditional herbal medicines are being used much more frequently as remedies for various medical conditions. **Because herbal products are not marketed as drugs, they are not subjected to rigorous safety and efficacy testing**. Their purchase in health food and vitamin stores carries with it an implicit assumption of safety, leading many users to ignore the potential for toxicity
- the use of herbal medicines should be a part of any clinical history-taking when considering obscure cases of acute hepatic injury
- ingestion of **pyrrolizidine alkaloids**, usually in the form of teas, has been well established as a cause of veno-occlusive disease. Other herbal products with hepatotoxic potential are listed in Table 8.7

K Other hepatotoxins

1 Amanita mushroom poisoning

- Western Europe, where amateur mushroom hunting is a popular pastime, has the highest incidence. In the USA most poisonings occur in the Pacific Northwest, though *Amanita* species have been identified in oak woodlands throughout the

Chinese herbal preparations
Jin Bu Huan
Fu-san-chi
medicinal teas

Chaparral leaf
Comfrey
Germander
Margosa oil
Pennyroyal oil
Mate tea
Senecio tea
Senna fruit extract
Preparation of mistletoe, motherwort, skullcap, and jalerian
Preparation of asafetida, hops, gentian, and skullcap

(Table 8.7: Herbal products with known hepatotoxic potential)

USA. *Amanita phalloides* accounts for more than 90% of fatalities. Consumption of a single mushroom can lead to fulminant hepatic failure and death

- *Amanita* mushrooms have no characteristic smell or taste and cooking does not destroy its toxin
- amatoxin interferes with mRNA synthesis and results in cell necrosis. *Amanita* poisoning has four characteristic phases:
  1. latent asymptomatic period ranging from 6 to 24 hours;
  2. gastrointestinal phase (mimicking viral gastroenteritis), lasting 12–24 hours, heralded by severe crampy abdominal pain, nausea, vomiting, and profuse watery diarrhea;
  3. another latent phase lasting 12–24 hours, in which clinical symptoms improve but liver dysfunction is first noted on laboratory testing;
  4. rapid progression to fulminant hepatic failure from massive hepatocellular necrosis
- **liver transplantation is almost always necessary, so early evaluation and referral to a transplant center is crucial**

2. **Aflatoxins**: produced by the fungus *Aspergillus flavus*; a contaminant of a variety of nuts, corn, wheat, barley, rice, cottonseed, and soy beans. A warm and moist environment favors production of the toxin. Epidemiologic studies point to an association between the quantity ingested (from contaminated food) and *the* incidence of hepatocellular carcinoma in Africa. The highest estimated daily ingestion of aflatoxins occurs in Mozambique, which also bears the highest incidence of primary hepatocellular carcinoma. May act as co-carcinogens with hepatitis B virus

3. **Arsenic**: used as pesticides and in the production of dyes, ceramics, paint, petroleum, and semi-conductors. Acute injury may result in hepatocellular necrosis; chronic exposure (first described in vineyard workers with insecticide exposure) has been linked to the development of hepatic angiosarcoma

4. **Carbon tetrachloride**: widely used in the production of solvents and as a grain fumigant, fire extinguisher, propellant, and cleaning agent. Poisoning usually follows

inhalation of the vapor in a poorly ventilated environment and bears significant neuro- and nephrotoxicity. It is a potent hepatotoxin. and a single exposure can lead to massive hepatocellular necrosis within 12 to 24 hours. Most deaths are due to renal failure occurring during the second week post intoxication; deaths due to liver failure occur within a week of exposure

5 **Vinyl chloride**: used as a solvent and in the production of polyvinyl chloride and resins. Chronic exposure may result in multicentric angiosarcoma, hepatic fibrosis, and noncirrhotic portal hypertension

6 Miscellaneous drugs: Table 8.8 shows additional drugs associated with liver toxicity

Omeprazole	Mild necroinflammatory hepatitis
Hydroxychloroquine	Fulminant hepatic failure
Propylthiouracil (PTU)	Hepatocellular damage
Terbutaline	Hepatocellular or granulomatous injury
Thiabendazole	Cholestasis, vanishing bile duct syndrome
Trazodone	Cholestasis, mixed cholestatic–hepatocellular injury
Ciprofloxacin	Cholestatic hepatitis
Clozapine	Mixed cholestatic–hepatocellular injury
Disulfiram	Necroinflammatory damage
Hydralazine	Granulomatous, hepatocellular, or cholestatic injury
Labetalol	Hepatocellular necrosis
Nitrofurantoin	Chronic hepatitis, acute cholestatic, or hepatocellular injury
Tacrine	Mild hepatocellular injury
Quinidine	Hepatocellular injury or granulomatous hepatitis
Ticlopidine	Cholestasis

(Table 8.8: Miscellaneous drugs associated with liver toxicity)

References

1   Lee WM. *Acute liver failure.* (N Engl J Med 1993) 329: 862–72

2   Zimmerman HJ, Maddrey WC. *Acetaminophen (paracetamol) hepatotoxicity with regular intake of alcohol: analysis of instances of therapeutic misadventure.* (Hepatology 1995) 22: 767–73

3   Whitcomb DC, Block GD. *Association of acetaminophen hepatotoxicity with fasting and ethanol use.* (JAMA 1994) 272: 1845–50

4   O'Grady JG, Alexander GJ, Hayllar KM, Williams R. *Early indicators of prognosis in fulminant hepatic failure.* (Gastroenterology 1989) 97: 439–45

5   Smilkstein MJ, Knapp GL, Kulig KW, Rumack BH. *Efficacy of oral N-acetylcysteine in the treatment of acetaminophen overdose. Analysis of the national multicenter study (1976 to 1985).* (N Engl J Med 1988) 319: 1557–62

6   Friis H, Andreasen PB. *Drug-induced hepatic injury: an analysis of 1100 cases reported to the Danish Committee on Adverse Drug Reactions between 1978 and 1987.* (J Intern Med 1992) 232: 133–8

7   Banks AT, Zimmerman HJ, Ishak KG, Harter JG. *Diclofenac-associated hepatotoxicity: analysis of 180 cases reported to the Food and Drug Administration as adverse reactions.* (Hepatology 1995) 22: 820–7

8   Tarazi EM, Harter JG, Zimmerman HJ, Ishak KG, Eaton RA. *Sulindac-associated hepatic injury: analysis of 91 cases reported to the Food and Drug Administration.* (Gastroenterology 1993) 104: 569–74

9   McKenzie R, Fried MW, Sallie R et al. *Hepatic failure and lactic acidosis due to fialuridine (FIAU), an investigational nucleoside analogue for chronic hepatitis B.* (N Engl J Med 1995) 333: 1099–1105

10 Gray DR, Morgan T, Chretien SD, Kashyap ML. *Efficacy and safety of controlled-release niacin in dyslipoproteinemic veterans.* (Ann Intern Med 1994) 121: 252–8

11 Ray DC, Drummond GB. *Halothane hepatitis.* (Br J Anaesth 1991) 67: 84–89

12 Dreifuss FE, Langer DH, Moline KA, Maxwell JE. *Valproic acid hepatic fatalities. US experience since 1984.* (Neurology 1989) 39: 201–7

13 Hagley MT, Benal RL, Hulisz DT. *Suspected cross-reactivity of enalapril- and captopril-induced hepatotoxicity.* (Ann Pharmacother 1992) 26: 780–1

14 Moertel CG, Fleming TR, Macdonald, Haller DG, Laurie JA. *Hepatic toxicity associated with fluorouracil plus levamisole adjuvant therapy.* (J Clin Oncol 1993) 11: 2386–90

15 Rummack BH, Matthews H. *Acetaminophen poisoining.* (Pediatrics 1975) 55: 871–6

16 Black M. *Acetaminophen hepatotoxicity.* (Gastroenterology 1984) 78: 382–9

17 DeLeve LD, Kaplowitz N. *Mechanisms of drug-induced liver disease.* (Gastroenterol Clin N Am 1995) 24: 787–810

18 Fry SW, Seeff LB. *Hepatotoxicity of analgesics and anti-inflammatory agents.* (Gastroenterol Clin N Am 1995) 24: 875–905

19 Lee WM. *Drug-induced hepatotoxicity.* (N Engl J Med 1995) 333: 1118–25

20 Lewis JH, Zimmerman HJ. *Drug-induced liver disease.* (Med Clin N Am 1989) 73: 775–92

21 Kremer JM, Alarcon GS, Lightfoot RW et al. *Methotrexate for rheumatoid arthritis: suggested guidelines for monitoring liver toxicity.* (Arthritis Rheum 1994) 37: 316–26

22 Schiano TD, Black M. *New developments in drug hepatotoxicity.* (Curr Opin Gastroenterol 1995) 11: 267–73

23 Watkins PB. *Role of cyctochromes P450 in drug metabolism and hepatotoxicity.* (Semin Liver Dis 1990) 10: 235–50

24 Westphal JF, Vetler D, Brogard JM. *Hepatic side-effects of antibiotics.* (J Antimicrob Chemother 1994) 33: 387–401

25 Zimmerman HJ, Ishak KG. *General aspects of drug-induced liver disease.* (Gastroenterol Clin North A 1995) 24: 739–57

CHAPTER 9

Cirrhosis and portal hypertension: an overview

CATHERINE ANN PETRUFF, M.D.

SANJIV CHOPRA, M.D.

Key Points

1 The major causes of cirrhosis include chronic hepatitis B, chronic hepatitis C, alcohol and hemochromatosis

2 An etiologic classification of cirrhosis is more useful than a morphologic one (micronodular, macronodular, mixed), because important management issues such as family counseling, vaccination, and specific therapy are best addressed once the etiology has been determined

3 Important and potentially life-threating complications of cirrhosis include ascites, spontaneous bacterial peritonitis, variceal hemorrhage, hepatic encephalopathy, hepatorenal syndrome, and primary hepatocellular carcinoma

4 The Child–Pugh classification is useful in assessing prognosis and estimating the potential risk of variceal bleeding and operative mortality

1   Cirrhosis

A   Definition

- the word "cirrhosis" is derived from the Greek word *kirrhos*, meaning orange or tawny, + -osis, meaning condition
- **World Health Organization definition of cirrhosis: a diffuse process characterized by fibrosis and the conversion of normal liver architecture into structurally abnormal nodules which lack normal lobular organization**
- may be associated with failure in the function of hepatic cells and interference with blood flow in the liver, frequently resulting in:
  - jaundice
  - portal hypertension and varices
  - ascites
  - hepatic encephalopathy
  - ultimately hepatic failure
- this definition distinguishes cirrhosis from certain other types of liver disease which have either nodule formation or fibrosis, but not both. These other hepatic disorders may be characterized by portal hypertension in the absence of cirrhosis. **Nodular regenerative hyperplasia**, for example, is characterized by diffuse nodularity without fibrosis, whereas chronic **schistosomiasis** is characterized by Symmes' pipestem fibrosis with no nodularity

B   Classification

1 Morphologic classification: less useful because of considerable overlap
  a Micronodular cirrhosis – uniform nodules < 3 mm in diameter: alcohol, hemochromatosis, biliary obstruction, hepatic venous outflow obstruction, jejunoileal bypass, Indian childhood cirrhosis
  b Macronodular cirrhosis – nodular variation > 3 mm in diameter: chronic hepatitic C, chronic hepatitis B, alpha-1 antitrypsin deficiency, primary biliary cirrhosis
  c Mixed cirrhosis – a combination of micronodular and macronodular cirrhosis. Micronodular cirrhosis frequently evolves into macronodular cirrhosis

2 Etiologic classification: preferred
  - this method of classification is the most useful clinically; by combining clinical, biochemical, histologic, and epidemiologic data, the likely etiologic agent can be ascertained
  - the two most common causes of cirrhosis are excessive alcohol use and viral hepatitis. Table 9.1 lists the etiologic classification

C   Pathology

A liver biopsy should be performed in all patients with suspected cirrhosis unless there are major contraindications

1 Gross examination: the liver surface is irregular, with multiple yellowish nodules.

1 Viral hepatitis (B, C, D, ?G)

2 Alcohol

3 Metabolic
  a Genetic hemochromatosis (iron overload)
  b Wilson's disease (copper overload)
  c Alpha-1 antitrypsin deficiency
  d Cystic fibrosis
  e Galactosemia
  f Glycogen storage disease
  g Hereditary tyrosinemia
  h Hereditary fructose intolerance
  i Hereditary hemorrhagic telangiectasia
  j Abetalipoproteinemia
  k Porphyria

4 Biliary disease
  a Extrahepatic biliary obstruction
  b Intrahepatic biliary obstruction
    • Primary biliary cirrhosis
    • Primary sclerosing cholangitis
  c Childhood biliary disease
    • Byler's disease (progressive childhood cholestasis)
    • Alagille's syndrome (arteriohepatic dysplasia)
    • Aagenaes' syndrome (cholestasis with lymphedema)
    • Zellweger's syndrome
    • Indian childhood cirrhosis

5 Venous outflow obstruction
  a Budd–Chiari syndrome
  b Veno-occlusive disease
  c Severe right-sided heart failure

6 Drugs, toxins, chemicals, e.g., methotrexate, amiodarone

7 Immunologic
  a Autoimmune hepatitis
  b Graft-versus-host disease

8 Miscellaneous
  a Other infections, e.g., syphilis, schistosomiasis
  b Sarcoidosis
  c Nonalcoholic steatohepatitis (NASH)
  d Jejunoileal bypass for obesity
  e Hypervitaminosis A
  f Cryptogenic

(Table 9.1: Etiologic classification of cirrhosis)

Depending on the severity of the cirrhosis, the liver may be enlarged due to multiple regenerating nodules or, in the final stages, small and shrunken

2 Pathologic criteria for diagnosis of cirrhosis
  a Nodularity (regenerating nodules)

    b Fibrosis (deposition of connective tissue creates pseudolobules)

    c Fragmentation of the sample

    d Abnormal hepatic architecture

    e Hepatocellular abnormalities

- pleomorphism
- dysplasia
- regenerative hyperplasia

3 Information obtained from histologic examination

    a Establishment of the presence of cirrhosis

    b Aid in determination of the etiology of the cirrhosis

    c Assessment of histologic activity

    d Determination of the stage of development, e.g., stages of primary biliary cirrhosis

    e Diagnosis of hepatocellular carcinoma

4 Specific histologic methods for determining etiology

    a Immunohistochemistry (e.g., hepatitis B virus)

    b Polymerase chain reaction (PCR) techniques (e.g., hepatitis C virus)

    c Quantitative copper measurement (Wilson's disease)

    d Quantitative iron measurement and calculation of Hepatic Iron Index

- can distinguish heterozygotes from homozygotes in (genetic) hemochromatosis

    e PAS-positive, diastase-resistant globules (alpha-1 antitrypsin deficiency)

D   Clinical features

There are protean manifestations of cirrhosis. In many cases cirrhosis is clinically silent. A patient with cirrhosis may present with none, some, or all of the findings listed below

1   General features
- fatigue
- anorexia
- malaise
- weight loss
- muscle wasting
- fever

2   Gastrointestinal
- parotid enlargement
- diarrhea
- cholelithiasis
- gastrointestinal bleeding
  - esophageal/gastric/duodenal/rectal varices
  - portal hypertensive gastropathy/colopathy
  - peptic ulcer disease
  - gastritis

3 Hematologic
- anemia
  - folate deficiency
  - spur cell anemia (hemolytic anemia seen in severe alcoholic liver disease)
  - splenomegaly with resultant pancytopenia
- thrombocytopenia
- leukopenia
- impaired coagulation
- disseminated intravascular coagulation
- hemosiderosis

4 Pulmonary
- decreased oxygen saturation
- altered ventilation–perfusion relationships
- primary pulmonary hypertension
- hyperventilation
- reduced pulmonary diffusion capacity
- hepatic hydrothorax
  - accumulation of fluid within the pleural space in association with cirrhosis and in the absence of primary pulmonary or cardiac disease
  - usually right sided (70%)
  - typically associated with clinically apparent ascites, but can be found in patients without ascites
- hepatopulmonary syndrome
  - triad of liver disease, an increased alveolar–arterial gradient while breathing room air, and evidence for intrapulmonary vascular dilatations
  - characterized by dyspnea, platypnea, orthodeoxia, digital clubbing, and severe hypoxemia

5 Cardiac: hyperdynamic circulation

6 Renal
- secondary hyperaldosteronism – leads to sodium and water retention
- hepatic glomerulosclerosis
- renal tubular acidosis (more frequent in alcoholic cirrhosis, Wilson's disease, and primary biliary cirrhosis)
- hepatorenal syndrome

7 Endocrine
- hypogonadism
  - males: loss of libido, testicular atrophy, impotence, decreased amounts of testosterone
  - females: infertility, dysmenorrhea, loss of secondary sexual characteristics
- feminization=acquisition of estrogen-induced characteristics:
  - spider telangiectases
  - palmar erythema

- gynecomastia
- changes in body hair patterns
- diabetes
- elevated parathyroid hormone levels – may be due to hypovitaminosis D and secondary hyperparathyroidism

8 Neurologic
- hepatic encephalopathy
- peripheral neuropathy

9 Musculoskeletal
- reduction in lean muscle mass
- hypertrophic osteoarthropathy: synovitis, clubbing, and periostitis
- hepatic osteodystrophy
- muscle cramps
- umbilical herniation

10 Dermatologic
- spider telangiectases
- palmar erythema
- nail changes: clubbing (esp. primary biliary cirrhosis), white nails, azure lunules (Wilson's disease)
- Dupuytren's contractures
- jaundice

E   Potential complications of cirrhosis

- ascites (see Ch. 11)
- spontaneous bacterial peritonitis (see Ch. 11)
- variceal hemorrhage (see Ch. 10)
- hepatic encephalopathy (see Ch. 13)
- hepatocellular carcinoma (see Ch. 27)
- hepatorenal syndrome (see Ch. 12)

F   Diagnosis of cirrhosis

1 Physical examination
- stigmata of chronic liver disease and/or cirrhosis
  - spider telangiectases
  - palmar erythema
  - Dupuytren's contractures
  - gynecomastia
  - testicular atrophy
- features of portal hypertension
  - ascites
  - splenomegaly

- caput medusae
- evidence of hyperdynamic circulation, e.g., resting tachycardia
- features of hepatic encephalopathy
  - confusion
  - asterixis
  - fetor hepaticus
- other
  - jaundice
  - bilateral parotid enlargement
  - scanty chest and axillary hair

2 Laboratory evaluation (see also Ch. 1)

- tests of hepatocellular necrosis
  - aminotransferases (AST, ALT)
  - lactate dehydrogenase (LDH) and LD5 isoenzyme
- tests of cholestasis
  - alkaline phosphatase
  - serum bilirubin (conjugated and unconjugated)
  - gamma glutamyltranspeptidase (GGTP)
  - 5′-nucleotidase
- tests of synthetic function
  - serum albumin
  - prothrombin time
- special tests to aid in diagnosis
  - viral hepatitis serology
  - PCR techniques for detecting viral genetic material
  - serum iron, total iron binding capacity (TIBC), ferritin (hemochromatosis)
  - ceruloplasmin (Wilson's disease)
  - alpha-1 antitrypsin level and protease inhibitor type
  - serum immunoglobulins
  - autoantibodies: anti-nuclear antibody (ANA), anti-mitochondrial antibody (AMA), anti-liver kidney microsomal antibody (LKM), anti-smooth muscle antibody (SMA)
- screening test for hepatocellular carcinoma: serum alpha fetoprotein

3 Imaging modalities (see also Ch. 1)

- abdominal ultrasound
  - noninvasive, relatively inexpensive
  - can easily detect ascites, biliary dilatation, hepatic masses
  - duplex–Doppler ultrasonography can further assess hepatic and portal vein patency
- computed tomography (CT)
  - noninvasive, more expensive
  - findings in cirrhosis are nonspecific

- may be helpful in the diagnosis of hemochromatosis; increased density of the liver is suggestive
- magnetic resonance imaging (MRI)
  - noninvasive, expensive, major recent advance
  - excellent for further evaluation of suspicious liver lesions; can help differentiate focal fat from a possible hepatic malignancy
  - can easily assess hepatic vasculature without the need for nephrotoxic contrast agents; probably more reliable than Doppler ultrasound
  - excellent modality for assessing iron overload states
  - magnetic resonance cholangiography (MRC), recently introduced as a noninvasive method to image the biliary tree
- radionucleotide studies
  - colloid liver spleen scan using ^{99m}Tc sulfur colloid may aid in the detection of cirrhosis; there is increased uptake of colloid in the bone marrow and spleen, with decreased uptake in the liver
  - seldom performed; supplanted by CT and MRI
- barium swallow: may aid in the detection of esophageal varices, although esophagoscopy is more accurate for detection of varices

4 Liver biopsy (see also Ch. 1)
  - the "gold standard" for the diagnosis of cirrhosis
  - usually performed percutaneously
  - relatively low-risk procedure
  - complications: bleeding, infection, pneumothorax

G Management

1 Specific treatments are available in certain instances,
  - phlebotomy for hemochromatosis
  - *d*-penicillamine for Wilson's disease
  - alcohol avoidance for alcohol-induced cirrhosis
  - antiviral agents such as interferon alpha for viral hepatitis

2 In most cases, management focuses on treatment of complications which arise in the setting of cirrhosis (e.g., variceal hemorrhage, hepatic encephalopathy, ascites, and spontaneous bacterial peritonitis)

3 Screening for hepatocellular carcinoma with serial ultrasound examination at frequent intervals (e.g., every 6 months) and serum alpha fetoprotein measurements should be performed in selected patients (e.g., patients with chronic hepatitis B, chronic hepatitis C, and hemochromatosis)

4 In end-stage cirrhosis orthotopic liver transplantation can be a life-saving procedure if the patient is an appropriate candidate

H Prognosis

- Depends on the development of cirrhotic-related complications
- a classification scheme proposed to assess survival, **Child's classification**, has

undergone various modifications. The system currently employed by many hepatologists is the **Child–Pugh modification** (Table 9.2)

Parameter	Numerical score		
	1	2	3
Ascites	None	Slight	Moderate/severe
Encephalopathy	None	Slight/moderate	Moderate/severe
Bilirubin (mg/dL)	<2.0	2–3	>3.0
Albumin (mg/L)	>3.5	2.8–3.5	<2.8
Prothrombin time (seconds increased)	1–3	4–6	>6.0

Total numerical score	Child–Pugh class
5–6	A
7–9	B
10–15	C

(Table 9.2: Modified Child–Pugh classification for cirrhosis)

- patients with compensated cirrhosis may have a relatively long life expectancy, if they do not exhibit evidence of decompensation. There is an estimated 47% 10-year survival in compensated patients, but only a 16% 5-year survival when decompensation occurs
- in patients with cirrhosis and varices who have not yet had their first variceal hemorrhage, the risk of bleeding from varices can be predicted based on a scoring system that incorporates the Child–Pugh classification, size of varices, and certain endoscopic stigmata such as red wale markings and cherry-red spots (see Ch. 10)
- In cirrhotics, the risk of general anesthesia and operative mortality is also dependent on the Child–Pugh classification (see Ch. 30)

I Evaluation

See Figure 9.1

2 Portal Hypertension

A Definition: An increase in portal venous pressure

- normal portal pressure: 5–10 mmHg
- portal hypertension: > 12 mmHg
- normal portal blood flow: 1–1.5 L/min
- elevated portal pressure increases the gradient between portal pressure and inferior vena caval pressure above the normal range of 2–6 mmHg
- increased resistance to portal blood flow leads to formation of portosystemic

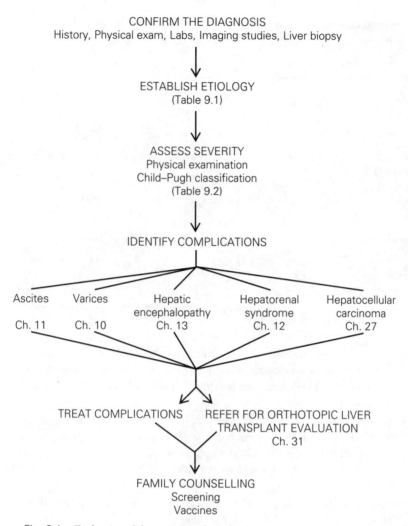

CONFIRM THE DIAGNOSIS
History, Physical exam, Labs, Imaging studies, Liver biopsy

ESTABLISH ETIOLOGY
(Table 9.1)

ASSESS SEVERITY
Physical examination
Child–Pugh classification
(Table 9.2)

IDENTIFY COMPLICATIONS

Ascites	Varices	Hepatic encephalopathy	Hepatorenal syndrome	Hepatocellular carcinoma
Ch. 11	Ch. 10	Ch. 13	Ch. 12	Ch. 27

TREAT COMPLICATIONS   REFER FOR ORTHOTOPIC LIVER TRANSPLANT EVALUATION
Ch. 31

FAMILY COUNSELLING
Screening
Vaccines

Fig. 9.1   Evaluation of the patient with cirrhosis

collaterals that divert portal blood flow to the systemic circulation, effectively bypassing the liver

B   Classification (Table 9.3)

- there are causes of portal hypertension other than cirrhosis
- the major classification scheme employed is based on the location of the block to portal flow: prehepatic, intrahepatic, and posthepatic. Intrahepatic causes are further separated into presinusoidal, sinusoidal, and postsinusoidal (Fig. 9.2). There is some overlap with this method of classification

C   Clinical consequences

1 Varices: gastroesophageal, anorectal, retroperitoneal, other
2 Portal hypertensive gastropathy

1 Prehepatic
- Portal vein thrombosis
- Cavernous transformation of the portal vein
- Splenic vein thrombosis
- Splanchic arteriovenous fistula
- Idiopathic tropical splenomegaly

2 Intrahepatic (some overlap exists)

a Presinusoidal: affects portal venule
- Schistosomiasis (most common cause of portal hypertension worldwide)
- Congenital hepatic fibrosis
- Sarcoidosis
- Chronic viral hepatitis
- Primary biliary cirrhosis (early)
- Myeloproliferative diseases
- Nodular regenerative hyperplasia
- Hepatoportal sclerosis (idiopathic portal hypertension)
- Malignant disease
- Wilson's disease
- Hemochromatosis
- Polycystic liver disease
- Amyloidosis
- Toxic agents: copper, arsenic, vinyl chloride, 6-mercaptopurine

b Sinusoidal: affects sinusoids
- All causes of cirrhosis (Table 9.1)
- Acute alcoholic hepatitis
- Severe viral hepatitis
- Acute fatty liver of pregnancy
- Vitamin A intoxication
- Systemic mastocytosis
- Peliosis hepatis
- Cytotoxic drugs

c Postsinusoidal: affects central vein
- Veno-occlusive disease
- Alcoholic central hyaline sclerosis

3 Posthepatic

a Hepatic vein thrombosis
- Budd–Chiari syndrome
- Vascular invasion by tumor

b Inferior vena caval obstruction
- Inferior vena cava web
- Vascular invasion by tumor

c Cardiac disease
- Constrictive pericarditis
- Severe tricuspid regurgitation

(Table 9.3: Classification of portal hypertension)

3 Caput medusae

4 Ascites

5 Congestive splenomegaly

6 Hepatic encephalopathy

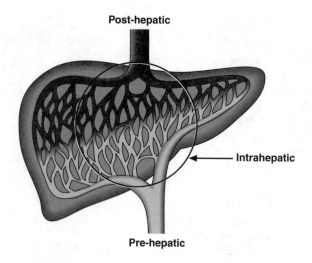

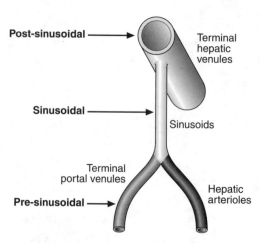

Fig. 9.2   Sites of block in portal hypertension

D   Measurement of portal pressure

- in most cases diagnosis of portal hypertension can be based on physical findings. However, there are instances where actual measurement of the portal pressure is required
- patency of the portal vein should be assessed prior to measurement of portal pressure. This may be accomplished by duplex–Doppler ultrasound or magnetic resonance angiography

1 Direct measurement of portal pressure: invasive, expensive, complicated, accurate

- operative portal vein measurement; requires laparotomy; affected by many variables including anesthesia

- percutaneous transhepatic measurement
- transjugular measurement

2 Indirect measurement of portal pressure: preferred method, less invasive, safer, less complicated

- hepatic vein catheterization
  - involves cannulation of the hepatic vein via a femoral approach, balloon occlusion of the hepatic vein, and measurement of the wedged hepatic vein pressure (WHVP)
  - portal venous pressure gradient obtained, defined as the **difference between the portal pressure and that in the inferior vena cava**
  - WHVP actually measures sinusoidal pressure, not portal pressure

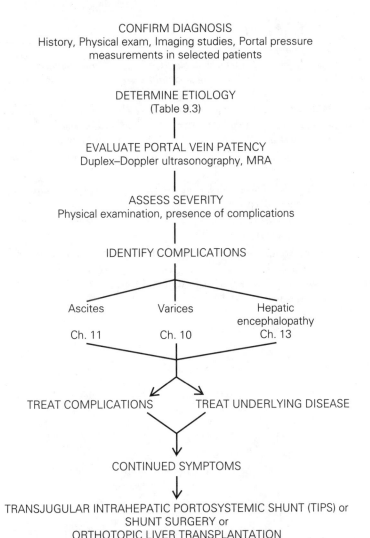

Fig. 9.3   Evaluation of the patient with portal hypertension

- portal pressure may be underestimated in cases of presinusoidal portal hypertension
- can measure hepatic blood flow
- intrasplenic measurement
  - involves percutaneous puncture of the spleen
  - not routinely performed

E Treatment of complications of portal hypertension

See Chapters 10–13 and 31

F Evaluation

See Figure 9.3

References

1 Albers I, Hartman H, Bircher J, Creutzfeldt. *Superiority of the Child–Pugh classification to quantitative liver function tests for assessing prognosis of liver cirrhosis.* (Scand J Gastroenterol 1989) 24: 269–76

2 Anthony PP, Ishak KG, Nayak NC, Poulsen HE, Scheuer PJ, Sobin LH. *The morphology of cirrhosis: recommendations on definition, nomenclature, and classification by a working group sponsored by the World Health Organization.* (J Clin Pathol 1978) 31: 395–414

3 Bosch J, Navasa M, Garcia-Pagan JC, DeLacy AM, Rodes J. *Portal hypertension.* (Med Clin North Am 1989) 73: 931–52

4 Christensen E, Schicting P, Fauerholdt L et al. *Prognostic value of Child–Turcotte criteria in medically treated cirrhosis.* (Hepatology 1984) 4(3): 430–5

5 D'Amico G, Pagliaro L, Bosch J. *The treatment of portal hypertension: a meta-analytic review.* (Hepatology 1995) 22: 332–51

6 Gines P, Quintero E, Arroyo V et al. *Compensated cirrhosis: natural history and prognostic factors.* (Hepatology 1987) 7: 122–8

7 McIntyre N, Benhamou J, Bircher J, Rizzetto M, Rodes J. *Oxford Textbook of Clinical Hepatology.* (Oxford: Oxford University Press) 1991

Portal hypertension and gastrointestinal bleeding

JAMES PULEO, M.D.   NORMAN D. GRACE, M.D.

▼

Key Points

1 Patients with cirrhosis who develop large esophageal varices as a consequence of portal hypertension have a 25–35% risk of a variceal hemorrhage and a 30–50% mortality rate associated with the bleeding episode. Mortality is dependent on the clinical status of the patient and the severity of the bleeding episodes

2 Nonselective beta adrenergic blockers are the only proven therapy for the prevention of first variceal hemorrhage in patients with cirrhosis

3 Both endoscopic therapy (sclerotherapy, variceal ligation) and pharmacologic therapy (vasopressin plus nitroglycerin, somatostatin, glypressin) are effective in controlling the acute bleeding episode. The combination of endoscopic and pharmacologic therapy offers advantages over the use of either therapy alone

4 Endoscopic variceal ligation is the endoscopic treatment of choice for the prevention of recurrent variceal bleeding

5 Nonselective beta adrenergic blockers or combinations of beta blockers and long-acting nitrates are effective in prevention of recurrent variceal bleeding. Serial measurement of portal pressure is helpful in assessing the effectiveness of therapy and making appropriate changes when indicated

▶

6 For patients failing medical therapy to prevent recurrent variceal hemorrhage, options include transjugular intrahepatic portosystemic stent shunts (TIPS), surgical shunts or liver transplantation. Selection of the appropriate rescue procedure is dictated by the clinical status of the patient, the availability of expertise in the procedure and, in the case of liver transplantation, appropriateness of the condition and availability of a donor organ

---

1   Portal Hypertension: Overview

A   Pathophysiology

1 Portal hypertension is defined as an increase in the portal venous pressure gradient (PVPG) and is a function of portal venous blood flow and hepatic and portocollateral resistance

2 In patients with cirrhosis, portal hypertension is initiated by an increase in hepatic and portocollateral resistance. This resistance is modulated by an increase in levels of intrahepatic endothelin, a potent vasoconstrictor, and a decrease in levels of intrahepatic nitric oxide, a vasodilator

3 Hepatic resistance may be modified by changes in perivenular and presinusoidal myofibroblasts as well as the smooth muscle component of portocollateral vessels

4 Portal hypertension is exacerbated by the development of systemic vasodilatation, which leads to plasma volume expansion, an increase in cardiac output, and a hyperdynamic circulation. Systemic vasodilatation is a result of an increase in systemic levels of nitric oxide and, to a lesser extent, increased circulatory levels of glucagon, prostaglandins, tumor necrosis factor (TNF) alpha, and other cytokines and alterations in the autonomic nervous system

5 **Any increase in portal blood flow and/or hepatic or portocollateral resistance will increase portal pressure. Conversely, any decrease in portal blood and/or hepatic resistance will decrease portal pressure. This forms the basis for the pharmacologic treatment of portal hypertension**

B   Pharmacotherapy

1 Two classes of drugs – vasoconstrictors and vasodilators – are used for treatment of portal hypertension

2 **Vasoconstrictors** (vasopressin, somatostatin, nonselective beta blockers) produce a decrease in splanchnic blood flow which leads to a decrease in portal venous blood flow and portal pressure

3 **Vasodilators** (nitroglycerin, long-acting nitrates, prazosin) alter resistance by inducing changes in the intrahepatic perivenular and perisinusoidal myofibroblasts as well as the smooth muscle component of portocollateral vessels

4 Combined use of vasoconstrictors and vasodilators offers the potential benefit of additive reductions in portal pressure, but their use may be limited by the side effects of treatment

C Epidemiology of esophagogastric variceal hemorrhage (EVH)

1 Fifty percent of patients with alcoholic cirrhosis will develop esophageal varices within 2 years of diagnosis, and 70–80% will do so within 10 years.[1] In patients with cirrhosis secondary to hepatitis C, the risk is somewhat less, 30% develop esophageal varices within 6 years of the initial diagnosis of cirrhosis.[2]

2 Twenty-five to thirty-five percent of patients with cirrhosis and large esophageal varices will experience an episode of variceal bleeding, the majority occurring within the first year after diagnosis of varices. Risk of first EVH decreases significantly after the first year

3 In patients with cirrhosis who survive the initial episode of EVH with conservative medical management, the risk of recurrent EVH is 65–70%, with most episodes occurring within 6 months of the index bleed

4 Treatment to prevent recurrent EVH needs to be initiated immediately following control of the acute EVH

5 EVH accounts for approximately one third of deaths in patients with cirrhosis and portal hypertension. The mortality rate for each episode of EVH is 30–50% depending on the clinical status of the patient

D Risk factors for first variceal hemorrhage (FVH)

1 Prospective studies have identified the following risk factors for EVH:
- large esophageal varices
- presence of endoscopic red color signs (red wales, cherry red spots, hematocystic spots); these are essentially small varices on the surface of large varices
- Child's classification, especially the presence of ascites (see Ch. 9)
- active alcohol consumption in patients with alcoholic liver disease

2 Gastroesophageal reflux does not play a role in initiating esophageal variceal hemorrhage

E Predictive value of portal hemodynamic measurements

1 Measurement of the **hepatic venous pressure gradient (HVPG)** is an easy and reproducible method for estimating PVPG. HVPG is the difference between the wedged or occluded hepatic venous pressure and the free hepatic venous pressure. HVPG has a high correlation with PVPG in patients with cirrhosis when hepatic resistance is sinusoidal or postsinusoidal, as in patients with alcoholic cirrhosis. HVPG tends to underestimate PVPG when the defect is presinusoidal, as in primary biliary cirrhosis

2 **An HVPG of ≥ 12 mmHg is necessary for esophageal varices to form and bleed.** However, the absolute level of HPVG does not correlate with risk of bleeding

3 According to LaPlace's law, variceal wall tension (T) is a function of the transmural pressure (TP) times the radius (r) of the varix divided by the variceal wall thickness (w)

$$T = (\text{TP}_1 - \text{TP}_2) \times r/w$$

This calculation combines measurements of variceal size and pressure and has the highest predictive value for determining the risk of EVH

4 Risk of recurrent EVH correlates with the level of HVPG; **the higher the HVPG, the greater the risk of recurrent EVH**

5 HVPG is also prognostic for survival; **the higher the HVPG, the worse the survival**

6 Serial measurements of HVPG are predictive of the risk of recurrent EVH. **Patients who have a decrease in HVPG to a level below 12 mmHg are not at risk for recurrent EVH. Patients in whom HVPG decreases by ≥20% over the first few months after the index bleed, usually in response to pharmacologic therapy, have a marked decrease in the risk of recurrent EVH, whereas patients who have less than a 20% decrease in HVPG while on pharmacologic therapy maintain a high risk of recurrent EVH**[3,4]

2 Prevention of Initial Variceal Hemorrhage

A Pharmacologic therapy

1 **For patients with large esophageal varices and no prior history of variceal hemorrhage, nonselective beta adrenergic blockers are the treatment of choice** and the only therapy that has been verified in well-designed prospective randomized controlled trials (RCTs).[5] Use of these drugs will decrease the risk of initial variceal bleeding by approximately 40%

2 Nonselective beta blockers (propranolol, nadolol, timolol) should be offered to patients who are deemed to be reasonably compliant in taking medication and who have no contraindications to the use of beta blockers, such as insulin-dependent diabetes mellitus, severe chronic obstructive lung disease, or congestive heart failure

3 For patients unable to tolerate beta blocker therapy, the use of long-acting nitrates (isosorbide 5-mononitrate) may be a reasonable alternative

4 In routine practice, dose of the nonselective beta blocker is determined by a 25% decrease in the resting heart, a decrease in the heart rate to 55/min, or the development of side effects of therapy. If portal hemodynamic studies are readily available, serial measurements of HVPG in response to beta blocker therapy may be of value in determining the therapeutic dose and potential clinical benefit of beta blockers

5 Although data on the long-term (greater than 2–3 years) use of these drugs to prevent first EVH are limited, treatment should probably be continued indefinitely

B Endoscopic therapy

1 Although early RCTs evaluating sclerotherapy for the prevention of FVH were encouraging, more recent studies have shown no benefit, and in two large studies a higher mortality was observed in patients treated with sclerotherapy. Limitations in

the quality of design, selection of patients, and determination of endpoints in the RCTs evaluating sclerotherapy preclude recommendation of this technique for the prevention of FVH

2 Data on the use of esophageal variceal ligation for prevention of FVH are very limited, and this technique also cannot be recommended at this time

3 Combined sclerotherapy and treatment with nonselective beta blockers offers no advantage over the use of beta blockers alone for prevention of FVH

C Surgical therapy

1 Although portosystemic shunt surgery markedly decreases the risk of FVH, RCTs have clearly demonstrated an increased incidence of hepatic encephalopathy and liver failure and a decrease in overall survival associated with such surgery. Therefore, prophylactic shunt surgery is not indicated for the prevention of FVH

2 Decisions about candidacy for liver transplantation should be dictated by the overall clinical status of the patient. The presence of varices by itself is not an indication for liver transplantation (see Ch. 31)

3 Management of Acute Variceal Hemorrhage

A Initial management

1 Resuscitation of the patient is critical in the management of the patient with cirrhosis and suspected variceal hemorrhage and should include the following measures:
- establish adequate venous access for blood and fluid replacement
- insert a nasogastric or Ewald tube to assess the severity of bleeding and to lavage gastric contents prior to endoscopy
- treat clotting factor deficiencies with fresh frozen plasma if indicated
- administer blood transfusions to establish hemodynamic stability. Caution should be taken not to overtransfuse the patient. In general, patients should be kept slightly undertransfused, usually with a hematocrit in the low 30s, so as not to increase portal pressure and exacerbate variceal bleeding
- establish airway protection in patients with massive bleeding or evidence of hepatic encephalopathy
- Initiate antibiotic treatment in patients who are potentially septic. Prior to treatment, blood cultures, a diagnostic paracentesis if ascites is present, and other studies as indicated should be performed

2 Endoscopy is the only reliable means for establishing the source of bleeding and should be performed as soon as the patient is adequately resuscitated. The diagnosis of esophagogastric variceal bleeding is determined either by direct visualization of bleeding or, more often, by evidence of recent bleeding in patients with varices and no other visible source of bleeding.

B Endoscopic therapy

1 **Sclerotherapy** is successful in controlling acute esophageal variceal bleeding in 80–90% of patients. Control should be obtained with one to two sessions. Additional

sessions are of minimal benefit. Patients continuing to bleed after two sessions of sclerotherapy should be considered sclerotherapy failures and alternative methods to control bleeding should be instituted

2 Variations in technique or the sclerosant employed have not been shown to influence outcome. In general, sodium tetradecylsulfate or sodium morrhuate has been employed in the USA, while polidocanol or ethanolamine has been more popular in Europe and absolute alcohol has been used in Asia

3 Serious complications related to sclerotherapy have been reported in 10–20% of patients, with an associated mortality rate of 2%. Severe mucosal ulceration causing bleeding is the most common of these complications, while esophageal perforation, mediastinitis, and pulmonary complications have also been reported. Longer-term complications include dysphagia secondary to stricture formation

4 **Endoscopic variceal ligation (banding)** has a success rate comparable with sclerotherapy for the control of acute variceal bleeding and has the potential advantages of far fewer side effects. Performance of this technique may be difficult in patients with massive variceal bleeding.

C Pharmacologic therapy

1 The use of vasoactive drugs for treatment of acute bleeding related to portal hypertension offers several advantages

- treatment can be started in the emergency room or even on the way to the hospital, when variceal bleeding is suspected

- unlike endoscopic therapy, in which the effects of treatment are local, vasoactive agents lower portal pressure

- use of vasoactive agents prior to endoscopy may offer the endoscopist a clearer view of the varices due to less active bleeding

- vasoactive agents are the only established treatment for sources of portal hypertensive bleeding other than esophageal varices, such as gastric varices more than 2 cm below the gastroesophageal junction or portal hypertensive gastropathy. Other therapies such as the use of thrombin or cyanoacrylate glue are still considered experimental

2 Currently available agents include vasopressin, nitroglycerin, somatostatin, octreotide and glypressin (not available in the USA) (see Table 10.1)

- **vasopressin** controls bleeding in about 50% of patients but has significant side effects (e.g., myocardial and mesenteric ischemia) that limit its use. Recurrent bleeding occurs in up to 45% of patients, and there is no survival benefit associated with its use

- the combination of **vasopressin and nitroglycerin** has been shown to control variceal bleeding in a higher percentage of patients than vasopressin alone. More importantly, addition of nitroglycerin ameliorates many of the systemic side effects of vasopressin, making its use more tolerable

- **somatostatin**, given intravenously by bolus followed by continuous infusion, has been effective in controlling variceal bleeding in 60–80% of patients and has practically no serious side effects associated with its use

- because somatostatin is not generally available in the USA, **octreotide**, its synthetic analog with a longer half-life, has been used in the USA in place of somatostatin. Data from RCTs of octreotide are more variable than those for somatostatin, but the drug is safe and has gained wide acceptance for this indication

- **glypressin**, a synthetic analog of vasopressin, has a longer half-life than vasopressin and, therefore, can be given by intravenous bolus infusion. RCTs have shown this drug to be more effective than vasopressin, with far fewer side effects. Although not available in the USA, it is used widely in Europe

Drug	Route	Administration	Dose
1 Vasopressin	i.v.	Continuous infusion	0.1–0.4 units/min
Nitroglycerin	i.v.	Continuous infusion	40–400 µg/min
2 Glypressin	i.v.	Initial bolus	2 mg/4 h
		Subsequent bolus	1–2 mg/4 h
3 Somatostatin	i.v.	Initial bolus	250–500 µg
		Continuous infusion	250–500 µg/h
4 Octreotide	i.v.	Initial bolus	25–50 µg
		Continuous infusion	25–50 µg/h

Treatment should be continued for 5 days

(Table 10.1: Pharmacologic treatment of acute variceal bleeding)

There is increasing evidence that the combination of endoscopic and pharmacologic therapy offers clinical advantages over the use of either therapy alone, with less rebleeding in the acute period (first 5 days) and lower transfusion requirements.[6] However, combination therapy has not been shown to improve survival

D   Balloon tamponade

- although endoscopic therapy has replaced balloon tamponade as initial therapy for variceal bleeding, balloon tamponade may still be of value as a temporizing treatment for failures of pharmacologic and endoscopic therapy, while more definitive treatment for the control of acute variceal bleeding is awaited
- success with balloon tamponade can often be achieved with inflation of just the gastric balloon, thereby avoiding the additional complications associated with use of the esophageal balloon
- complication rates with the use of balloon tamponade relate to the experience of the team using the balloon. Very specific precautions are required to minimize the risk of aspiration and asphyxiation. The balloon should not be kept inflated for more than 24 hours

E   Treatment for failures of medical therapy

1 A recent National Institutes of Health consensus conference supported the use of the percutaneous transjugular intrahepatic stent shunt (TIPS) for the rescue of the 10–20% of patients who fail medical therapy for the control of acute variceal hemorrhage.[7]

2 In experienced hands, TIPS is successfully placed in 90–95% of patients, with relatively low immediate mortality compared with the use of surgical shunts

3 Rebleeding and/or hepatic encephalopathy are long-term complications of the procedure

4 In a few selected centers, the early use (within 12 hours of diagnosis) of portosystemic shunt surgery has been advocated, with excellent results reported. However, this approach has not gained widespread acceptance

4 Prevention of Recurrent Variceal Hemorrhage

Because of the high recurrence rate of variceal bleeding after control of initial bleeding, it is not surprising that medical therapy for the control of acute variceal bleeding has not been associated with improved survival. Treatment to prevent recurrent variceal bleeding has a greater potential to influence long-term survival

- the high-risk period for recurrent variceal bleeding is the first 6 months and especially the first few weeks after the index bleed
- it is crucial that therapy to prevent recurrent bleeding be initiated as soon as the acute bleeding episode is adequately controlled

A Endoscopic therapy

1 Endoscopic variceal ligation (EVL) has replaced sclerotherapy (EST) as the endoscopic therapy of choice for the prevention of recurrent variceal bleeding. When compared to EST, EVL is associated with lower rates of recurrent bleeding, mortality, and complications and requires fewer sessions for variceal obliteration

2 The combination of EVL and EST offers no advantage over EVL alone.

3 With the development of multiple banding devices (e.g., the "six shooter"), use of an overtube is not necessary, thereby avoiding a significant complicating factor for this procedure.

B Pharmacologic therapy (see Table 10.2)

1 Nonselective beta adrenergic blockers (propranolol, nadolol) have been shown to reduce the risk of recurrent variceal bleeding and to reduce mortality associated with bleeding. A significant overall survival benefit has not been demonstrated, perhaps because of a type 2 error

2 Beta blocker therapy is indicated for patients:
- with good hepatic function (Child's classes A and B)
- deemed to be compliant with taking medication
- with no contraindications to use of beta blockers (e.g., insulin-dependent diabetes, congestive heart failure, severe chronic lung disease)

3 The therapeutic dose of beta blockers is determined by a 25% reduction in resting heart rate, a decrease in heart rate to 55/min, or the development of side effects

4 In centers where hepatic hemodynamic measurements are readily available, serial measurements (baseline and at 3 months) of the HVPG is predictive of the efficacy of treatment. Recurrent variceal bleeding is significantly reduced when:

- HVPG decreases below 12 mmHg
- there is at least a 20% decrease in HVPG from baseline

5 If therapy with beta blockers does not achieve one of these endpoints, addition of a second drug (e.g., a long-acting nitrate) should be considered in an attempt to reduce HVPG further. Alternatively, the patient might be switched to endoscopic therapy

6 Although data are limited, patients who have contraindications to or develop severe side effects from nonselective beta blockers might be treated with long-acting nitrates

Drug	Initial dose	Therapeutic dose (range/day)
1 Propranolol	40 mg b.i.d.	40–400 mg
2 Nadolol	40 mg q.d.	40–160 mg
3 Timolol	10 mg q.d.	5 mg q.o.d. to 40 mg
4 Isosorbide 5-mononitrate	20 mg b.i.d.	20 mg t.i.d.–20 mg q.i.d.

(Table 10.2: Pharmacologic treatment for prevention of variceal bleeding)

C Combined endoscopic and pharmacologic therapy

1 Although the published RCTs have problems with design and follow-up has been short, there appears to be an advantage to the combination of sclerotherapy and beta blockers when compared with sclerotherapy alone for the prevention of recurrent bleeding but not for a reduction in mortality

2 Based on data from 2 RCTs, the combination of sclerotherapy and beta blockers is superior to sclerotherapy alone for both the prevention of recurrent variceal bleeding and for improved survival.[8]

3 There are insufficient data to evaluate the combination of endoscopic variceal ligation and pharmacologic therapy for the treatment of recurrent variceal bleeding

D TIPS

Although several RCTs have shown TIPS to be superior to sclerotherapy in the prevention of recurrent variceal bleeding, its use is associated with a higher frequency of hepatic encephalopathy. At present, TIPS should be reserved for failures of medical therapy, except in highly selected patients, e.g., those awaiting liver transplantation

E Treatment for failures of medical therapy

1 TIPS is very effective at reducing portal pressure and is currently the preferred treatment for patients failing initial medical therapy, especially for those patients who are poor operative risks

2 For good-risk patients (Child's A), shunt surgery remains an attractive alternative. In patients with nonalcoholic cirrhosis, a distal splenorenal shunt is preferable to a portosystemic shunt because of the lower frequency of hepatic encephalopathy associated with the selective shunt

3 Liver transplantation should always be considered for patients with end-stage liver disease. Selection of candidates is dictated by the patient's clinical status, the etiology of cirrhosis, abstinence from alcohol in patients with alcoholic cirrhosis, and the availability of a donor organ

4 For patients who are candidates for liver transplantation, a TIPS procedure or distal splenorenal shunt is preferable to a portosystemic shunt so that surgical anatomy is preserved

5 Management of Nonesophageal Variceal Sources of Bleeding Related to Portal Hypertension

A Gastric varices

1 Gastric varices that extend more than 5 cm below the gastroesophageal junction or isolated to the fundus are at high risk for bleeding

2 Neither sclerotherapy nor endoscopic variceal ligation is effective for the control of acute gastric variceal bleeding or the prevention of recurrent variceal bleeding. The efficacy of thrombin or cyanoacrylate glue needs to be tested in RCTs before their use can be recommended

3 Pharmacologic therapy should be considered for initial treatment of acute bleeding and prevention of recurrent bleeding

4 Patients who fail pharmacologic therapy should be considered for TIPS, shunt surgery, or liver transplantation

B Portal hypertensive gastropathy

1 This is a common complication of cirrhosis and portal hypertension, but significant gastrointestinal bleeding from this source is relatively uncommon

2 Endoscopically, portal hypertensive gastropathy ranges from a mild form characterized by a diffuse mosaic mucosal pattern to more severe forms characterized by brown spots, cherry red spots, a granular mucosa and diffuse mucosal hemorrhages

3 Prior treatment of esophageal varices with sclerotherapy has been associated with an increase in the severity of portal hypertensive gastropathy

4 Pharmacologic therapy is the only medical option for treating acute bleeding or preventing recurrent bleeding from portal hypertensive gastropathy. Endoscopic therapy has no role

5 For the uncommon failures of medical therapy, TIPS, surgical shunts, or liver transplantation are the options for rescue

References

1 Cales P, Desmorat H, Vinel JP, et al. *Incidence of large esophageal varices in patients with cirrhosis: application to prophylaxis of first bleeding.* (Gut 1990) 31: 1298–1302

2 Pagliaro L, D'Amico G, Pasta L, et al. *Portal hypertension in cirrhosis: natural history.* In: Bosch J, Groszmann RJ, (eds). *Portal Hypertension: Pathophysiology and Treatment.* (Oxford: Blackwell Scientific Publications, 1994) 72–92

3 Villanueva C, Balanzo J, Novella MT, et al. *Nadolol plus isosorbide mononitrate compared with sclerotherapy for the prevention of variceal bleeding.* (N Engl J Med 1996) 334: 1624–9

4 Feu F, Garcia-Pagan JC, Bosch J, Luca A, Teres J, Escorsell A, Rodes, J. *Relationship between portal pressure response to pharmacotherapy and risk of recurrent variceal hemorrhage in patients with cirrhosis.* (Lancet 1995) 346: 1056–9

5 Grace ND. *Management of portal hypertension.* (Gastroenterologist 1993) 1: 39–58

6 Besson I, Ingrand P, Person B, et al. *Sclerotherapy with or without octreotide for acute variceal bleeding.* (N Engl J Med 1995) 333: 555–60

7 Shiffman ML, Jeffers L, Hoofnagle JH, Tralka TS. *The role of transjugular intrahepatic portosystemic shunt for treatment of portal hypertension and its complications: a conference sponsored by the National Digestive Diseases Advisory Board.* (Hepatology 1995) 22: 1591–7

8 Grace ND. *Nonsurgical therapy of hemorrhage from esophageal varices.* In: Conn HO, Palmaz JC, Rosch J, Rossle M, (eds). *Tranjugular Intrahepatic Portosystemic Shunts.* (New York: Igaku-Shoin, 1996) 15–34

9 Grace ND, Conn HO, Groszmann RJ, Richardson CR, Matloff DM, Garcia-Tsao G, et al. Propranolol for preventation of first variceal hemorrhage: A life-time commitment? (Hepatology, 1990) 12: 407(A)

Ascites and spontaneous bacterial peritonitis

DONALD J. HILLEBRAND, M.D.
BRUCE A. RUNYON, M.D.

▼

Key Points

1 Chronic parenchymal liver disease (e.g., cirrhosis, alcoholic hepatitis) is the most common cause of ascites; the development of ascites portends a poor prognosis with a 50% 2-year survival

2 Evaluation of the patient with ascites begins with a thorough history and physical examination aimed at detecting clinical clues as to the underlying disease process

3 Abdominal paracentesis with careful ascitic fluid analysis is a safe and cost-effective tool in the differential diagnosis of ascites. Indications include new-onset ascites, symptoms or signs suggestive of ascitic fluid infection, encephalopathy, and azotemia; paracentesis should also be part of the routine admission evaluation in patients with cirrhotic ascites. Routine ascitic fluid tests include cell count, culture in blood culture bottles, albumin, and total protein, with additional testing dictated by the clinical setting

4 Treatment of cirrhotic ascites involves a stepwise approach including dietary sodium restriction and combination diuretic therapy (spironolactone and furosemide). Second-line therapies include intermittent large-volume paracenteses, peritoneovenous shunting, and transjugular intrahepatic portosystemic shunting (TIPS)

▶

5 Spontaneous bacterial peritonitis (SBP) is the prototypic ascitic fluid infection and most commonly develops in the setting of pre-existing cirrhotic ascites. The significant morbidity and mortality of this infection demands prompt detection by paracentesis and ascitic fluid analysis and appropriate non-nephrotoxic antibiotic treatment

6 Norfloxacin has been advocated for the prophylaxis of SBP in high-risk groups of patients with ascites and has been shown to decrease the incidence of infection; however, prophylaxis does not decrease overall mortality

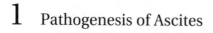

1 Pathogenesis of Ascites

Ascites is the term used to describe the condition of pathological accumulation of fluid (ascitic fluid) within the peritoneal cavity

A Overview

1 In the USA, chronic parenchymal liver disease is the leading cause of ascites; cirrhosis and alcoholic hepatitis account for the majority of cases (see Table 11.1)

2 The "overflow" and "underfill" theories (including a modification of the underfill theory – "peripheral arterial vasodilatation" theory) have been proposed to explain the pathogenesis of cirrhotic ascites

3 Malignancy may lead to ascites formation by peritoneal carcinomatosis, vascular involvement (either lymphatic or venous), or massive liver replacement

4 Peritoneal infections such as tuberculous peritonitis result in exudation of protein-rich fluid into the peritoneal cavity in a manner similar to peritoneal carcinomatosis

Cause[a]	Percentage
Chronic parenchymal liver disease (cirrhosis and alcoholic hepatitis)	81.4
Malignancy	10.0
Heart failure	3.0
Tuberculosis	1.7
Nephrogenous ("dialysis ascites")	1.0
Pancreatic, biliary, lymphatic tear, fulminant hepatic failure, chlamydia, and nephrotic syndrome	Each <1.0

[a]Adapted from Runyon (1995)[1]

(Table 11.1: Causes of ascites in the USA)

B Theories for the pathogenesis of cirrhotic ascites

1 Portal hypertension leads to excess formation of fluid within the congested hepatic

sinusoids which overwhelms the intra hepatic lymphatics and weeps across the liver capsule, pooling within the peritoneal cavity as ascites

2 Cirrhotics with ascites often demonstrate increased levels of:

- renin
- aldosterone
- angiotensin
- vasopressin
- sympathetic nervous system activity

3 The **overflow theory** proposes that a stimulus arising from the liver results in a *primary* increase in plasma volume through increased renal sodium retention, while the **underfill theory** proposes that when ascites formation begins there is a contraction of the intravascular fluid compartment with an increase in the plasma oncotic pressure and decrease in portal venous pressure which results in a *secondary* increase in renal sodium retention in an attempt to compensate.

4 The **peripheral arterial vasodilatation theory** is a modification of the underfill theory and proposes that peripheral arterial vasodilatation results in an increase in vascular capacitance and a decrease in effective plasma volume, which results in the secondary increase in renal sodium retention

C   Ascites development in malignancy and infection

Peritoneal carcinomatosis and peritoneal infections lead to ascites formation by the exudation of proteinaceous fluid into the peritoneal cavity. Extracellular fluid then follows, attempting to re-establish the oncotic gradient in the peritoneal cavity

- Malignancy can lead to ascites by several mechanisms:
  - peritoneal carcinomatosis
  - lymphatic invasion/obstruction
  - major vessel involvement (i.e., Budd–Chiari syndrome)
  - massive liver replacement by tumor

2   Evaluation of the Patient with Ascites

A   History and physical examination marks the starting point (see Ch. 9)

1 Historical clues can reveal chronic liver disease as the cause of the ascites

- alcoholic liver disease is the most common setting for ascites; quantifying alcohol intake is crucial. Estimate amount/duration of alcohol intake, screen for alcoholism (e.g., with CAGE [*C*ut down, *A*nnoyed/angered, *G*uilt, *E*ye openers?] or BUMP [*B*lack outs, *U*nplanned drinking, *M*edicinal drinking, *P*rotected alcohol supply?] acronyms), and question regarding family history of alcoholism and/or liver disease (see also Ch. 6)

- also question thoroughly for common risk factors for chronic viral liver disease, e.g., intravenous drug use, transfusions, tattoos, multiple sexual partners

2 Examination findings suggestive of chronic liver disease as the cause of ascites are:
  - hepatic encephalopathy
  - jaundice
  - gynecomastia
  - altered hair distribution
  - parotid gland enlargement
  - Terry's nails
  - abdominal wall collaterals
  - fetor hepaticus
  - spider telangiectases
  - proximal muscle wasting
  - splenomegaly
  - palmar erythema
  - testicular atrophy

3 Noncirrhotic causes of ascites are also often evident from clinical clues (see Table 11.2)

Cause of ascites	Clinical clues
Cardiac ascites	Setting and examination findings suggestive of congestive heart failure
Malignant ascites	Setting of known malignancy and absence of stigmata of liver disease; often abdominal pain and profound weight loss
Tuberculous ascites	Persistent abdominal pain and fever; often extraperitoneal tuberculosis
Nephrotic syndrome	Anasarca and substantial proteinuria in a diabetic
Pancreatic ascites	Follows episode of acute hemorrhagic pancreatitis or occurs in setting of chronic pancreatitis

(Table 11.2: Clinical clues to a noncirrhotic cause of ascites)

3   Ascitic Fluid Analysis in the Differential Diagnosis of Ascites

A   Diagnostic paracentesis

The diagnostic paracentesis is crucial; careful ascitic fluid analysis is cost effective and efficient in the differential diagnosis of ascites

1 Indications
  - new-onset ascites
  - *routinely* upon hospital admission in patient with ascites
  - symptoms or signs suggestive of ascitic fluid infection (i.e., fever, abdominal pain, elevated WBC count, encephalopathy, and renal impairment)

2 Diagnostic paracentesis technique involves passing a steel 22-gauge needle, via a Z-tract technique, below the level of percussed dullness, either in the midline between the symphysis pubis and the umbilicus or in either lower quadrant

3 Complications include abdominal wall hematoma (0.9% of paracenteses require blood transfusions), fluid leak at the site, and inadvertent bowel perforation by the paracentesis needle

B   Ascitic fluid analysis

Ascitic fluid tests commonly ordered are shown in Table 11.3

Routine	Optional	Occasional	Unhelpful
Cell count	Glucose	TB smear/culture	pH
Culture[a]	LDH	Cytology	Lactate
Albumin[b]	Amylase	Triglyceride	CEA
Total protein	Gram stain	Bilirubin	AFP
			Cholesterol

[a]Blood culture bottles (2) inoculated at bedside (10 ml each)
[b]Required on initial ascitic fluid analysis only
 LDH, lactate dehydrogenase; TB, tuberculosis; CEA, carcinoembryonic antigen; AFP, alpha
 fetoprotein

(Table 11.3: Commonly ordered ascitic fluid tests)

1 Ascitic fluid cell count is the most important test
  - **fluid with $\geq$250 neutrophils/mm³ and a predominance of neutrophils is presumed infected**
  - any inflammatory cause or complication of ascites can lead to neutrocytic ascites ($\geq$250 neutrophils/mm³)

2 **Culture results are optimized by immediate inoculation of aerobic and anaerobic blood culture bottles with 10 mL of ascitic fluid at the bedside (sensitivity approximately 90%) (Runyon 1991)[1]**

3 Ascitic fluid albumin measurement is necessary to calculate the serum – ascites albumin gradient (SAAG)
  - **SAAG = serum albumin – ascites albumin**
  - **A SAAG $\geq$ 1.1 g/dL is 96.7% accurate in detecting portal hypertension (Runyon et al 1992)[2] and narrows the differential diagnosis (Table 11.4)**

4 Ascitic fluid total protein measurement assists in determining the cause of ascites (Table 11.5) and the risk of ascitic fluid infection (values <1.0 g/dL indicate a high risk)

4   Treatment of Cirrhotic Ascites

A   General considerations

1 Establish diagnosis of the underlying liver disease to determine available treatment and prognosis

High gradient (≥1.1 g/dL)	Low gradient (<1.1 g/dL)
Cirrhosis	**Peritoneal carcinomatosis**
Alcoholic hepatitis	**Tuberculosis (w/o cirrhosis)**
Cardiac ascites	Pancreatic ascites
Massive liver metastases	Biliary ascites
Fulminant hepatic failure	Nephrotic syndrome
Budd–Chiari syndrome	Connective tissue diseases
Portal vein thrombosis	Bowel obstruction/infarction
Veno-occlusive disease	
Acute fatty liver of pregnancy	
Myxedema	
"Mixed ascites"	

Source: Runyon (1995)[1]

(Table 11.4: Differential diagnosis of ascites based on SAAG)

Cause of ascites	Ascitic fluid clues
Cirrhotic ascites	SAAG ≥ 1.1 g/dL AFTP < 2.5 g/dL (usually)
Cardiac ascites	SAAG ≥ 1.1 g/dL AFTP > 2.5 g/dL
Peritoneal carcinomatosis	SAAG < 1.1 g/dL; AFTP > 2.5 g/dL Cytology generally yields malignant cells
Tuberculous ascites	SAAG < 1.1 g/dL (w/o cirrhosis)[a] AFTP > 2.5 g/dL (w/o cirrhosis)[a] WBC > 500/mm³ with lymphocyte predominance
Chylous ascites	SAAG < 1.1 g/dL AFTP > 2.5 g/dL Triglycerides in ascites > serum (usually > 200 mg/dL)
Nephrotic syndrome	SAAG < 1.1 g/dL AFTP < 2.5 g/dL
Pancreatic ascites	SAAG < 1.1 g/dL AFTP > 2.5 g/dL Amylase in ascites > serum (often > 1000 U/L)

[a]Cirrhosis present in half of cases
SAAG, serum – ascites albumin gradient; AFTP, ascitic fluid total protein

(Table 11.5: Ascitic fluid clues regarding the cause of ascites)

2 Identify possible precipitating factors of the ascites decompensation:
- dietary indiscretion
- gastrointestinal bleeding
- hepatocellular carcinoma
- nonsteroidal anti-inflammatory drugs (NSAIDs)
- iatrogenic (i.e., saline administration)
- medical noncompliance
- infection (e.g., spontaneous bacterial peritonitis)
- portal vein thrombosis

3 Sodium balance concept is the key to management

Net Na^+ balance = Na^+ intake – Na^+ loss

Na^+ intake = dietary + intravenous + medication related

Na^+ loss = insensible + fecal + urinary excretion

a No added salt diet: 2 g (88 mmol/day) Na^+ restriction

b Urine collections to assess net urinary excretion
- 24-hour urine collection for Na^+ and creatinine (in *complete* collection expect 15–20 mg/kg/day creatinine excretion in males and 10–15 mg/kg/day in females)
- serial monitoring determines optimal diuretic doses (Table 11.6)

Physical examination	Urine output (24-hour collection)	Laboratory studies
Weight	Volume	Sodium
Ascitic fluid volume	Sodium excretion	Potassium
Peripheral edema		Creatinine
Encephalopathy		

(Table 11.6: Parameters to follow in determining diuretic regimen)

- a negative sodium balance with a weight loss of 0.5 kg per day is a reasonable goal; however, patients with peripheral edema can tolerate greater rates of sodium excretion and more rapid weight loss
- urinary Na^+ excretion exceeding the prescribed dietary intake in a patient failing treatment indicates dietary noncompliance as the cause
- increase diuretics after 3 days if there has been no increase in urinary sodium excretion or decrease in body weight
- painful muscle cramps (in calves) may result from diuretics. Oral quinine sulfate up to 200 mg t.i.d. usually alleviates them

c Complications limiting diuretic management of ascites include:
- azotemia (most common limiting factor)

- potassium abnormalities
- alkalosis
- hypovolemia
- hyponatremia
- encephalopathy

B   Stepwise diuretic approach

1   **Spironolactone** (potassium-sparing diuretic which acts at the aldosterone-sensitive sodium channels in the distal nephron and collecting ducts) is the diuretic of choice for single-agent therapy of ascites

- less potent natriuretic than furosemide; however, hypokalemia is less likely to develop in patients taking spironolactone
- prolonged half-life of spironolactone and its metabolities (up to 5–7 days) allows once-daily dosing
- maximum daily dose is 400 mg

2   Combination diuretic regimens

The combination of **spironolactone and furosemide** is the most effective regimen for managing cirrhotic ascites in terms of shortest hospitalization times and avoidance of abnormal potassium levels[3]

- starting doses: spironolactone 100 mg + furosemide 40 mg once daily. This ratio of potassium-sparing/wasting diuretics leads to fewest potassium difficulties
- increase doses of both drugs while maintaining this ratio (e.g., spironolactone 200 mg + furosemide 80 mg daily)
- maximum doses: spironolactone 400 mg + furosemide 160 mg once daily
- ninety percent of cirrhotics with ascites will respond to regimen of sodium-restricted diet, spironolactone, and furosemide[4]
- liver transplantation should be considered in appropriate candidates

C   Refractory ascites

1   **Definition**: ascites that cannot be mobilized or the early recurrence of ascites which (i.e., after therapeutic paracentesis) cannot be satisfactorily prevented by medical therapy[5]

- lack of response to dietary sodium restriction and intensive diuretic treatment (spironolactone 400 mg and furosemide 160 mg daily) (*diuretic resistant*)
- diuretic-induced complications preclude use of effective diuretic doses (*diuretic intractable*)

2   A poor prognosis accompanies its development; approximately one quarter of patients survive an additional year.[3] Liver transplantation should be considered in appropriate candidates

3   **Treatment options**

a   **Large-volume paracentesis** is a safe and effective treatment. Associated with more rapid resolution of tense ascites during initial hospitalization and fewer electrolyte abnormalities and azotemia when combined with simultaneous volume expansion with intravenous administration of albumin.[6] Concerns remain regarding the depletion of the ascitic fluid's opsonic capacity, risk of ascitic fluid infection, procedure-related complications, and effect on nutritional status

b **Extracorporeal ultrafiltration of ascitic fluid with intravenous reinfusion of the protein concentrate** has been tried but has been limited by fever and worsening of baseline coagulopathy. Intraperitoneal reinfusion is being investigated to avoid these complications

c **Peritoneovenous shunting (PVS)** may offer improved long-term ascites management but does not change rates of total hospitalization or patient survival. Complications, including bacterial infections, congestive heart failure, gastrointestinal bleeding from ruptured gastroesophageal varices, disseminated intravascular coagulation (DIC), and shunt thrombosis or malfunctioning, have relegated these shunts to a select group of patients

d **Transjugular Intrahepatic Portosystemic Shunt (TIPS)** has recently been advocated for the management of refractory ascites. Its advantages include decompression of the underlying portal hypertension and a lower risk of variceal hemorrhage. Its disadvantages include significant procedure-related complications and long-term risk of hepatic encephalopathy in up to 25% of patients and significant rates of stent stenosis or occlusion (see also Ch. 10)

5   Spontaneous Bacterial Peritonitis and Ascitic Fluid Infections

1 Ascitic fluid infections develop primarily in patients with pre-existing cirrhotic ascites and less commonly in those with subacute liver disease, e.g., alcoholic hepatitis. Risk factors for the development of infection have been identified

2 Clinical presentation is variable. SBP is the most common type of ascitic fluid infection. A high index of suspicion is necessary to ensure early detection and initiation of antibiotics

3 SBP variants may have different prognostic significance and require different management strategies

4 Early initiation of appropriate broad-spectrum non-nephrotoxic antibiotics has decreased the mortality associated with ascitic fluid infections. Knowledge of the causative bacterial flora is key

5 Prophylactic antibiotics have been targeted to patients at high risk for the development of ascitic fluid infections. Despite decreasing the incidence of infection, these regimens have not yet demonstrated an ability to decrease mortality

A   Pathogenesis of ascitic fluid infection

1 Bacterial seeding of ascitic fluid is the initiator of ascitic fluid infections; however, the route that the bacteria take leading to seeding is controversial. The two most likely routes include translocation and hematogenous spread

a **Translocation** (passage of bacteria through the intestinal wall with culture positivity of mesenteric lymph nodes) as the route of access has support

- enteric organisms account for over 70% of ascitic fluid infections
- abnormal gut mucosal edema and permeability, in addition to bacterial overgrowth within the intestine of cirrhotics, promotes translocation
- passage of bacteria from the large intestine to mesenteric lymph nodes has been well demonstrated in rat models

  b **Hematogenous seeding** of the ascitic fluid also has support

  - half of SBP episodes are accompanied by bacteremia involving the same organism isolated from the ascitic fluid
  - the causative organism can often be cultured from a focus remote from the peritoneum (e.g., urinary or respiratory tract infection)

2 Colonization of ascitic fluid ("bacterascites") may lead to two different outcomes: clearance by intraperitoneal phagocytic cells or progressive bacterial growth with peritonitis (i.e., SBP). Bacterascites normally resolves as a result of opsonization of the bacteria and subsequent clearance by intraperitoneal phagocytic cells

- an ascitic fluid total protein < 1.0 g/dL carries an increased risk of infection. Below this level of ascitic fluid protein, opsonic activity is negligible. SBP develops 10 times more frequently in hospitalized cirrhotics with low-protein ascites than with high protein ascites.
- gastrointestinal bleeding (specifically, variceal hemorrhage) is a major risk factor for ascitic fluid infection. Gastrointestinal hemorrhage with shock has been shown to promote translocation of bacteria in the rat model
- a prior episode of SBP is the most important risk factor; two thirds of these patients will develop a recurrence of infection within the following year

B   Clinical features

1 The evolution of our understanding of the incidence and clinical presentation of ascitic fluid infection has contributed to improved outcomes[7]

- approximately 11% of cirrhotic patients with ascites will develop SBP each year. Ascitic fluid infection occurs in up to one quarter of patients with cirrhotic ascites upon hospital admission
- early studies found that three quarters of infected patients did not survive to be discharged from hospital. More recent studies suggest an in-hospital mortality rate of one third, while the infection-related mortality rate has fallen to under 10%[7]
- clinical presentation is variable; one third of patients are without the classical symptoms and signs (Table 11.6) of abdominal pain, fever, and hypotension
- Occurrence of any of these symptoms and/or signs in a patient with ascites should prompt a diagnostic paracentesis to exclude ascitic fluid infection
- overwhelming infection usually results in early death, while in-hospital death reflects mortality from gastrointestinal bleeding and liver and/or kidney failure

C   Spontaneous bacterial peritonitis and variants

1 *Spontaneous bacterial peritonitis* **(SBP) is defined as a positive ascitic fluid culture (usually of a single organism) and a polymorphonuclear neutrophil count in ascites ≥ 250 cells/mm³ in the absence of a known or suspected intra-abdominal surgical source of the infection**

Symptoms	Signs
Abdominal pain	Abdominal tenderness
Nausea	Fever
Vomiting	Hypotension
Rigors	Tachycardia
Diarrhea	Leukocytosis
Encephalopathy	Azotemia
Malaise	Increasing bilirubin

(Table 11.6: Clinical picture of ascitic fluid infections)

2 ***Culture-negative neutrocytic ascites* (CNNA) is defined as a negative ascitic fluid culture, an ascitic fluid neutrophil count ≥ 250 cells/mm^3, and no apparent intra-abdominal source of infection***

- occurs most commonly in the setting of suboptimal culture technique
- an elevated ascitic fluid neutrophil count with a negative culture despite sensitive technique most commonly represents the resolution of transient bacterial colonization of the ascitic fluid because of the fluid's inherent antibacterial properties (complement, opsonins, immunoglobulins, etc.). However, in some cases bacterial growth may continue, leading to SBP and positive ascitic fluid culture
- the decision to initiate antibiotic treatment for ascitic fluid infections is usually prompted by an elevated ascitic fluid neutrophil count (≥ 250 cells/mm^3) and/or the overall clinical setting (see below). CNNA and SBP have comparable mortality rates; therefore, similar management is warranted
- recent antibiotic exposure may suppress the ascitic fluid culture, given the relatively low bacterial load (approximately 1 organism per ml)
- causes other than SBP should be kept in mind (see Table 11.7)

Peritoneal carcinomatosis
Pancreatitis
Tuberculous peritonitis
Connective tissue disease-related peritonitis
Hemorrhage into ascitic fluid

(Table 11.7: Non-SBP causes of neutrocytic ascites)

3 ***Monomicrobial non-neutrocytic bacterascites* (MNB) is a variant of SBP defined by a positive ascitic fluid culture (single organism) associated with a normal ascitic fluid neutrophil count (<250 cells/mm^3)***

- although patients with MNB generally having less severe liver disease than those with SBP, there is *no* difference in ascitic fluid total protein compared with SBP

- the outcome of bacterascites is determined by the presence or absence of associated clinical symptoms or signs. **Asymptomatic bacterascites** typically resolves spontaneously without antibiotic treatment, while progression to SBP (neutrocytic response) is predicted by the presence of characteristic symptoms and/or signs. **Symptomatic bacterascites should be managed in the same manner as SBP.**
- when an ascitic fluid culture unexpectedly yields an organism, prompt repeat paracentesis is mandatory to evaluate for the development of a neutrocytic response, which would mandate antibiotic treatment. Several exceptions exist:
  - *Staphylococcus epidermidis* and other coagulase-negative staphylococci should be considered contaminants unless a foreign body is present (e.g., peritoneovenous shunt).
  - *Staphylococcus aureus* and alpha-hemolytic streptococci should also be considered skin contaminants unless associated with a neutrocytic response

4 *Polymicrobial bacterascites* **indicates inadvertent perforation of the bowel by the paracentesis needle and is defined by an ascitic fluid culture demonstrating multiple organisms in the setting of a normal neutrophil count (<250 cells/mm^3)**

- inadvertent bowel perforation by paracentesis occurs rarely, typically in the setting of an extremely difficult paracentesis, and may be obvious when air or stool is aspirated during the tap; a Gram stain revealing multiple organisms despite a normal ascitic fluid neutrophil count is also a clue to its occurrence
- the majority of inadvertent bowel perforations resolve spontaneously without development of secondary peritonitis; however, a repeat paracentesis should be performed to evaluate for a neutrocytic response and the need for antibiotics
- management of patients who develop a neutrocytic ascitic fluid response involves empiric broad-spectrum antibiotics to cover Gram-negative enteric, Gram-positive, and anaerobic organisms. Repeat paracentesis after 48 hours of antibiotic treatment should be considered to confirm response to antibiotic management

5 *Secondary bacterial peritonitis* **is differentiated from SBP in that a known or suspected primary intra-abdominal source of infection exists (e.g., perforated viscus or intra-abdominal abscess). With an ascitic fluid neutrophil count ≥250 cells/mm^3 associated with a positive culture (often with multiple gut organisms)**

- differentiating secondary (surgical) bacterial peritonitis from SBP may be difficult. Clinical clues include multiple organisms on Gram stain or culture (particularly anaerobes and/or fungi) and free intraperitoneal air on radiographic studies
- ascitic fluid clues aid in the differentiation; if two of these three ascitic fluid criteria exist then a secondary peritonitis should be suspected and sought (see Table 11.8)
- in addition, if a repeat paracentesis performed after 48 hours of appropriate antibiotic treatment reveals an ascitic fluid neutrophil count *above* the baseline (pretreatment) value, secondary peritonitis should be suspected

Secondary bacterial peritonitis
Total protein > 1.0 g/dL
Glucose < 50 mg/dL
LDH > upper limit of normal for serum

(Table 11.8: Ascitic fluid findings in surgical peritonitis)

- management involves empiric broad-spectrum antibiotics to include coverage of Gram-negative enteric, Gram-positive, and anaerobic bacteria. Surgical consultation and water-soluble contrast studies of the upper (in younger patients who are more likely to have perforated peptic ulcer disease) or lower (in older patients who are more likely to have perforated colonic divertula) gastrointestinal tract are necessary to localize the perforation
- prompt surgical intervention is mandatory; medical therapy alone is not sufficient

D   Treatment

A clinical diagnosis of ascitic fluid infection alone is not sufficient; the diagnosis must be supported by ascitic fluid cell counts and culture. Therefore, a paracentesis <u>must</u> be performed

> Empiric treatment is strongly recommended based on an ascitic fluid neutrophil count ≥ 250 cells/mm³ <u>prior to</u> the availability of culture results

1 Knowledge of the bacterial flora responsible for ascitic fluid infections is critical in determining an appropriate empiric treatment regimen. The most common causative organisms include *Escherichia coli* (43%), *Klebsiella pneumoniae* (11%), and *Streptococcus* species (23%)
   - anaerobic organisms rarely lead to ascitic fluid infections except in secondary peritonitis
   - the flora responsible for ascitic fluid infections continues to change, presumably as a result of antibiotic pressures and improved cultivation techniques
   - organisms which usually demand treatment with an aminoglycoside agent (i.e., *Enterococcus* or *Pseudomonas*) are unusual pathogens in SBP

> Aminoglycosides carry an unacceptable risk of nephrotoxicity and, when compared with cephalosporin-containing regimens, have resulted in only fair infection cure rates and poor survival rates. Aminoglycosides are considered contraindicated in cirrhotics with ascites

   - fungi do not cause spontaneous bacterial peritonitis; they are cultured from ascitic fluid only in cases of secondary (e.g., surgical) peritonitis
2 Third-generation cephalosporins are recommended as treatment.

> Cefotaxime, a non-nephrotoxic broad-spectrum third-generation cephalosporin, provides coverage for over 94% of the flora responsible for SBP and is the antibiotic of choice for empiric treatment. Recommended dose is 2 g i.v. every 8 hours

Other antibiotic regimens studied have not yet been shown to be superior to cefotaxime

- ascitic fluid cultures rapidly become sterile with even the first dose(s) of antibiotics
- the antibiotic spectrum may be narrowed once culture results become available and the sensitivities of the causative organism are known
- short-term (5 days) and long-term (10 days) treatment regimens with cefotaxime have been compared and offer equivalent efficacy and rates of cure, relapse, and reinfection in addition to overall morbidity and mortality[7]
- **follow-up paracentesis** is indicated whenever secondary (surgical) bacterial peritonitis is suspected or the typical clinical response to cefotaxime (i.e., fall in serum white cell count, defervesence, etc.) does not occur. Secondary bacterial peritonitis or SBP caused by an organism resistant to cefotaxime will yield persistently positive ascitic fluid cultures and ascitic fluid neutrophil counts above the baseline (pretreatment) values

3 Increased ability to diagnose SBP, more appropriate use of non-nephrotoxic broad-spectrum antibiotics such as cefotaxime, and overall improvement in the care of these critically ill patients have led to improved infection-related survival rates in SBP

6 Prophylaxis

1 The fluoroquinolone antibiotic **norfloxacin** has been the primary antibiotic utilized for SBP prophylaxis. While norfloxacin has been effective, other agents are also being investigated

2 Patients at high risk for development of SBP include hospitalized cirrhotics with low-protein ascites (ascitic fluid total protein < 1.5 g/dL), gastrointestinal hemorrhage, and a previous episode of SBP. Prophylactic therapy to prevent SBP has been suggested in these situations

3 Concerns exist regarding the routine use of antibiotic prophylaxis for SBP

A Prophylactic antibiotic regimens

1 Initial studies demonstrated decreased episodes of bacteremia and peritonitis when multiple oral nonabsorbable antibiotics were utilized; however, the considerable cost, significant side effects, and poor palatability limited their use

2 Norfloxacin, a poorly absorbed fluoroquinolone, has been utilized in order to achieve *selective intestinal decontamination* in cirrhotics. Norfloxacin has several characteristics that make it suitable for prophylaxis:

- poor absorption when taken orally (approximately 30%)
- effectiveness against enteric Gram-negative organisms which are the principal flora of SBP

- sparing of Gram-positive and anaerobic organisms so as to maintain their protective role in the normal gut flora. Other agents studied include ciprofloxacin and trimethoprim–sulfamethoxasole

B Patient groups at high risk for SBP

1 Hospitalized patients with low-protein ascites (ascitic fluid total protein < 1.5 g/dL) are at particular risk of developing SBP because of invasive access lines, monitors, bladder catheters, etc.

- prophylaxis with norfloxacin 400 mg orally daily (while hospitalized) has been shown to eliminate SBP and decrease the overall incidence of infection without an effect on in-hospital mortality[7]

2 Cirrhotic patients with gastrointestinal hemorrhage are at high risk for SBP due to increased bacterial translocation resulting from the hemorrhage and associated shock

- prophylaxis with norfloxacin 400 mg orally twice daily started immediately after emergent endoscopy and continued for 7 days has been shown to decrease the incidence of bacteremia and/or SBP, the overall incidence of infection and the cost of antibiotic treatment without significantly reducing mortality[7]

3 Patients recovering from an episode of SBP have an extremely high recurrence rate of infection. The associated mortality is considerable

- norfloxacin 400 mg orally daily following recovery from an episode of SBP has been shown to decrease the probability of recurrent SBP from 68% to 20% at 1 year without altering the overall mortality[7]

C Concerns about routine antibiotic prophylaxis for SBP

1 Routine long-term use of prophylactic norfloxacin leads to the development of quinolone-resistant organisms in the fecal flora in half of patients treated.[9] Gram-positive organisms including *Enterococcus* have arisen as causative organisms in the era of norfloxacin prophylaxis. Concerns remain regarding the possible emergence of other resistant organisms (i.e., *Pseudomonas* and/or fungal superinfection)

2 Despite the significant reduction in overall infection and incidence of SBP, routine norfloxacin prophylaxis has not yet improved overall mortality associated with the underlying liver disease in these high-risk groups of patients. With the dramatic improvement in infection-related mortality resulting from prompt diagnosis and initiation of non-nephrotoxic broad-spectrum antibiotics such as cefotaxime for SBP, whether prophylaxis is able to decrease morbidity and mortality associated with SBP further remains to be determined

3 The cost of norfloxacin is significant. To date no randomized trials have prospectively compared the cost of prophylaxis versus surveillance and prompt paracentesis when clinical changes suggest the possibility of infection

4 Norfloxacin prophylaxis may induce allergic reactions, renal dysfunction (interstitial nephritis), gastrointestinal side effects (nausea, vomiting, dysgeusia, and/or diarrhea), oral candidiasis, and *Clostridium difficile* colitis.

References

1 Runyon BA. *Approach to the patient with ascites*. In: Yamada T, Alpers D, Wyang O, Powell CD, Silversteen F, (eds). *Textbook of Gastroenterology*. (New York: Lippincott-Raven, 1995) 927–52

2 Runyon BA, Montano AA, Akriviadis EA, Antillon MR, Irving MA, McHutchison JG. *The serum – ascites albumin gradient is superior to the exudate – transudate concept in the differential diagnosis of ascites.* (Ann Intern Med 1992) 117: 215–20

3 Arroyo V, Gines P, Gerbes AL et al. *Definition and diagnostic criteria of refractory ascites and hepatorenal syndrome in cirrhosis.* (Hepatology 1996) 23: 164–76

4 Stanley MM, Ochi S, Lee KK, et al. *Peritoneovenous shunting as compared with medical treatment in patients with alcoholic cirrhosis and massive ascites.* (N Engl J Med 1991) 321: 1632–8

5 Arroyo V, Gines P, Gerbes AL, et al. *Definition and diagnostic criteria of refractory ascites and hepatorenal syndrome in cirrhosis.* (Hepatology 1996) 23: 164–176

6 Gines P, Arroyo V, Quintero E, et al. *Comparison of paracentesis and diuretics in the treatment of cirrhotics with tense ascites: results of a randomized study.* (Gastroenterology 1987) 93: 234–41

7 Guarner C, Runyon BA. *Spontaneous bacterial peritonitis: pathogenesis, diagnosis.* (Gastroenterologist 1995) 3: 311–28

8 Wang SS, Tsai YT, Lee SD, et al. *Spontaneous bacterial peritonitis in patients with hepatitis B-related cirrhosis and hepatocellular carcinoma.* (Gastroenterology 1991) 101: 1656–62

9 Dupeyron C, Mangeney N, Sedrati L, Campillo B, Fouet P, Leluan G. *Rapid emergence of quinolone resistance in cirrhotic patients treated with norfloxacin to prevent spontaneous bacterial peritonitis.* (Antimicrob Agents Chemother 1994) 38: 340–4

CHAPTER 12

Hepatorenal syndrome

JOHN PYNE, M.D.   TIMOTHY R. MORGAN, M.D.

Key Points

1 Hepatorenal syndrome (HRS) is a syndrome of progressive renal failure occurring in a patient with advanced liver disease and portal hypertension in the absence of specific causes of renal failure

2 The syndrome is associated with activation of endogenous vasoactive systems and changes in arterial circulation, including reversible renal arterial vasoconstriction and vasodilation of the splanchnic arterial system.

3 There are two types of HRS. In type I HRS, renal failure develops within 2 weeks. In type I HRS, renal failure develops after 2 or more weeks

4 All patients should receive a fluid challenge of at least 1.5 L to reverse undiagnosed intravascular volume depletion. Liver transplantation can reverse HRS and may be considered in suitable patients. Otherwise, prognosis is poor, with most patients dying within 2 months

1 Historical Overview

- 1863 – Austin Flint showed that most cases of renal failure in cirrhosis occur in the absence of significant histologic changes in the kidney at autopsy
- 1877 – Frerichs described oliguria in patients with ascites and suggested it is related to underfilling of the arterial circulation secondary to portal hypertension
- 1956 – Hecker and Sherlock gave first detailed description of hepatorenal syndrome (HRS). They described nine patients with liver disease associated with renal failure characterized by a lack of proteinuria and low urinary sodium excretion
- 1960s–1970s – kidneys from patients with HRS successfully transplanted to patients with chronic renal failure. HRS reversed by liver transplantation, confirming the functional nature of the renal failure

2 Definitions

A Hepatorenal syndrome

A syndrome consisting of progressive renal failure (see below) occurring in a patient with advanced liver disease and portal hypertension.[1] Characteristics include:

- absence of other identifiable causes of renal failure
- activation of endogenous vasoactive systems (see below)
- abnormalities in the arterial circulation: vasodilation of the splanchnic system associated with vasoconstriction of the brachial, femoral, and renal arteries. Renal arterial vasoconstriction leads to decreased renal blood flow and a consequent decrease in glomerular filtration rate (GFR)

B Progressive renal failure

- a doubling of serum creatinine to a level greater than 2.5 g/dL or
- a 50% reduction of the initial 24-hour creatinine clearance to a level lower than 20 mL/min

C Two types of hepatorenal syndrome

1 Acute HRS (type I HRS)

- rapid and progressive increase in blood urea nitrogen (BUN) and creatinine over a period of 1–14 days, with BUN usually between 60 and 120 mg/dL and creatinine between 2 and 8 mg/dL
- associated with anuria, oliguria, and hyponatremia
- associated with jaundice, encephalopathy, and coagulopathy
- typically seen in patients with severe alcoholic hepatitis or fulminant hepatic failure
- patients often admitted to hospital with normal serum creatinine; renal failure develops during hospitalization

- about half the time associated with a complication (e.g., infection, GI bleed) or a therapeutic maneuver (paracentesis)
- poor prognosis: median survival time less than 2 weeks

2 Chronic HRS (type II HRS)

- slowly progressive renal failure with BUN and creatinine increasing over weeks to months, with BUN between 30 and 80 mg/dL and creatinine between 2 and 4 mg/dL
- associated with far advanced, but relatively stable, chronic liver disease (e.g., hepatitis B, C, primary biliary cirrhosis)
- responds temporarily to volume expansion
- associated with diuretic-resistant ascites
- survival longer than for acute HRS, but shorter than in patients with ascites without renal failure

3 Hemodynamic and Renal Abnormalities in HRS

A Hemodynamic abnormalities in severe liver disease (see also Ch. 11)

- increase in cardiac output – often in excess of 10 L/min
- decrease in systemic vascular resistance – often less than 500 dyne s/cm^5
- decrease in blood pressure – mean blood pressure often less than 85 mmHg
- increase in renal vascular resistance, due to renal artery vasoconstriction with subsequent decrease in renal blood flow (RBF) and GFR

B Sodium retention, water retention, decreased RBF

Chronologically, patients with severe liver disease and ascites (patients at highest risk for HRS) develop several types of renal functional abnormalities prior to the development of HRS. These abnormalities are most severe in HRS

1 Sodium retention

- earliest and most common change in renal function in cirrhosis
- in experimental animals with cirrhosis, sodium retention precedes ascites formation
- in most patients with cirrhosis, initial sodium retention occurs in the setting of a normal GFR and is due to excess sodium reabsorption in both the proximal and distal tubules of the kidney
- probably due to overactivity of renin–angiotensin–aldosterone system and the sympathetic nervous system

2 Water retention

- occurs after the onset of sodium retention
- due to impaired ability to excrete free water, causing increased total body water relative to sodium and leading to dilutional hyponatremia (seen in 35% of patients with cirrhotic ascites)
- free water clearance is usually normal in patients with cirrhosis without ascites

(compensated cirrhosis), but is abnormal in most patients with cirrhosis and ascites
- pathogenesis of impaired water excretion:
  - increased plasma level of vasopressin (primary cause)
  - reduced renal synthesis of prostaglandins
  - decreased delivery of filtrate to ascending limb of Henle (diluting segment of nephron), due to increased proximal sodium absorption and decreased GFR

3 Renal vasoconstriction

- chronologically, the final abnormality in renal function in cirrhotic patients
- leads to decreased RBF and decreased GFR, without significant anatomical abnormalities of the kidney
- moderate degrees of renal vasoconstriction are seen in nonazotemic patients with cirrhosis and ascites, implying that renal vasoconstriction occurs before the development of HRS
- numerous studies and techniques have demonstrated marked renal vasoconstriction leading to a preferential reduction in renal cortical perfusion in patients with HRS
  - renal arteriography reveals marked beading and tortuosity of interlobar and arcuate arteries and absence of cortical nephrograms. Postmortem nephrograms are normal
  - ^{133}Xe washout technique
  - Doppler ultrasound
  - p-aminohippuric acid excretion

4 Pathogenic Factors Involved in HRS

A Overview

1 HRS results from a progressive change in the systemic circulation which occurs in patients with cirrhosis and worsens with the onset of ascites.[2] These changes include increased blood flow through the splanchnic circulation, decreased RBF, decreased systemic vascular resistance, and increased cardiac output. **There are significant changes in every known regulator of vascular tone (both vasodilator and vasoconstrictor) and regulators of sodium and water excretion.** A brief review of abnormalities in these neurohumoral systems is given in Table 12.1

B Renin–angiotensin–aldosterone system (RAAS)

1 Important regulator of intravascular volume and arterial pressure
- plasma renin activity (PRA) and aldosterone are elevated in patients with cirrhosis and ascites and especially in those with HRS
- increased aldosterone results from increased production of renin by the kidney and not from decreased aldosterone catabolism

2 Renin
- synthesized by juxtaglomerular apparatus (JGA) of kidneys

	Cirrhosis, early ascites	Cirrhosis, advanced ascites	HRS
PRA/aldo/NE	nl, ↑	↑↑	↑↑↑
AVP	nl, ↑	↑↑	↑↑↑
Urinary prostaglandins (PGE$_2$, 6-keto PGF$_1$ alpha)	nl, ↑	↑↑	↓
Urinary thromboxane (TXB2)	nl, ↑	↑↑	?
Splanchnic vasodilation	↑	↑↑	↑↑↑
Renal arterial blood flow	nl, ↓	↓↓	↓↓↓
Blood pressure	nl, ↓	↓↓	↓↓↓
Cardiac output	nl, ↑	↑↑	↑↑↑
Systemic vascular resistance	nl, ↓	↓↓	↓↓↓
Urine sodium excretion	↓	↓↓	↓↓↓

(Table 12.1: Neurohormonal and vascular changes in liver disease)

- three mechanisms regulate renin release: 1 decreased renal perfusion pressure, 2 decreased NaCl concentrations sensed in *macula densa*, 3 sympathetic nervous system stimulation via beta-1 adrenoceptor in JGA

3 Angiotensin II
- causes smooth muscle contraction and vasoconstriction
- directly inhibits tubular sodium absorption

4 Aldosterone
- enhances sodium reabsorption in collecting tubules
- levels are more elevated in patients with ascites and marked sodium retention (those at highest risk of HRS) than in ascitic patients with mild sodium retention
- aldosterone implicated in pathogenesis of sodium retention:
  - inverse correlation between urinary sodium excretion and plasma aldosterone level
  - hyperaldosteronism precedes sodium retention in experimental animals with cirrhosis
  - spironolactone can reverse sodium retention
- about 30% of patients with cirrhosis and ascites have normal aldosterone levels despite sodium retention
- activation of RAAS helps maintain blood pressure in patients with severe liver disease. Administration of an angiotensin-converting enzyme inhibitor or an angiotensin receptor antagonist (saralasin) is followed by a dramatic drop in systemic blood pressure and systemic vascular resistance in patients with cirrhosis and ascites

C Sympathetic nervous system (SNS)

1 Important in the control of intravascular volume and arterial pressure. A decrease in intravascular volume causes stimulation of both low-pressure receptors (in atria and pulmonary arteries) and high-pressure receptors (in carotid arteries, JGA, and aorta), resulting in increased SNS activity

2 Progressively increasing SNS activity causes the following to occur in a stepwise manner:
- increased renin release: mediated by beta-1 adrenoceptors
- increased sodium reabsorption in proximal tubules (due to a direct tubular effect as well as decreased RBF and GFR): mediated by alpha-1 adrenoceptors
- renal vasoconstriction with a decrease in RBF and GFR: mediated by alpha-1 adrenoceptors

3 Plasma norepinephrine (NE) levels are normal to minimally elevated in cirrhotics without ascites but increased in cirrhotics with ascites, with highest levels seen in those with HRS

4 There is an association between circulating NE levels and severity of liver disease as measured by:
- Child's classification (higher NE levels in patients with higher Child's score) (see Ch. 9)
- portal hypertension (higher NE levels with higher portal pressure)
- sodium and water retention (higher NE levels with more severe sodium and water retention)
- RBF and GFR (higher NE levels with decreased RBF and GFR)

5 Elevated NE levels are due to enhanced SNS activity and not to decreased metabolism

6 Experimental studies support SNS overactivity as a mediator of sodium and water retention as well as a pathogenic factor in HRS:
- bilateral renal denervation in experimental animals increases urinary volume and sodium excretion
- lumbar sympathetic block improves sodium excretion and RBF in patients with HRS
- inhibition of SNS with clonidine (a central alpha-adrenergic blocker) is associated with reduced renal vascular resistance and increased GFR

7 Increased SNS activity in patients with decompensated cirrhosis is a baroreceptor-mediated response to decreased effective circulating volume (see below) and probably not a "hepatorenal" reflex due to portal hypertension
- central blood volume correlates inversely with SNS activity
- SNS can be suppressed by measures that increase the effective arterial volume (head-out water immersion) but have minimal or no effect on hepatic sinusoidal pressure

D Arginine vasopressin (AVP) (or antidiuretic hormone (ADH))

1 Under physiologic conditions, AVP is released from the neurohypophysis in response to osmotic stimuli (increased serum osmolality increases serum AVP level).

However, in pathologic conditions, AVP secretion is influenced mainly by changes in blood pressure

2 Increased secretion of AVP is nonosmotic in origin in patients with cirrhosis and ascites and responds to changes in systemic hemodynamics, not to changes in serum osmolality

• plasma AVP level correlates with elevated PRA and NE levels in decompensated cirrhosis and is highest in patients with HRS

• AVP level is reduced by maneuvers that increase effective arterial blood volume (head-out water immersion)

3 AVP has a major role in water retention in cirrhotic patients with ascites. Elevated levels of AVP correlate with reduced free water excretion

• Brattleboro rats (rats with congenital deficiency of AVP) with cirrhosis have no impairment of water excretion

• Antagonists to the AVP receptor can restore the ability of kidneys to excrete water in cirrhotic rats with ascites

4 AVP may contribute to HRS by causing renal vasoconstriction and decreased renal blood flow and GFR; plasma AVP levels correlate inversely with RBF and GFR

E Prostaglandins and other eicosanoids

1 In normal conditions, prostaglandin production is not an important mediator of renal hemodynamics. In patients with renal vasoconstriction, however, prostaglandins have a critical role:

• compensatory protective effect on renal circulation by causing arterial vasodilation

• modulation of tubular effect of AVP: increased PGE_2 levels in nonazotemic patients with cirrhosis and ascites antagonize effects of AVP on collecting tubules and help maintain free water excretion

2 PGE_2 and PGI_2 (prostacyclin) are renal vasodilators, while thromboxane A_2 is a renal vasoconstrictor

3 Prostaglandins probably have a major role in homeostasis of renal circulation in patients with decompensated cirrhosis with ascites

• urinary excretion of PGE_2 and 6-keto PGF_1 alpha (metabolite of PGI_2) is increased in patients without renal failure compared with healthy controls

• Nonsteroidal anti-inflammatory drug (NSAID) administration to cirrhotics with ascites causes decreased RBF and GFR in patients with high levels of NE/RAAS/AVP (marked elevations of vasoconstrictor systems), but has little effect in patients with no activation of these systems

4 In patients with HRS, some studies have shown decreased urinary excretion of PGE_2 and 6-keto PGF_1 alpha compared with patients without renal failure, suggesting decreased renal synthesis of prostaglandins as a factor in HRS

5 There are conflicting reports on whether the ratio of urinary PGE_2 to thromboxane B_2 (metabolite of thromboxane A_2) is important in HRS

F Atrial natriuretic peptide

1 Released into the circulation in response to atrial distention or elevated levels of vasoactive substances such as AVP, angiotensin II, and endothelin

2 Causes vasodilation of the afferent arteriole and vasoconstriction of the efferent arteriole leading to increased GFR as well as inhibition of sodium reabsorption by suppressing release of renin from the JGA and release of aldosterone from the *zona glomerulosa* of the adrenal gland

3 ANP levels are elevated in decompensated cirrhotics, with HRS patients having the highest levels. Therefore, renal resistance to ANP is most marked in HRS
- ascitic patients with marked activation of RAAS/SNS (i.e., patients at highest risk for HRS) are resistant to the natriuretic effects of pharmacologic doses of ANP
- bilateral renal denervation restores the natriuretic response to ANP in cirrhotic rats

G   Nitric oxide

1 Effects
- potent systemic vasodilator via relaxation of vascular smooth muscle
- an antagonist of the vasoconstrictor effects of angiotensin II and endothelin 1

2 Nitric oxide synthase: nitric oxide is formed by the action of the enzyme nitric oxide synthetase (NOS), which converts L-arginine to L-citrulline and nitric oxide. There are two forms of NOS.

a   Constitutive NOS
- an isoform present in endothelial cells which constantly produces nitric oxide
- present under basal conditions; has a short half-life
- produces small amounts of nitric oxide (compared with inducible form)

b   Inducible NOS
- activated under certain pathologic conditions, such as stimulation by endotoxins or certain cytokines
- when activated, releases large amounts of nitric oxide and for longer periods (many hours) than constitutive isoform

3 Increased production of nitric oxide could be involved in the pathogenesis of the hyperdynamic circulation seen in patients with cirrhosis and ascites. Several experimental findings support this hypothesis:
- inhibition of NOS with *N*G-monomethyl L-arginine causes greater blood pressure increase in cirrhotic rats with ascites than in normal control rats
- NOS inhibition in cirrhotic animals causes a marked increase in splanchnic vascular resistance, implying local release of nitric oxide in maintaining splanchnic vasodilation
- in cirrhotic patients with ascites, the serum concentrations of nitrite and nitrate (metabolites of nitric oxide) are increased compared with cirrhotics without ascites and healthy control patients
- decreased responsiveness in vitro of aortic rings from cirrhotic animals to vasoconstrictors can be corrected by *N*G-monomethyl-L-arginine. This implicates nitric oxide as a factor in causing decreased vascular reactivity to vasoconstrictors

H   Endothelin

1 A 21-amino acid molecule that is a potent vasoconstrictor

2 Synthesized mainly by endothelial cells and causes contraction of vascular smooth muscle

3 The most important effect of endothelin in the kidney is renal vasoconstriction, which can decrease RBF and GFR

4 Cirrhotic patients have elevated endothelin 1 plasma levels compared with controls. Patients with ascites have higher levels than those without ascites. Patients with HRS have the highest levels of endothelin 1

I   Renal kallikrein–kinin system

1 Activation of kinins via the enzyme kallikrein causes renal vasodilation, increasing RBF. Kinins also inhibit the renal tubular absorption of sodium

2 Activity of the kinin system is assessed by measurement of urinary kallikrein excretion, which estimates renal kallikrein production

3 In patients with ascites, urinary kallikrein excretion is increased, but in HRS it is reduced

4 The decrease in urinary kallikrein excretion seen in HRS suggests that renal kallikrein depletion may contribute to the development of renal failure

5 There are many complex interactions of this system with other systems, such as the vasodilatory prostaglandins; therefore, it is difficult to establish the role of kinins in the maintenance of renal function in cirrhosis

J   Endotoxemia

1 Potent renal vasoconstrictors; can produce vasodilation in other circulatory beds

2 Endotoxin produced in the intestinal lumen can bypass Kupffer's cells (liver cells responsible for removing endotoxin) through portosystemic shunts and enter the systemic circulation

3 The data are conflicting on the role of endotoxemia in contributing to HRS, because endotoxemia is common in patients with chronic liver disease. Some studies suggest that endotoxemia is more common in cirrhotics with HRS than in those without renal failure

4 Endotoxins stimulate the production of nitric oxide by increasing inducible NOS. Elevated nitric oxide levels may be another way that endotoxemia may contribute to the hyperdynamic circulation

K   Leukotrienes

1 Intravenous administration of leukotriene C_4 to normal rats increases renal vascular resistance, causing decreased RBF and GFR

2 Urinary excretion of leukotrienes in HRS is higher than in controls or in patients with cirrhosis without HRS

L   Calcitonin gene-related peptide (CGRP)

1 Formed by alternative splicing of the primary calcitonin gene transcript

2 Found throughout the neural, vascular, and endocrine systems and in perivascular nerve fibers in the liver, mesenteric blood vessels, and the kidney

3 A potent vasodilator; mediates vasodilation of the mesenteric blood vessel and acts as a vasodilator of renal arteries

4 Plasma levels of CGRP are significantly higher in patients with HRS than in healthy controls

5 Theories Proposed to Explain Sodium Retention and Ascites Formation in Cirrhosis (see also Ch. 11)

Three theories have been proposed to explain sodium retention in cirrhosis:

- underfill theory
- overflow theory
- peripheral arterial vasodilation theory

A Underfill theory

1 Classical, oldest theory

2 Proposes that ascites formation results in loss of intravascular volume, leading to activation of sodium-retaining systems (e.g., SNS, RAAS)

3 Urinary sodium retention is secondary, occurring in response to activated SNS, RAAS, etc.

4 Theory is consistent with activation of vasoconstrictor and sodium-retaining neurohumoral systems

5 Theory is inconsistent with presence of increased cardiac output, decreased peripheral resistance, and lack of an increase in intravascular volume during spontaneous diuresis

B Overflow theory

1 Proposed by Lieberman and colleagues (1969)[3]

2 Proposes primary abnormality is urinary sodium retention (i.e., increased sodium reabsorption in the kidney). The mechanism of urinary sodium retention is unknown

3 Urinary sodium retention leads to intravascular volume expansion. The overexpanded intravascular volume "overflows" into the extravascular space (e.g., hepatic lymphatics (ascites), peripheral edema)

4 Theory explains increased intravascular space, increased cardiac output, and decreased peripheral resistance

5 Theory does not explain activation of SNS, RAAS, and other sodium-retaining and vasoconstrictor systems. These neurohumoral systems should be suppressed by excess sodium retention. Blood pressure should be increased by volume expansion, but is decreased in cirrhosis

C Peripheral vasodilation theory

1 Primary (unexplained) abnormality is dilation of peripheral arterial system, possibly a result of portal hypertension and splanchnic arterial vasodilation[4]

2 Arterial baroreceptors sense arterial dilation as decreased "effective arterial blood volume". Body responds by increasing cardiac output and activating sodium-retaining and vasoconstrictor systems (e.g., SNS, RAAS) until equilibrium is achieved

3 Theory explains increased cardiac output, decreased peripheral resistance, and activation of vasoconstrictor and sodium-retaining retaining hormonal systems in cirrhosis

4 Experimental studies support peripheral arterial vasodilation as an early event in cirrhosis, occurring prior to, or coincident with, sodium retention

6   Predictive Factors for Development of HRS

HRS develops in approximately 15% of patients within 6 months of first hospitalization with ascites and in 40% within 5 years.[5] Factors correlated with higher probability of developing HRS in patients hospitalized with ascites are shown in Table 12.2. Factors not predictive of development of HRS include liver function tests, etiology of liver disease, and Child–Pugh score

	Univariate	Multivariate
Serum sodium < 134 mEq/L	<0.005	<0.0001
Hepatomegaly	<0.05	<0.03
Plasma renin activity > 3.5 ng/mL/h	<0.0003	<0.05
Serum creatinine > 0.9 mg/dL	<0.05	NS
Poor nutritional status	<0.005	NS
Mean arterial pressure < 86 mmHg	<0.05	NS
Serum osmolality < 280 mOsm/kg	<0.05	NS

(Table 12.2: Factors that correlate with increased probability of HRS in patients hospitalized with ascites)[5]

7   Differential Diagnosis (see Table 12.3)

A   Acute tubular necrosis (ATN)

Occurs with a relatively high frequency in patients with cirrhosis and ascites, perhaps because they are frequently exposed to hypotension (e.g., GI bleeding), sepsis, or nephrotoxic drugs. Differentiating ATN from HRS can be difficult. Patients with ATN usually have an active urinary sediment (granular casts) and a urine sodium excretion greater than 10 mEq/L (often close to 30 mEq/L). Urinary sodium excretion cannot be used as a major diagnostic criterion to separate ATN from HRS since sodium excretion can be greater than 10 mEq/L in patients with HRS and less than 10 mEq/L in ascites and ATN. Urinary enzymes (gamma glutamyltranspeptidase, leucine aminopeptidase) or beta-2 microglobulin may be useful in differentiating ATN from HRS. The prognosis of ATN in patients with cirrhosis and ascites is poor but better than the prognosis of HRS

Liver previously normal

Heart failure
Shock
Syndrome of hemolysis, elevated liver tests, and low platelets (HELLP)
Infection (leptospirosis, tuberculosis, yellow fever, malaria)
Sickle cell disease
Connective tissue diseases
Reye's syndrome

Diseases affecting liver and kidney

Polycystic kidney, Caroli's syndrome
Amyloidosis
Sarcoidosis
Cryoglobulinemia due to chronic hepatitis C
Polyarteritis nodosa due to chronic hepatitis B
IgA nephropathy in alcoholic liver disease

Renal failure in chronic liver disease

Drug induced
Toxins (e.g., carbon tetrachloride)
Intravascular volume depletion
Hepatorenal syndrome
  acute
  chronic

(Table 12.3: Differential diagnosis of renal failure in liver disease)

B Drug-induced renal failure

1 **NSAIDs**: because prostaglandins, primarily PGI_2, are important in maintaining renal artery dilation in patients with ascites, blocking prostaglandin synthesis with NSAIDs (e.g., aspirin, ibuprofen, piroxicam, indomethacin) results in marked arterial vasoconstriction and consequent reduction in RBF and GFR. Within 1 hour of NSAID administration, creatinine clearance and RBF are markedly reduced. Urine output decreases and remains low for several hours

2 **Antibiotics**: aminoglycosides (e.g., gentamicin) are the archetypical drug-induced cause of renal failure. In cirrhosis with ascites, susceptibility of the kidney to gentamicin-induced ATN is increased. Standard doses of aminoglycosides can cause renal failure in patients with ascites. Consequently, **aminoglycosides are relatively contraindicated in patients with ascites**. If used, blood levels should be monitored frequently. Therapeutic blood levels will not guarantee against development of ATN

3 **Intravenous radiographic contrast agents**

4 **Diuretics**: most patients with ascites are treated with diuretics. Occasionally, diuretic use leads to excess renal sodium and water loss with consequent volume depletion and prerenal azotemia. **Diuretics should be stopped in all patients in whom the diagnosis of hepatorenal syndrome is considered.** However, there is no clear evidence that diuretic use, particularly diuretic use which raises the serum creatinine (up to 2.0–2.5 mg/dL), causes or predisposes to HRS

5 Table 12.4 compares urinary findings in various disease states.

	Cirrhosis with ascites	Prerenal azotemia	HRS	ATN
Urine sodium (mEq/L)	Variable, usually <40	<10	<10	>30
FENa[a] (%)	<1	<1	<1	>1
Urine output	Normal	Decreased	Decreased	Variable
Urine sediment	Normal	Normal	Normal	Casts, cell debris
Urine osmolality	Variable, Usually <serum	>Serum	>Serum	=Serum
Urine : plasma creatinine ratio		<30 : 1	>30 : 1	<20 : 1
GFR response to volume expansion	None	Improved	None to temporary improvement	Variable

[a]FENa, fractional excretion of sodium.

(Table 12.4: Urinary findings in various disease states)

C   Glomerulopathies

Immune complex disease (e.g., cryoglobulinemia) and IgA nephropathy

D   Prerenal azotemia

Intravascular volume depletion can lead to prerenal azotemia. Causes of intravascular volume depletion include diuretic use, vomiting, diarrhea, and paracentesis without intravascular volume replacement. It is difficult to differentiate prerenal azotemia from HRS based on the urinary sodium, urinary volume, or creatinine clearance. An inciting event (e.g., vomiting) and evidence of volume depletion (e.g., orthostatic change in blood pressure or heart rate, increase in hematocrit and plasma proteins) suggest the diagnosis of prerenal azotemia, which improves with volume replacement

8   Diagnostic Criteria for HRS

1 A panel of international experts recently published criteria for the diagnosis of hepatorenal syndrome.[1] Major Criteria must be present for the diagnosis of HRS, and Additional Criteria are usually, but not invariably, present.

2 **Major Criteria:** all of the following major criteria must be present:
- chronic or acute liver disease with advanced hepatic failure and portal hypertension
- low glomerular filtration rate, as indicated by serum creatinine of >1.5 mg/dL or 24-hour creatinine clearance < 40 mL/min

- No other explanation for the renal insufficiency. In particular: absence of shock, ongoing bacterial infection, and current or recent treatment with nephrotoxic drugs. Absence of gastrointestinal fluid losses (repeated vomiting or intense diarrhea) or renal fluid losses (weight loss > 500 g/day for several days in patients with ascites without peripheral edema or 1000 g/day in patients with peripheral edema)
- no sustained improvement in renal function (decrease in serum creatinine to 1.5 mg/dL or less or increase in creatinine clearance to 40 mL/min or more) following diuretic withdrawal and expansion of plasma volume with 1.5 L of isotonic saline
- proteinuria < 500 mg/dL and no ultrasonographic evidence of obstructive uropathy or parenchymal renal disease

3 **Additional Criteria:** these are typically present in patients with HRS and describe typical findings in the urine and blood:
   - urine volume < 500 mL per 24 hours
   - urine sodium < 10 mEq/L
   - urine osmolality > plasma osmolality
   - urine red blood cells < 50 per high-power field
   - serum sodium concentration < 130 mEq/L

9 Diagnostic Work-up for HRS (see Table 12.5)

A General

1 Diagnostic evaluation consists primarily of exclusion of other causes of renal failure. The diagnosis of advanced chronic liver disease should be obvious from the long history of liver disease and the presence of hypoalbuminemia, prolonged prothrombin time, and portal hypertensive ascites. Patients with HRS following acute liver injury have signs of liver failure (e.g., altered mental status)

2 Measurement of serum creatinine is usually sufficient to diagnose renal insufficiency. Because of the severe muscle wasting in patients with advanced liver

---

1 History and physical examination: GI bleeding, sepsis (e.g., blood, urine, ascites), vomiting, diarrhea, shock, heat failure, disseminated intravascular coagulation

2 Medications: review current and recent (e.g., acetaminophen, aminoglycosides, halothane) drug use; stop diuretics

3 Laboratory tests: serum creatinine, BUN, sodium, osmolality, urinalysis, 24-hour urine collection for volume, sodium, creatinine, protein and osmolality

4 Ultrasound of kidneys to exclude obstructive uropathy

5 Intravenous volume challenge with 1.5 L of fluid

6 Review specific causes of renal failure in liver disease (see Table 12.4) and order specific tests, as appropriate

(Table 12.5: Diagnostic work-up in patients with liver disease and renal failure)

disease, serum creatinine levels may significantly underestimate GFR (e.g., serum creatinine of 1.5 mg/dL might signify a GFR of 60 mL/min in a healthy 40-year-old man and a GFR of 30 mL/min in a patient with cirrhosis and ascites). Consequently, measurement of creatinine clearance on an accurately collected 24-hour urine specimen is a better estimate of the severity of renal insufficiency

B   Exclusion of other causes of renal disease

- history and physical examination: exclude nephrotoxic drug use, vomiting, diarrhea, excess diuresis, sepsis, and shock
- urine tests: urinalysis should exclude ATN (absence of casts), significant proteinuria, and significant red blood cells. Urinary sodium is usually less than 10 mEq/mL, and 24-hour urine volume is less than 500 mL, with urine osmolality higher than serum osmolality
- renal ultrasound: excludes obstructive uropathy and evidence of intrinsic renal disease (e.g., polycystic kidney, small kidneys suggestive of chronic renal disease)

C   Plasma volume expansion

Should be given to all patients before the diagnosis of HRS is made. In general, 1.5 L of normal saline can be given intravenously over several hours while the patient is hospitalized. Some physicians prefer to administer a different plasma volume expander (e.g., hespan, albumin, blood), under more intensive nursing supervision (e.g., intensive care unit) or with monitoring of central venous pressures. Serum creatinine should be checked 6–12 hours after finishing the i.v. infusion. In patients with volume depletion, serum creatinine improves significantly, although it may not return to normal for several days

10   Treatment (see Table 12.6)

A   Standard treatment

- consider liver transplant evaluation. Renal function often returns to normal following liver transplantation. Usually, patients with HRS have had advanced liver disease for months and have been candidates for liver transplant evaluation. The mortality rate after liver transplantation is higher in patients with ascites and HRS than in patients with ascites and normal serum creatinine[6]

1 Restrict sodium intake to 2 g/day
2 If serum sodium < 125 mEq/L, then restrict fluid intake to 1500 mL/day
3 Treat infection, GI bleeding
4 Tell patient and/or family of poor prognosis
5 Consider liver transplant evaluation
6 Intravenous fluid challenge with at least 1.5 L (if not previously given)

(Table 12.6: Treatment of patients with hepatorenal syndrome)

- the patient and family should be told that the prognosis is extremely poor
- restrict dietary sodium intake to 2 g (88 mEq) or less per day. Because patients excrete almost no sodium in their urine, all ingested sodium remains in the body, primarily in the extracellular space (edema and ascites). Patients ingesting 88 mEq sodium per day gain approximately 2/3 kg (1.5 pounds) in weight per day
- if patient is severely hyponatremic (serum sodium less than 125 mEq/mL), restrict fluid intake to less than 1.5 L per day
- treat sepsis, gastrointestinal bleeding. Avoid placing a chronic indwelling catheter in the urinary bladder
- as stated previously, patients should receive an i.v. fluid challenge with at least 1.5 L of normal saline to reverse unsuspected volume depletion

B Specific treatments

1 The following treatments should be considered in all patients with HRS:
- liver transplantation[7]
- specific treatment of liver disease which will improve liver function

2 The following treatments were hopeful in preliminary studies but should not be considered standard in patients with HRS:
- ornipressin (vasopressin analog): i.v. administration reversed the hyperdynamic circulation, increased GFR and urinary sodium excretion.[8] Mechanism of action is presumed to be vasoconstriction of splanchnic circulation. Potential problem is systemic vasoconstriction (ischemic necrosis). Hemodynamic and renal improvement reverses when ornipressin is stopped, unless liver function improves
- aprotinin: i.v. administration improved natriuresis. Mechanism of action may be inhibition of kallikrein–kinin system, resulting in vasoconstriction of the splanchnic circulation and increased renal blood flow[9]
- transjugular intrahepatic portosystemic shunt (TIPS): TIPS insertion in eight patients with HRS reduced serum creatinine by 50% and improved urinary sodium excretion from 2 mEq/day to 75 mEq/day

3 The following treatments are considered ineffective in the treatment of HR:
- hemodialysis, peritoneal dialysis: hypotension, bleeding, and infection are problems. Hemodialysis may be useful in patients with acute liver failure who are awaiting liver transplantation
- lumber sympathectomy
- plasma volume expansion
- intrarenal vasodilators: prostaglandin A_1 or E_1, misoprostol (PGE_1 analog), alpha-adrenergic blockers, beta-adrenergic agonists, acetylcholine, papaverine
- systemic vasoconstrictors or vasodilators: calcium channel blockers, dopamine
- surgical portosystemic shunts
- peritoneovenous shunts (e.g., LeVeen shunt, Denver shunt)
- paracentesis
- thromboxane synthase inhibitors: dazoxiben, OKY 046
- ex vivo baboon liver perfusion
- head-out water immersion

11   Prognosis

1   The prognosis of HRS is extremely poor. Median survival is 10–14 days; 75% of patients are dead by 3 weeks and 90% by 8 weeks. Survival is somewhat longer in patients with type II (slow-onset) HRS, but overall survival remains extremely poor

2   Approximately 4–10% of patients may recover significant renal function and have prolonged survival[5]

References

1   Arroyo V, Gines P, Gerbes AL, et al. *Definition and diagnostic criteria of refractory ascites and hepatorenal syndrome in cirrhosis.* (Hepatology 1996) 23: 164–76

2   Fernandez-Seara J, Prieto J, Quiroga J, et al. *Systemic and regional hemodynamics in patients with liver cirrhosis and ascites with and without functional renal failure.* (Gastroenterology 1989) 97: 1304–12

3   Lieberman FL, Denison EK, Reynolds TB. *The relationship of plasma volume, portal hypertension, ascites and renal sodium retention in cirrhosis: the "overflow" theory of ascites formation.* (Ann NY Acad Sci 1970) 170: 202–12

4   Schrier RW, Arroyo V, Bernardi M, Epstein M, Henriksen JH, Rodes J. *Peripheral arterial vasodilation hypothesis: a proposal for the initiation of renal sodium and water retention in cirrhosis.* (Hepatology 1988) 8: 1151–7

5   Gines A, Escorsell A, Gines P, et al. *Incidence, predictive factors and prognosis of the hepatorenal syndrome in cirrhosis with ascites.* (Gastroenterology 1993) 105: 229–36

6   Cuervas-Mons V, Millan I, Gavaler JS, Starzl TE, Van Thiel DH. *Prognostic value of preoperatively obtained clinical and laboratory data in predicting survival following orthotopic liver transplantation.* (Hepatology 1986) 6: 922–7

7   Iwatsuki S, Popovtzer MM, Corman JL, et al. *Recovery from "hepatorenal syndrome" after orthotopic liver transplantation.* (N Engl J Med 1973) 289: 1155–9

8   Lenz K, Hortnagl H, Druml W, et al. *Beneficial effect of 8-ornithine vasopressin on renal dysfunction in decompensated cirrhosis.* (Gut 1989) 30: 90–6

9   Brensing KA, Textor J, Raab P, et al. *Sustained improvement of hepatorenal syndrome after TIPS-insertion in patients with terminal liver cirrhosis not eligible for transplantation.* (Gastroenterology 1996) 110: 1158A

10 Wong F, Blendis L (eds). *Hepatorenal disorders.* (Semin Liver Dis 1994) 14: 1–105

Hepatic encephalopathy

KEVIN D. MULLEN, M.B., F.R.C.P.I.

▼

Key Points

1 The key to the diagnosis of hepatic encephalopathy is recognition that significant liver disease is present

2 The occurrence of any neuropsychiatric symptoms or signs in a patient with significant liver dysfunction should be considered hepatic encephalopathy until proven otherwise

3 Patients with suspected overt hepatic encephalopathy are managed by a three-pronged strategy: other causes for encephalopathy are ruled out, precipitating factors are corrected, and empirical therapy is instituted

4 Acute liver failure-associated hepatic encephalopathy (ALFA-HE) is rare, and its clinical course and treatment are distinct from those seen in chronic liver disease

5 There are many hypotheses regarding the pathogenesis of hepatic encephalopathy. However, operationally the ammonia concept is perfectly suited for the clinician caring for patients with hepatic encephalopathy

6 The diagnosis of hepatic encephalopathy is clinical and not based on blood ammonia levels

▲

1   Definition

A wide spectrum of neuropsychiatric abnormalities occurring in patients with significant liver dysfunction due to an as yet uncertain mechanism
   Significant liver dysfunction implies one of the following:

- acute liver failure
- cirrhosis with or without major portosystemic shunting
- major portosystemic shunting without cirrhosis

2   Basic Theories of Pathophysiology

- reduced hepatic production of compounds which maintain normal central nervous system (CNS) function
- failure of hepatic detoxification of neuroactive compounds arising from the gut. Cross-circulation experiments in animal model favor this theory

A   Failure of hepatic detoxification due to:

1   Loss of function or mass of hepatocytes
2   Intrahepatic and extrahepatic splanchnic blood bypass of hepatocytes

Note: clinically evident or overt hepatic encephalopathy (HE) is generally seen only when obvious loss of hepatic function has occurred

B   Specific hypothesis of hepatic encephalopathy

1   Direct ammonia neurotoxicity
2   Multiple synergistic neurotoxins: ammonia, mercaptans, octanoic acid
3   Synthesis of false neurotransmitters and plasma amino acid imbalance
4   Alterations in CNS tryptophan metabolites, such as serotonin
5   Excess gamma aminobutyric acid (GABA)
6   Presence of "endogenous" or "natural" benzodiazepines

Ammonia neurotoxicity is not only the simplest hypothesis but has the most support. Whether partially or totally correct (or not), it conceptually is easy to understand. Most effective therapy for HE reduces ammonia in some fashion

3   Clinical Presentations

A   Acute liver failure-associated hepatic encephalopathy (ALFA-HE) (fulminant hepatic failure (see Ch. 2))

B   Associated with chronic liver disease and/or portosystemic shunting

1   Subclinical HE

2 Single or recurrent episodes of overt HE

3 Chronic overt HE

4 Acquired hepatocerebral degeneration[1]

5 Spastic paresis[2]

Last two are very rare and are the exceptions to the rule that HE is usually reversible. Generally occur in background of fluctuating HE

4 Diagnosis

Consideration of the possibility of HE only arises when significant liver dysfunction is known or suspected to be present. Frequently, clinical or laboratory evidence of liver failure and/or portal hypertension is obvious. However, in a significant minority of patients evidence of significant liver dysfunction may be subtle, as in the following conditions:

- well-compensated cirrhosis, e.g., hepatitis C, remote alcohol abuse
- non-cirrhotic portal hypertension:
  - splanchnic vein thrombosis
  - schistosomiasis
  - noncirrhotic portal fibrosis
  - idiopathic
- congenital hepatic fibrosis
- congenital intrahepatic and extrahepatic portosystemic shunts

A Historical points suggesting occult liver disease and/or portosystemic shunting (see also Ch. 9)

- past history of i.v. drug use (hepatitis B or C)
- family history of cirrhosis (hemochromatosis)
- residence in areas endemic for schistosomiasis
- umbilical sepsis (splanchnic vein thrombosis)
- history of pancreatitis (splenic vein thrombosis)
- past history of hepatitis (hepatitis B or C, alcoholic hepatitis)
- past history of use of hepatotoxic drugs, e.g., methotrexate, nitrofurantoin

B Physical signs suggesting underlying significant liver disease

- fetor hepaticus
- spider telangiectases (especially in men)
- gynecomastia
- loss of body hair (in men)
- testicular atrophy
- loss of muscle mass
- jaundice
- Kayser–Fleischer rings

- splenomegaly
- ascites
- amenorrhea
- caput medusae
- hepatomegaly
- scratch marks
- edema
- ecchymoses

C Laboratory test abnormalities

- elevated blood ammonia levels
- hypergammaglobulinemia
- thrombocytopenia
- leukopenia
- pancytopenia
- elevated cerebrospinal fluid (CSF) glutamine levels
- decreased plasma branched-chain/aromatic amino acid ratio
- hepatitis C antibody
- hepatitis B serology

The above listed historical points, physical signs, and laboratory tests can individually or in combination indicate the presence of underlying liver dysfunction even when traditional tests of hepatic function, such as serum albumin and prothrombin times, are normal. It should be emphasized that patients with well-preserved synthetic function of the liver uncommonly develop overt HE. Usually a very major precipitating factor is needed to induce an episode in such patients (see below)

D Subclinical HE

Defined and diagnosed by subnormal performance on at least one of the following selected psychometric tests but with a normal routine neurological examination:

- Reitan Trail Test A or B
- Digit Symbol Test
- Block Design Test
- Purdue Peg Board Test

Subclinical HE is a real entity, but its impact of the quality of life for patients is uncertain. It is present in 60–70% of cirrhotic patients even if their disease is well compensated. The natural history of progression to overt HE appears most closely related to worsening liver function. It responds to standard HE treatment (see below).

E Overt HE

A clinical diagnosis made when alterations in consciousness and a generalized movement disorder occur in a patient with known or suspected significant liver dysfunction.

1 Alterations in consciousness

Stage I	mild confusion, personality change, sleep disturbance
Stage II	drowsiness, intermittent disorientation, short attention span
Stage III	somnolent but arousable, gross disorientation
Stage IVa	coma, arousable by painful stimuli
Stage IVb	unresponsive

Stages III–IV can also be assessed by the Glasgow Coma Scale (maximum score 15, the lower the score, the more severe the HE) (see Table 13.1)

			Score
Eyes	Open	Spontaneously	4
		To verbal command	3
		To pain	2
		No response	1
Best motor response	To verbal commands	Obeys	6
	To painful stimulus	Localizes pain	5
		Flexion	3
		Extension	2
		No response	1
Best verbal response		Oriented and talking	5
		Disoriented and talking	4
		Inappropriate speech	3
		Incomprehensible speech	2
		No response	1

(Table 13.1: Glasgow Coma Scale)

2 Generalized movement disorder

- asterixis
- hyperreflexia
- muscular rigidity
- extensor plantar response
- slow monotonous speech
- immobile facies
- parkinsonian features
- decerebrate posturing

None of the above signs is specific for HE. Indeed, virtually any neuropsychiatric abnormality in a patient with significant liver dysfunction can be HE

5 Additional Diagnostic Tests

A Blood ammonia test

1 Elevated blood level *not* diagnostic of HE
2 Normal level does *not* rule out HE
3 Very high level may indicate unsuspected urea cycle enzyme deficiency
4 Major value is to suggest HE when cause for encephalopathy is very obscure
5 Clinical evaluation (not blood ammonia monitoring) should be basis for assessing response to treatment
6 If blood ammonia testing is done:

- arterial, arterialized or capillary blood better than venous
- needs prompt assay or else ammonia level will be increased artefactually
- unreliable after major muscle activity, like seizure
- reliance on ammonia level for diagnosis is unwise

B Electrophysiological assessment

1 Electroencephalography (EEG) (standard or computer-assisted analysis): rarely utilized clinically. Some value in research setting
2 Sensory evoked potentials

- early latency or exogenous evoked potentials
- late latency or endogenous

3 Reaction time devices

All of the above have been studied, particularly as measures of subclinical HE. They are excellent research tools but are still undergoing validation. They have not entered the clinical arena to any extent

C Cerebral morphology

1 CT and MRI

- evidence of cortical atrophy common
- worse in alcoholic liver disease (but not dependent only on alcohol)
- not synonymous with hepatocerebral atrophy
- relationship of observed abnormalities to HE uncertain
- findings have no direct bearing on liver transplant suitability

2 T1-weighted hyperintensity of basal ganglia on MRI

- commonly seen in cirrhosis
- correlates best with severity of liver disease
- relationship to HE uncertain
- in part related to brain manganese deposition
- reverses after liver transplantation
- not synonymous with hepatocerebral atrophy

6   Immediate Management

Response to management confirms diagnosis post hoc

A   Three-pronged strategy for acute management

1 Rule out other causes of encephalopathy. If any present, treat

2 Identify and treat correctable precipitating factors

3 Initiate empirical treatment

B   Exclude other causes of encephalopathy

Patients with significant liver dysfunction are susceptible to many causes of encephalopathy other than HE:

- sepsis
- hypoxia
- hypercapnia
- acidosis
- uremia
- sensitivity to CNS drugs
- gross electrolyte changes
- postictal confusion
- delirium tremors
- Wernicke–Korsakoff syndrome
- intracerebral hemorrhage
- CNS sepsis
- cerebral edema/intracranial hypertension*
- hypoglycemia*
- pancreatic encephalopathy
- drug intoxication

Many patients will simultaneously have other causes of encephalopathy as well as HE, contributing to difficulty in diagnosing HE

C   Identify precipitating factors

Most patients with significant liver disease (except for ALFA-HE) have an identifiable precipitating factor responsible for inducing the onset of an episode of HE. Correcting these are a key aspect of the management of HE. The list has arisen from years of clinical observation. Some can be easily envisaged to enhance production and/or absorption of gut compounds. Others are less obvious but may act by reducing hepatic function. Sepsis and CNS-active drugs can independently cause encephalopathy or precipitate HE:

- gastrointestinal hemorrhage

*Usually seen only in acute liver failure

- sepsis
- constipation
- dietary protein overload
- dehydration
- CNS-active drugs
- hypokalemia/alkalosis
- poor compliance with lactulose therapy
- postanesthesia
- postportal decompression procedure*
- bowel obstruction or ileus*
- uremia
- superimposed hepatic injury*
- development of hepatocellular carcinoma*

D   Empiric therapy for HE

1 Gut cleansing with enemas and gastric aspiration or lavage
2 Low or zero protein diet
3 Delivery of lactulose 50 ml po or via nasogastric tube every 2 h until loose bowel movements passed. Then titrated from 30 ml po q.i.d. down to point that 2–3 loose bowel movements a day are passed. Lower doses may suffice if patient not comatose

Empiric therapy may be effective by correcting precipitating factors. However, because there is no way of predicting the response to correcting precipitating factors, all patients should receive full empiric therapy

E   Response to management

In virtually every case of overt HE in chronic liver disease, it should be possible to reverse encephalopathy. Failure to reverse HE after 72 hours of treatment may indicate that:

1 A cause of encephalopathy has been missed or treated inadequately
2 A precipitating factor has been missed, treated inadequately, or remains uncorrected
3 Effective empirical therapy has not been instituted

The commonest reason for ineffective empiric therapy is lack of delivery of lactulose into the small intestine or right colon. Only intestinal obstruction or ileus should prevent this. Reluctance to use nasogastric tube delivery of lactulose in the comatose patient because of fear of precipitating a variceal bleed is unwarranted

4 Second-line therapy may be needed:
- neomycin 500 mg po q.i.d. (use higher doses with caution)
- metronidazole 250 mg po q.i.d. (recommend only short-term use)[3]
- vancomycin[4] 250 mg po q.i.d.

*May be difficult or impossible to correct

- sodium benzoate (not approved for use in the USA)[5]
- flumazenil (may be effective but very short length of action)[6]

7 Problems Peculiar to ALFA-HE (see also Ch. 2)

1 Accounts for small fraction of HE cases/year (?2%)
2 Treatment follows the same principles as in chronic liver disease, but:
   - precipitating factors are often not obvious and, even if present, correction is usually not effective
   - overall response to empiric therapy is poor
   - if deep coma occurs, the prognosis is poor without liver transplantation
   - cerebral edema and intracranial hypertension are common and often lethal
   - other concurrent causes of encephalopathy are common, e.g., hypoglycemia, acidosis, sepsis
   - about 20% of cases have agitated delirium or seizure phase

8 Long-term Treatment of HE

1 Lactulose (30 ml twice to four times a day), lactitol (12 g four times a day) or lactose (15–20 g four times a day) (in lactose-deficient patients) by mouth in doses sufficient to induce one to two loose bowel movements per day
2 Neomycin 2 g/day (concern: risk of ototoxicity)
3 Vegetable-based protein diet
4 Branched-chain amino acid-enriched oral diet
5 Bromocriptine[7]
6 Zinc repletion[8]
7 Sodium benzoate (5 g po b.i.d.)*
8 Ornithine aspartate (6 g po t.i.d.)*

The above therapies are usually used for maintenance therapy. Failure of one generally leads to trying the next listed treatment. Long-term low-protein diet is not ideal if protein restriction to avoid HE is insufficient for maintaining nitrogen balance

9 Other Options for Intractable or Recurrent HE

A Orthotopic liver transplantation (see also Ch. 31)

1 Clearly indicated for intractable HE
2 Also indicated for recurrent HE or HE only responsive to low-protein diet

Indication for liver transplantation usually takes into account other factors as well as HE.

---

*Not usually available in the USA

B   Modification of existing portosystemic shunts

Surgical or transjugular intrahepatic portosystemic stent (TIPS)-created shunts may be amenable to:

- closure, possibly in combination with other measures to prevent recurrent variceal bleeding
- reduction in shunt diameter[9]

The above can be achieved in selected cases by radiological and/or surgical interventions. Usually only attempted if the patient is not a liver transplant candidate

- acquired spontaneous portosystemic shunts are occasionally amenable to occlusion (by embolization) or reduction in flow (e.g., splenic artery embolization)
- congenital portosystemic shunts are amenable in some cases to closure

C   Others

- colonic exclusion – virtually abandoned
- arterialization of portal venous stump – ?abandoned
- radiological portal vein thrombolysis + TIPS[10]
- TIPS in Budd–Chiari syndrome

References

1   Victor M, Adams RD, Ede M. *The acquired (non-Wilsonian) type of chronic hepatocellular degeneration*. (Medicine (Baltimore) 1965) 44: 345–96

2   Mendoza G, Marti-Fabergas J, Kulisevsky J, Escartin A. *Hepatic myelopathy: a rare complication of portacaval shunt*. (Eur Neurol 1994) 34: 209–12

3   Morgan HH, Read AE, Spellac DCE. *Treatment of hepatic encephalopathy with metronidazole*. (Gut 1982) 23: 1–7

4   Tarda K, Ikeda T, Hayashi K et al. *Successful use of vancomycin hydrochloride in the treatment of lactulose resistant hepatic encephalopathy*. (Gut 1990) 31: 702–6

5   Sushma S, Dasarathy S, Tandon RK et al. *Sodium benzoate in the treatment of acute hepatic encephalopathy: a double blind randomized trial*. (Hepatology 1992) 16: 138–44

6   Pomier-Layrargues JF, Giguère J, Lavoie J et al. *Flumazemil in cirrhotic patients in hepatic coma: a randomized double-blind placebo-controlled crossover trial*. (Hepatology 1994) 19: 31–7

7   Morgan M, Jakobovitz AW, James M, Sherlock S. *Successful use of bromocriptine in the treatment of hepatic encephalopathy*. (Gastroenterology 1980) 78: 663–5

8   Van der Rijt CC, Schalm SW, Schat H et al. *Overt hepatic encephalopathy precipitated by zinc deficiency*. (Gastroenterology 1991) 100: 1074–118

9   Hauenstein KH, Haag K, Ochs A, Langer M, Rössle M. *Reducing stent for TIPS-induced refractory hepatic encephalopathy and liver failure*. (Radiology 1994) 194: 175–9

10   Blum U, Haag J, Rössle M et al. *Noncavernomatous portal vein thrombosis in hepatic cirrhosis: treatment with transjugular intrahepatic portosystemic shunt and local thrombolysis*. (Radiology 1995) 195: 155–7

11   Adams RD, Foley JM. *The neurological disorder associated with liver disease*. (Res Publ Assoc Nerv Ment Dis 1953) 32: 198–237

12   Basile AS, Jones EA, Skolnick P. *The pathogenesis and treatment of hepatic encephalopathy:*

evidence for the involvement of benzodiazepine receptor ligands. (Pharmacol Rev 1991) 43: 27–71

13   Conn HO, Lieberthal MM. *The Hepatic Coma Syndromes and Lactulose.* Baltimore: Williams & Wilkins, 1978)

14   Crossley IR, Williams R. *Progress in the treatment of chronic portosystemic encephalopathy.* (Gut 1984) 25: 85–98

15   Ferenci P, Puspok A, Steindl P. *Current concepts in the pathophysiology of hepatic encephalopathy.* (Eur J Clin Invest 1992) 22: 573–81

16   Gitlin N. *Subclinical portal-systemic encephalopathy.* (Am J Gastroenterol 1988) 83: 8–11

17   Krieger D, Kreiger S, Jansen O, et al. *Manganese and chronic hepatic encephalopathy.* (Lancet 1995) 346: 270–4

18   Kugler CFA, Lotterer E, Petter J, et al. *Visual event-related P300 potentials in early portosystemic encephalopathy.* (Gastroenterology 1992) 103: 302–310

19   Plum F, Hindfelt B. *The neurological complications of liver disease.* In: Vanicu PJ, Bruyn GA, (eds). *Handbook of Clinical Neurology.* (New York: Elsevier, 1986) 349–77

20   Sherlock S, Summerskill WHJ, White LP, Phear EA. *Portal-systemic encephalopathy: neurological complications of liver disease.* (Lancet 1956) 2: 453–7

Primary biliary cirrhosis

YOUNG-MEE LEE, M.D.
MARSHALL M. KAPLAN, M.D.

Key Points

1 Primary biliary cirrhosis (PBC) is a chronic cholestatic liver disease that usually affects middle-aged women

2 The cause of PBC remains unknown, although genetic and immunologic factors appear to play a role

3 PBC is divided into four histologic stages

4 Many patients are asymptomatic at the time of diagnosis. The signs and symptoms of cholestasis develop as the disease progresses

5 The diagnosis of PBC should be considered in patients with unexplained cholestasis or elevation of serum alkaline phosphatase. A percutaneous liver biopsy should be performed to confirm the diagnosis and to determine the prognosis

6 There is no proven medical treatment for the underlying disease, although drugs such as ursodeoxycholic acid, colchicine, and methotrexate are promising and their use is associated with improvement of histology in some patients. Liver transplantation has improved the survival of the patients with liver failure from primary biliary cirrhosis

1   Epidemiology and Genetics

A   Epidemiology

1 Primary biliary cirrhosis (PBC) is found in all races
2 It accounts for almost 2% of deaths worldwide from cirrhosis
3 Estimates of prevalence range from 19 to 151 per million population, while estimates of annual incidence range from 3.9 to 15 cases per million population per year
4 Approximately 90–95% of patients are female
5 Age of onset typically ranges from 30 to 70

B   Genetics

1 Genetic factors appear to play a role in PBC, although the disorder is not inherited in a simple recessive or dominant pattern
2 Familial occurrences of PBC have been observed. The prevalence of PBC in families with one affected member is estimated to be 1000 times greater than that in the general population
3 The lack of concordance of PBC in identical twins suggests that some triggering event is required to initiate PBC in a genetically susceptible individual[1]
4 There is a weak association between PBC and human leukocyte antigen (HLA) DR8 and the DQB1 gene[2]

2   Immunological Abnormalities and Pathogenesis

A   Immunologic abnormalities

- the large number of immunologic abnormalities in PBC suggests that the disease is caused by some abnormality of immune regulation; however, there is no direct proof of this hypothesis
- some of the immunologic abnormalities which are present in patients with PBC are as follows:

1 Antimitochondrial antibody (AMA)

- detected in 95% of patients with PBC
- does not affect the course of PBC
- not specific for PBC and is found in a small percentage of patients with autoimmune and drug-induced hepatitis
- not one antibody but a family of antibodies that react with different antigens within the mitochondria
- anti-M2:
  - the major autoantibody found in PBC
  - directed principally against the dihydrolipoamide acyltransferase component (E2) of the ketoacid dehydrogenase complexes on the inner mitochondrial membrane. Pyruvate dehydrogenase is the best known of these enzyme complexes (Fig. 14.1)

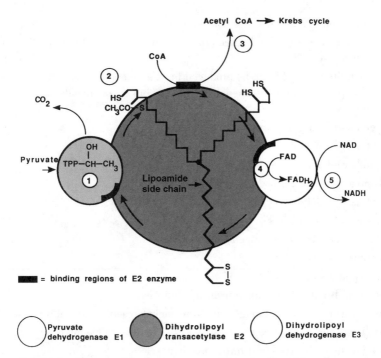

Fig. 14.1   Pyruvate dehydrogenase, one of the mitochondrial antigens against which antimitochondrial antibody (AMA) is directed. The M2 AMA bind primarily to the epitope within the lipoamide side chain of the large E2 unit and, to a lesser extent, to sites on E1 and E3 subunits. (Courtesy of M. Eric Gershwin, M.D.)

- anti-M4, anti-M8 and anti-M9
  - other AMA described in PBC
  - their existence could not be confirmed in recent studies which employed highly purified cloned human mitochondrial proteins as antigens; they may represent artifacts of previously used methodology
- role of AMA
  - the relationship between AMA and immunologic bile duct injury remains unclear
  - E2 antigens of pyruvate dehydrogenase complex stimulate interleukin 2 production by peripheral blood mononuclear cells and T cells cloned from liver biopsies of PBC patients
  - a molecule with some antigenic features of the E2 subunit of pyruvate dehydrogenase is aberrantly expressed on the luminal surface of biliary epithelial cells from PBC patients but not control subjects or patients with primary sclerosing cholangitis[3]
  - recent data demonstrate that pyruvate dehydrogenase E2 is expressed in bile duct epithelial cells before two other antigens that are also required for T lymphocyte cytotoxicity: HLA class II antigens and another recognition factor, BB1/B7[4]

- mitochondrial antigens are not tissue specific
- there is no correlation between the presence or titer of AMA and the severity of the course of PBC
- high titers of AMA can be produced in experimental animals by immunizing with pure human pyruvate dehydrogenase, but these animals have no liver disease

2 Other circulating autoantibodies
- antinuclear antibodies
- antithyroid antibodies
- lymphocytotoxic antibodies
- anti-acetylcholine receptor antibodies
- antiplatelet antibodies
- antiribonucleoprotein antigen Ro antibodies
- antihistone antibodies
- anticentromere antibodies

3 Increased levels of serum immunoglobulins
- increased levels of a serum IgM which are immunoreactive and highly cryoprecipitable
- may cause false-positive results with assays to detect immune complexes

4 Association with other autoimmune diseases
- thyroiditis, hypothyroidism
- rheumatoid arthritis
- CREST syndrome (calcinosis, Raynaud's phenomenon, esophageal dysmotility, sclerodactyly, telangiectases)
- Sjögren's syndrome
- scleroderma

5 Abnormalities of cellular immunity
- impaired T cell regulation
- decreased numbers of circulating T lymphocytes
- sequestration of T lymphocytes within hepatic portal triads
- negative delayed hypersensitivity skin tests

B Pathogenesis

1 There are two related processes which appear to cause hepatic damage and result in the clinical features of PBC (Fig. 14.2)
2 The first process is the chronic destruction of small bile ducts, presumably mediated by activated lymphocytes. It seems likely that the initial destructive bile duct lesion in PBC is caused by cytotoxic T lymphocytes
   - bile duct cells in patients with PBC express increased amounts of the Class I histocompatibility complex antigens HLA-A, HLA-B, and HLA-C, and Class II HLA-DR antigens, in contrast to normal bile duct cells
   - the bile duct lesion resembles disorders that are known to be mediated by cytotoxic T lymphocytes, such as that seen in graft-versus-host disease and in rejection of allografts

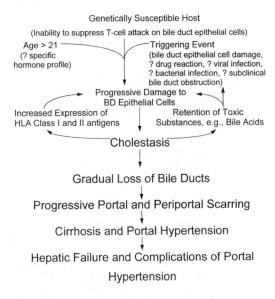

Fig. 14.2   The cause of PBC remains unknown, although genetic and immunologic factors appear to play a role. Possible pathogenesis of PBC is summarized in this figure
BD = bile duct

3 The second process is chemical damage to hepatocytes in areas of liver where bile drainage is impeded by the destruction of the small bile ducts and results in a diminished number of bile ducts within the liver

- there is retention of bile acids, bilirubin, copper, and other substances that are normally secreted or excreted into bile
- the increased concentration of some of these substances, such as bile acids, may cause further damage to liver cells
- the signs and symptoms of PBC are due to long-standing cholestasis
- the destruction of bile ducts eventually leads to portal inflammation and scarring, and ultimately to cirrhosis and liver failure

3   Pathology

A   Gross findings

1 Liver is enlarged, smooth, and bile stained in late stages of the disease
2 With progression of the disease, the liver enlarges further, becoming nodular and grossly cirrhotic
3 There is an increased prevalence of gallstones, approximately 40%
4 There is an increased prevalence of nodular regenerative hyperplasia in the early stage of PBC, which may account for high prevalence of portal hypertension in some patients early in the course of PBC[5]
5 Enlarged lymph nodes due to benign reactive hyperplasia may be seen in the porta hepatitis and around the aorta and inferior vena cava

B Hepatic histology

1 Four histological stages of PBC have been identified

2 With the progression of the disease, the stages advance over time from the initial lesion of stage I to stage IV (frank cirrhosis)

3 Considerations in liver biopsy staging:

  a Liver may not be uniformly affected; thus, liver biopsy may be subject to sampling variation

  b Several stages may be seen on one biopsy specimen. By convention, staging is based on the most advanced lesion seen on the biopsy specimen

  c Histological stages

   • **stage I**
      – damaged bile ducts are usually surrounded by a dense infiltrate of mononuclear cells, most of which are lymphocytes (Figs 14.3 and 14.4, see plate section)
      – these florid, asymmetric destructive lesions of interlobular bile ducts are irregularly scattered throughout the portal triads and are often seen only on large surgical biopsies of the liver
      – inflammation is confined to the portal triads

   • **stage II**
      – the lesion is more widespread but less specific
      – there may be reduced numbers of normal bile ducts within portal triads and increased numbers of atypical, poorly formed bile ducts with irregularly shaped lumina (Figs 14.5 and 14.6, see plate section)
      – there is diffuse portal fibrosis and mononuclear cell infiltrates within triads
      – inflammation may spill into the surrounding periportal areas

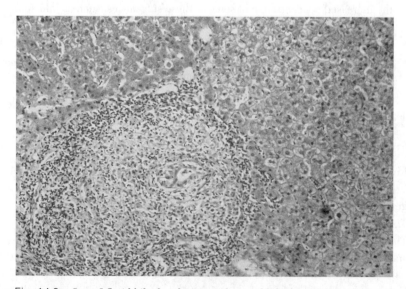

Fig. 14.3   Stage I florid bile duct lesion. A damaged bile duct is at the center of the lymphocytic granulomatous reaction (Masson trichrome, ×372). See page xvii.

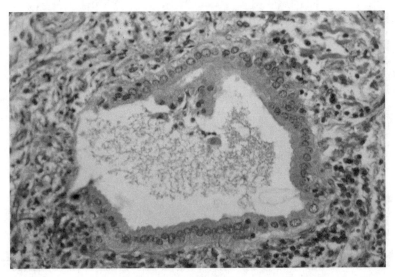

Fig. 14.4   Stage 1 florid bile duct lesion. The epithelial cell lining of a small duct is infiltrated with lymphocytes (H&E, ×930). See page xvii.

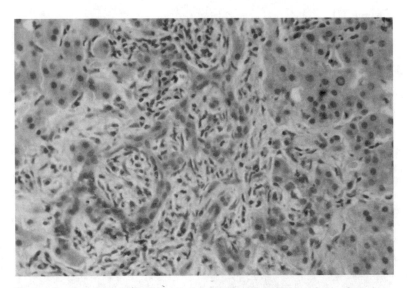

Fig. 14.5   Stage II primary biliary cirrhosis. Atypical bile duct hyperplasia is seen. There are tortuous bile ducts with inflammatory cell infiltrate consisting of primarily lymphocytes and few neutrophils (H&E, ×930). See page xviii.

> − a diminished number of bile ducts in an otherwise unremarkable appearing needle biopsy of the liver should alert one to the possibility of primary biliary cirrhosis

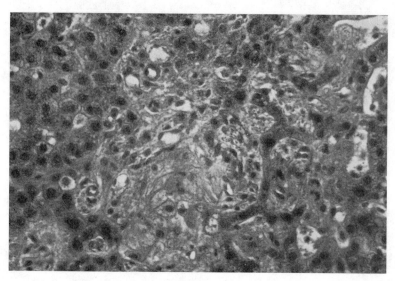

Fig. 14.6   Stage II primary biliary cirrhosis. There are no recognizable bile ducts in this portal triad (Masson trichrome, ×930). See page xviii.

- **stage III**
    - similar to stage II except that fibrous septa extend beyond triads and form portal-to-portal bridges (Fig. 14.7, see plate section)
- **stage IV**
    - represents the end stage of the lesion, with frank cirrhosis and regenerative nodules (Fig. 14.8, see plate section)

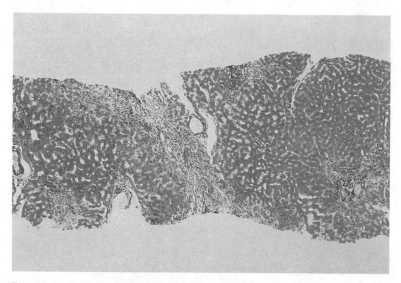

Fig. 14.7   Stage III primary biliary cirrhosis. Portal-to-portal fibrous septum is shown (Masson trichrome, ×162). See page xix.

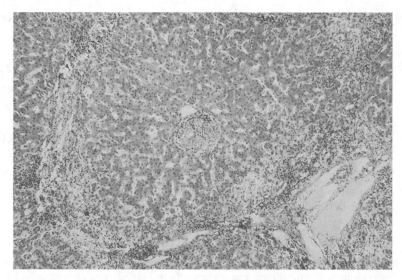

Fig. 14.8   Stage IV primary biliary cirrhosis. There is a noncaseating granuloma in the center of a nodule. Portal triads are linked by bands of connective tissue and inflammatory cells. (Masson trichrome, ×162). See page xix.

     – the findings may be indistinguishable from other types of cirrhosis. However, **a paucity of normal bile ducts in areas of scarring should alert one to the possibility of PBC**

4   Clinical Features

A   Symptoms

- about 48–60% of patients are asymptomatic at the time of diagnosis
- the signs and symptoms of PBC are due to long-standing cholestasis

1   Fatigue

- most common symptom
- noted up to 78% of patients at presentation
- nonspecific and not always recognized as a symptom of PBC

2   Pruritus

- etiology is unknown. Itching is not due to retention of the naturally occurring primary and secondary bile acids but of another substance which is normally secreted into bile and which binds to cholestyramine and colestipol
- more recently, increased opioidergic tone related to chronic cholestasis has been suggested as a potential cause[6]
- the earliest specific complaint of PBC is pruritus; it is characteristically worse at bedtime
- pruritus may initially occur during the third trimester of pregnancy and persist after delivery

- it rarely resolves spontaneously until late-stage cirrhosis, when the only possible treatment is liver transplantation

3 Malabsorption

- impaired secretion of bile causes a diminished concentration of bile acids within the intestinal lumen. Bile acid concentration may fall below the critical micellar concentration and be inadequate for complete digestion and absorption of neutral triglycerides in the diet
- patients complain of nocturnal diarrhea, frothy, bulky stools, or weight loss in the face of a voracious appetite and increased caloric intake
- there may be malabsorption of the fat-soluble vitamins A, D, E and K, and calcium
- pancreatic insufficiency may also contribute to malabsorption. This is most likely to occur in patients with concomitant sicca syndrome

4 Osteoporosis

- osteopenic bone disease occurs in at least 25% of PBC patients. The pathogenesis is still unclear
- osteomalacia is uncommon and occurs only in home-bound patients who have advanced PBC and little exposure to sunlight
- clinical symptoms of osteoporosis:
  - bone pain
  - spontaneous collapse of vertebral bodies and hairline fractures of ribs
  - fractures of long bones are less common

B Physical examination

1 Findings may vary and depend on the stage of the disease; may be normal in asymptomatic patients
2 Hepatomegaly is found in approximately 70%
3 Splenomegaly is present in 35%
4 Skin abnormalities:
- increased skin pigmentation that resembles tanning is due to melanin, not bilirubin, in early-stage PBC
- excoriations may be diffuse due to intractable pruritus
- jaundice usually presents later in the course of the disease
- xanthelasma and xanthomata correlate with hypercholesterolemia. Xanthelasmas are more common than xanthomata (Fig. 14.9 and 14.10, see plate section)
  - approximately 10% of patients will eventually develop xanthomata
  - xanthomata are found on the palms of the hands and soles of the feet, over extensor surfaces of the elbows and knees, in tendons of the ankles and wrists, and on buttocks
5 Eyes: Kayser–Fleischer rings are rare and result from copper retention
6 End-stage PBC: spider telangiectases, temporal and proximal limb muscle wasting, ascites, and edema imply cirrhosis

C Natural history and prognosis

1 Asymptomatic patients have longer life expectancies than symptomatic patients

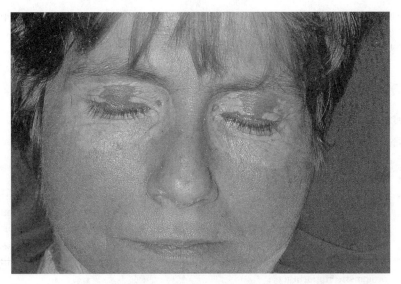

Fig. 14.9   Middle-aged woman with extensive bilateral xanthelasmas. See page xx.

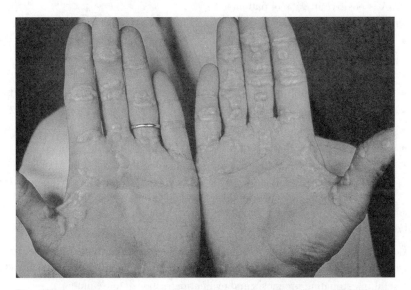

Fig. 14.10   Bilateral plantar xanthomas in the palms of a patient with PBC. See page xx.

2 Median survival for symptomatic patients ranges from 7½ to 10 years in different studies and is 7 years for histologic stages III and IV

3 Median survival of asymptomatic patients ranges from 10 to 16 years in various studies

4 Most asymptomatic patients develop symptoms, usually within 2–4 years

5 The presence or titer of AMA does not influence survival

6 Although virtually all published studies provide survival data, the more appropriate measurement today is "time of referral for liver transplantation". This can usually be estimated by subtracting 1–2 years from the number of years of survival

5 Diagnosis

A Laboratory tests

1 Liver function tests:
  - cholestatic pattern
  - biochemical tests are suggestive but rarely diagnostic of PBC
  - alkaline phosphatase and gamma glutamyltranspeptidase elevations are earliest abnormalities. These enzymes remain disproportionately elevated throughout the course of PBC, but the degree of elevation has little if any prognostic importance
  - serum aminotransferases are slightly elevated early in the course of the disease. They fluctuate at these levels during the course of disease and are also of little prognostic importance
  - serum bilirubin is usually normal early in the course, but becomes elevated as the disease progresses

2 AMA is positive in 95% of patients

3 Other associated findings:
  - serum albumin and prothrombin concentrations are normal in early stages and decreased in the late stage. Their decrease is a poor prognostic sign
  - elevated serum IgM
  - elevated cholesterol in at least 50% of patients
  - elevated high-density lipoproteins (HDL)
  - elevated hepatic and urinary copper
  - elevated serum ceruloplasmin
  - may be associated with hypothyroidism: elevated thyroid-stimulating hormone (TSH) is the best way to detect this. T4 levels may be factitiously normal because of increased serum concentrations of thyroid-binding globulin

B Liver biopsy

1 Confirms the diagnosis and provides an estimate of the duration of disease. In general, the more advanced the histologic stage, the longer the duration of disease

2 Useful in estimating prognosis and evaluating response to treatment

C Imaging tests

Useful to rule out bile duct obstruction

1 Ultrasound: noninvasive and usually adequate to rule out bile duct obstruction

2 Computed tomography in patients in whom ultrasound examination is technically not feasible

3 Endoscopic cholangiography: usually not needed except in AMA-negative patients in whom primary sclerosing cholangitis may be a possible diagnosis

D Diagnosis

1 Based on history, physical findings, blood tests, and liver biopsy

2 Primary biliary cirrhosis is likely if there are elevated alkaline phosphatase and serum IgM levels and positive antimitochondrial antibody

3 Diagnosis should be confirmed by liver biopsy in order to provide histologic staging and aid in prognosis

6 Treatment

A Management of symptoms of chronic cholestasis

1 Pruritus

- cholestryramine
  - the nonabsorbed resin will relieve pruritus in more than 90% of patients
  - therapy should be directed at symptomatic relief, with a usual dose of 4 g t.i.d.; best with meals
  - depending on the severity of cholestasis, it will take 1–4 days from the initiation of cholestyramine treatment before the itching remits
- antihistamines
  - occasionally helpful early in the course of PBC when itching is not severe; most likely acts by inducing sleep
- colestipol hydrochloride (ammonium resin)
  - as effective as cholestyramine and may be used in patients who find cholestyramine unpalatable. Some find colestipol equally unpalatable
- other antipruritogenic agents which may control itching in some patients (listed in order of suggested use):
  - ursodeoxycholic acid
  - phenobarbital
  - prednisone
  - cimetidine
  - rifampin
  - methyltestosterone
  - naloxone (opioid antagonist): based on recent data suggesting itching may be mediated by opioidergic neurotransmission
  - phototherapy with ultraviolet B light
  - large-volume plasmapheresis is almost always helpful but is inconvenient and expensive

2 Malabsorption of fat-soluble vitamins

- incidence is roughly proportional to the severity of cholestasis
- vitamins A, D, E, and K levels should be measured in jaundiced PBC patients; those with low levels should be treated

- treatment: vitamins should be administered orally as far apart from cholestyramine as possible, because it may bind and inhibit their absorption in the intestinal tract
  - oral vitamin K: 5 mg/day
  - vitamin A: 10,000–25,000 units/day
  - 25-OH vitamin D 20 μg t.i.w.; check serum levels of 25-OH vitamin D after several weeks
  - supplemental calcium
  - vitamin E: 400–1000 units/day

3 Steatorrhea

- treated by a low-fat diet supplemented with medium-chain triglycerides (MCT) to maintain a reasonable caloric intake
- most patients will tolerate 60 mL of MCT oil per day
- some patients with PBC and the sicca syndrome may have concomitant pancreatic insufficiency. This can be evaluated with the bentiromide test and treated with pancreatic replacement therapy
- PBC patients may develop iron-deficient anemia, reflecting unrecognized GI blood loss. Upper endoscopy is indicated to detect gastroesophageal varices or congestive gastropathy

4 Osteoporosis

- there is no effective medical treatment for the osteoporosis
- ineffective treatments: vitamin D, calcium, calcitonin, ursodeoxycholic acid
- proven treatment: liver transplantation has resulted in increased bone mineral density, but improvement is rarely noted until 1 year after transplantation. Bone mineral density decreases for up to 6 months after transplantation because of immunosuppression with glucocorticoids and physical inactivity

B Medical treatment of the underlying disease process (Table 14.1)

1 Corticosteroids

- do not alter the course of the disease and will accelerate the onset of osteoporosis
- bone thinning outweighs the transient improvement in serum enzyme tests

2 Azathioprine

- limited efficacy: safe but failed to improve biochemical tests or histology in prospective trials

Ineffective and/or toxic	Promising/in trial
Glucocorticoids	Colchicine
Azathioprine	Ursodeoxycholic acid (ursodiol)
D-Penicillamine	Methotrexate
Chlorambucil	
Cyclosporine	

(Table 14.1: Drug treatment of PBC)

3   D-Penicillamine

- a cupriuretic agent with some anti-inflammatory actions
- ineffective
- associated with greater than 25% frequency of toxic side effects in PBC patients

4   Chlorambucil

- improved bilirubin, albumin, IgM, and IgG and appeared to decrease hepatic inflammation in a short-term pilot study
- bone marrow toxicity and the risk of an untreatable type of leukemia with chronic usage preclude its prolonged use

5   Colchicine

- colchicine (oral 0.6 mg b.i.d.) has been evaluated in five prospective double-blind trials in PBC; three compared it with placebo, one with placebo and ursodeoxycholic acid, and one (in progress) with methotrexate
- there was significant improvement in bilirubin, albumin, alkaline phosphatase, cholesterol, alanine aminotransferase (ALT), and aspartate aminotransferase (AST) levels and survival in one study; improvement in ALT, AST, and alkaline phosphatase in two studies; and lesser improvements in these parameters in two studies. Biochemical improvement was less striking with colchicine than ursodeoxycholic acid or methotrexate
- diarrhea occurred in about 10% of patients; this cleared with lowering the dose from 0.6 mg b.i.d. to 0.6 mg q.d.
- there was no improvement in histology and symptoms
- a meta-analysis of the first three published studies indicates that colchicine decreases mortality due to liver failure
- colchicine is not a cure, but seems to slow the rate of progression

6   Ursodeoxycholic acid

- in four controlled trials, ursodeoxycholic acid (ursodiol), 12–15 mg/kg body weight/day orally, improved the serum bilirubin, alkaline phosphatase, aminotransferase, and IgM levels
- in some studies, it decreased pruritus and prolonged the time before clinical deterioration and referral for liver transplantation
- when data were pooled in three of these studies, ursodiol clearly prolonged the time before liver transplantation was required compared with placebo, but the improvement was modest, an increase from a mean of 3.45 years to 3.66 years until referral for liver transplantation
- in a fourth, multicenter study done in the USA, efficacy was limited to a subgroup of patients with stage I and II disease whose initial serum bilirubin level was less than 2 mg/dL
- preliminary data suggest an additive effect if ursodiol is used together with colchicine
- it is safe and well tolerated

7   Cyclosporine

- initial report of improved biochemical tests and symptoms and stabilization of liver histology was not confirmed in a subsequent 6-year 349-patient multicenter European study

- there was no effect on survival until the Cox multihazards correction method was used. The survival benefit was modest and less than that observed with azathioprine. Symptoms and histology were minimally improved
- side effects: hypertension and impaired renal function are common
- not used alone as treatment for PBC at this time

8 Methotrexate

- In a pilot study, low-dose oral pulse methotrexate has improved symptoms, biochemical tests, and histology.
- however, interstitial pneumonitis occurred in approximately 15% of patients with PBC, an incidence higher than that observed in rheumatoid arthritis patients (3–5%) and much higher than that seen in patients with psoriasis and malignancies. Symptomatic pneumonitis responds rapidly to cessation of methotrexate and starting corticosteroids
- in one recent study the efficacy of the combination of ursodiol plus methotrexate in a group of PBC patients was compared with that of an earlier group of patients who had received ursodiol alone. There was no added beneficial effect of methotrexate
- in two other studies, methotrexate was added to ursodiol only in patients whose blood tests had not normalized on ursodiol alone. In these studies, the effect of methotrexate was clearly additive to that of ursodiol
- we have now observed normalization of symptoms, blood tests and, most importantly, liver histology in some precirrhotic PBC patients in response to methotrexate alone or methotrexate combined with ursodiol and colchicine. Our recent data suggest that PBC may be effectively treated with the combination of these drugs and that the disease may go into remission if these drugs are used judiciously. It is important that drug use and dose be titrated in individual patients. This is done by monitoring the response of liver function tests and liver histology in individual patients

9 Conclusions

- diverse approach to the medical therapy reflects lack of understanding of pathogenesis of PBC

- although no medical therapy has been proven to alter the natural history of PBC, the benefit–risk ratio of ursodiol, methotrexate, and colchicine appears to be more favorable than that of the alternative, no treatment (with eventual referral to liver transplantation)

- studies evaluating the efficacy of combination agents such as ursodiol, colchicine and methotrexate, and cyclosporine and tacrolimus are in progress (Figure 14.11).

C Liver transplantation

1 Patients with end-stage PBC are excellent candidates for liver transplantation. End-stage PBC is defined as cirrhosis complicated by:

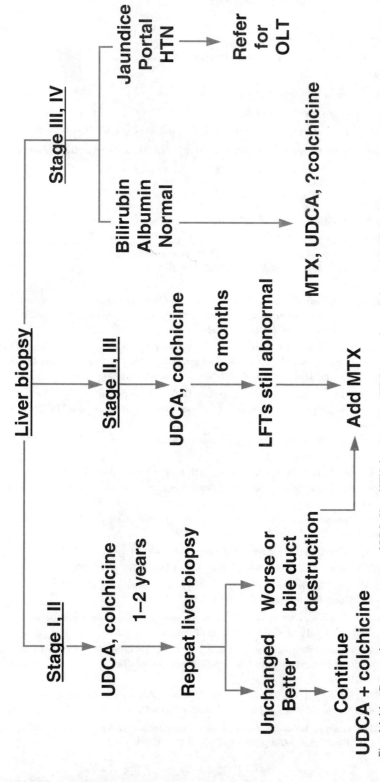

Fig. 14.11   Proposed treatment strategy of PBC. Key: HTN, hypertension; UDCA, ursodeoxycholic acid; LFT, liver function test; MTX, methotrexate; OLT, orthotopic liver transplantation

- gastroesophageal variceal hemorrhage
- intractable ascites
- hepatic encephalopathy
- severe osteoporosis with spontaneous bone fractures
- cachexia
- serum albumin less then 2.8 g/dL
- serum bilirubin greater than 10 mg/dL

2 One-year survival after transplantation in PBC patients is 85–90%

3 With adequate immunosuppression, recurrence of PBC after liver transplantation is rare

References

1 Kaplan MM, Rabson AR, Lee Y-M, Williams DL, Montaperto PA. *Discordant occurrence of primary biliary cirrhosis in monozygotic twins.* (N Engl J Med 1994) 331: 952

2 Underhill J, Donaldson P, Bray G, Doherty D, Portmann B, Williams R. *Susceptibility to primary cirrhosis is associated with the HLA-DR8-DQB1*0402 haplotype.* (Hepatology 1992) 16: 1404–8

3 Van de Water J, Turchany J, Leung PS et al. *Molecular mimicry in primary biliary cirrhosis: evidence for biliary epithelial expression of a molecule cross with pyruvate dehydrogenase complex-E2.* (J Clin Invest 1993) 91: 2653–64

4 Tsuneyama K, Van de Water J, Leung PS et al. *Abnormal expression of E2 component of the pyruvate dehydrogenase complex on the luminal surface of biliary epithelium occurs before major histocompatibility complex class II and BB1/B7 expression.* (Hepatology 1995) 21: 1031–7

5 Colina F, Pinedo F, Solis JA, Moreno D, Nevado M. *Nodular regenerative hyperplasia of the liver in early histological stages of primary biliary cirrhosis.* (Gastroenterology 1992) 102: 1319–24

6 Jones EA, Bergasa NV. *The pruritus of cholestasis: from bile acids to opiate agonists.* (Hepatology 1990) 11: 884–7

7 Balasubramaniam K, Grambsch PM, Wiesner RH, Lindor KD, Dickson ER. *Diminished survival in asymptomatic primary biliary cirrhosis: a prospective study.* (Gastroenterology 1990) 98: 1567–71

8 Dickson ER, Fleming TR, Wiesner RH, et al. *Trial of penicillamine in advanced primary biliary cirrhosis.* (N Engl J Med 1985) 312: 1011–15

9 James OFW. *D-Penicillamine for primary biliary cirrhosis.* (Gut 1985) 26: 109–13

10 Kaplan MM. *Primary biliary cirrhosis.* (N Engl J Med 1996) 335: 1570–80

11 Kaplan MM, Knox TA. *Treatment of primary biliary cirrhosis with low-dose weekly methotrexate.* (Gastroenterology 1991) 101: 1332–8

12 Kaplan MM, Alling DW, Zimmerman HJ, et al. *A prospective trial of colchicine for primary biliary cirrhosis.* (N Engl J Med 1986) 315: 1448–54

13 Lombard M, Portmann B, Neuberger J, et al. *Cyclosporine A treatment in primary biliary cirrhosis: results of a long-term placebo controlled trial and effect on survival.* (Gastroenterology 1993) 104: 519–26

14 Markus BH, Dickson ER, Grambsch PM, et al. *Efficacy of liver transplantation in patients with primary biliary cirrhosis.* (N Engl J Med 1989) 320: 1709–13

15 Poupon RE, Poupon R, Balkau B. *Ursodiol for the long term treatment of primary biliary cirrhosis: UDCA-PBC Study Group.* (N Engl J Med 1994) 330: 1342–7

Primary sclerosing cholangitis

RUSSELL H. WIESNER, M.D.

Key Points

1 Primary sclerosing cholangitis (PSC) is a chronic cholestatic disease which occurs most commonly in middle-age males and is frequently found in association with inflammatory bowel disease, most commonly ulcerative colitis

2 The diagnosis of PSC is based on clinical, biochemical, and most importantly, cholangiographic findings. The exclusion of identifiable causes of secondary sclerosing cholangitis is important

3 Diagnosis is often made on the basis of a cholestatic biochemical profile found in a patient with long-standing ulcerative colitis. The gradual onset of progressive fatigue and pruritus followed by jaundice represents the most frequent symptom complex which leads to the diagnosis

4 The etiology of PSC remains unknown, but evolving evidence points to autoimmune mechanisms

5 PSC is usually slowly progressive, leading to significant complications, some of which are specific to the syndrome, such as formation of dominant biliary strictures, choledocholithiasis, and cholangiocarcinoma. Several survival models have been formulated which can be used to estimate survival for the individual patient

6 Medical approaches to the treatment of PSC have focused principally on the use of cuprruretic, antifibrogenic, immunosuppressive, and choleretic agents. To date, none of these therapies has been shown to have a major impact on survival or the prevention of complications

7 Surgical therapy includes biliary tract reconstruction and proctocolectomy for ulcerative colitis. Neither of these procedures has been shown to halt the progression of PSC. Indeed, these procedures have been associated with increased morbidity and mortality in patients undergoing liver transplantation. The results of liver transplantation have been quite good with 5-year survival rates of 75–80%. Recurrence of PSC after liver transplantation has been described but appears to be infrequent and often clinically insignificant

1   Overview

- primary sclerosing cholangitis (PSC) is a chronic cholestatic liver disease characterized by fibrosing inflammation of both the intrahepatic and extrahepatic biliary tree
- the histopathologic evolution of PSC results in irreversible damage to the bile ducts, which ultimately leads to cholestasis, cirrhosis, liver failure, and premature death from liver failure unless liver transplantation is performed
- long-term follow-up of patients with PSC has revealed a high incidence of colon and bile duct cancers, both of which are likely to be related to chronic inflammation of the colon and bile ducts
- although several medical and surgical therapies have been evaluated for PSC, there is currently no therapy which achieves a complete clinical, biochemical, and histologic remission. Liver transplantation continues to be an important therapeutic intervention for the management of patients with end-stage PSC

2   Terminology and Diagnostic Criteria

- the term "primary sclerosing cholangitis" implies that the syndrome is idiopathic and distinguishes this entity from secondary sclerosing cholangitis resulting from identifiable causes (see Table 15.1)
- cholestatic biochemical profile (alkaline phosphatase level >1.5 times the upper limits of normal for 6 months)
- **cholangiographic findings** of irregularity of the intrahepatic and extrahepatic biliary tree. **This is the most important finding for the diagnosis of PSC**
- a liver biopsy compatible with the diagnosis of PSC and excluding other etiologies of chronic liver disease
- exclusion of secondary sclerosing cholangitis

	Primary	**Secondary**
Clinical setting	With or without inflammatory bowel disease	Biliary surgery Choledocholithiasis Trauma Ischemia Chemical therapy Infectious agents Congenital anomalies AIDS Malignancy Idiopathic adulthood ductopenia Amyloidosis
Ducts involved	Intrahepatic and extrahepatic ("classic" or global) Intrahepatic (small duct) Extrahepatic (large duct)	Perihilar and extrahepatic

(Table 15.1: Primary versus secondary sclerosing cholangitis)

3   Clinical Features and Presentation

- PSC is predominantly a disease of middle-age males; approximately 67% of patients are male, with a mean age of approximately 40 years at the time of diagnosis. There are no known race predilections
- PSC usually presents insidiously and in a variety of ways.

Modes of clinical presentation
- asymptomatic with abnormal liver tests
- pruritus, fatigue, jaundice
- recurrent cholangitis
- complications of chronic liver disease
- incidental discovery at laparotomy

Table 15.2 shows the frequency of signs and symptoms at the time of diagnosis of PSC, while Table 15.3 shows the frequency of abnormal biochemical tests at diagnosis

- histologic findings: virtually all patients have histologic abnormalities on liver biopsy. The main features include periductal fibrosis, inflammation, and bile duct proliferation alternating with ductal obliteration and ductopenia.

Table 15.4 shows the Ludwig staging system for classifying the severity of PSC

- radiologic features
  - widespread use of endoscopic and transhepatic cholangiography has been the major reason for the increased frequency of the diagnosis of PSC

Symptoms	Frequency (%)
Fatigue	75
Pruritus	70
Jaundice	65
Weight loss	40
Fever	35
Signs	**Frequency (%)**
Hepatomegaly	55
Jaundice	50
Splenomegaly	30
Hyperpigmentation	25
Xanthomas	4

(Table 15.2: Symptoms and signs of PSC diagnosis)

Test	Patients with abnormal results (%)
Serum alkaline phosphatase	99
Serum aminotransferase	95
Serum bilirubin	65
Serum albumin	20
Prothrombin time	10
Serum copper	50
Serum ceruloplasmin	75
Urine copper	65

(Table 15.3: Biochemical tests at diagnosis)

Stage I – portal stage	Portal hepatitis, bile duct abnormalities, or both; fibrosis or edema may be present; abnormalities do not extend beyond limiting plate
Stage II – periportal stage	Periportal fibrosis with or without inflammation extending beyond the limiting plate; piecemeal necrosis may be present
Stage III – septal stage	Septal fibrosis, bridging necrosis, or both
Stage IV – cirrhotic stage	Biliary cirrhosis

(Table 15.4: Ludwig staging system)

– the radiologic features most commonly seen in PSC include **1** diffusely distributed multifocal annular strictures with intervening segments of normal or slightly ectatic ducts; **2** short band-like strictures, and **3** diverticulum-like outpouchings

4 Associated Diseases

A variety of diseases are associated with PSC. Inflammatory bowel disease is the most common and most important of these:

Diseases associated with PSC
- inflammatory bowel disease
- celiac sprue
- sarcoidosis
- chronic pancreatitis
- rheumatoid arthritis
- retroperitoneal fibrosis
- thyroiditis
- Sjögren's syndrome
- autoimmune hepatitis
- systemic sclerosis
- lupus erythematosus
- vasculitis
- Peyronie's disease
- membranous nephropathy
- bronchiectasis
- autoimmune hemolytic anemia
- immune thrombocytopenic purpura
- histiocytosis X
- cystic fibrosis
- eosinophilia

Primary sclerosing cholangitis is associated with inflammatory bowel disease in over 75% of cases

1 The diagnosis of inflammatory bowel disease usually precedes that of PSC; however, PSC may occur prior to the diagnosis of inflammatory bowel disease or it can occur years following proctocolectomy. Furthermore, inflammatory bowel disease can develop following liver transplantation for PSC
2 No difference has been found in the course or severity of PSC with or without inflammatory bowel disease
3 Inflammatory bowel disease is usually quiescent and mild but at times can be severe, and a proctocolectomy may be required

5 Etiopathogenesis

The cause of PSC is unknown; genetic factors, acquired factors, or both may be involved in the etiology

Potential etiopathogenic factors
- portal bacteremia
- absorbed colon toxins
- toxic bile acids
- copper toxicity
- viral infection
- genetic predisposition
- immunologic mechanisms
- ischemic arteriolar injury

Currently, the pathogenesis of PSC is felt to be most closely linked to alterations in immune mechanisms:

- PSC is associated with other diseases thought to be of an autoimmune etiology, such as chronic ulcerative colitis and celiac sprue
- PSC is associated with human leukocyte antigen (HLA)-B8 and HLA-DR3, which are frequently noted in other autoimmune diseases
- immunologic abnormalities found in patients with PSC include elevated IgM levels, circulating immune complexes, decreased clearance of immune complexes, increased complement metabolism, enhanced autoreactivity of suppressor/cytotoxic T lymphocytes from peripheral blood, and expression of HLA class II antigens on biliary epithelial cells

The most likely scenario for the etiopathogenesis of PSC involves exposure of a genetically predisposed individual to an acute insult to the biliary system, perhaps a transient viral infection. It is proposed that an alteration in the bile ducts marks them as foreign and leads to destruction by autoimmune mechanisms

6 Natural History

- PSC is most often a slowly progressive disease
- in a study of 174 patients with a follow-up of 6 years, the median survival from the time of diagnosis was 11.9 years
- of a subgroup of 45 patients with PSC who were asymptomatic at the time of diagnosis and were followed for a mean of 6.25 years, 76% experienced progression of liver disease based on clinical and pathologic findings, and 31% developed liver failure
- by establishing the natural history of PSC we have been able to utilize the Cox multivariate regression analysis to develop a prognostic model based on four independent variables (see Table 15.5), estimate survival for an individual with PSC at any time during the course of the disease (see Fig. 15.1), and determine accurately the rate of disease progression

These models have been used to help in the selection and timing of liver transplantation in patients with PSC

| Serum bilirubin level |
| Histologic stage |
| Patient age |
| Splenomegaly |

(Table 15.5: Independent variables associated with survival in patients with PSC)

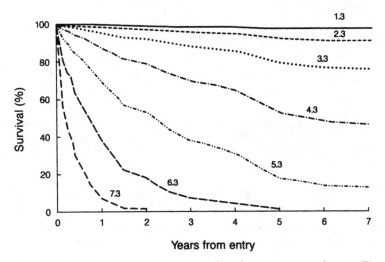

Fig. 15.1   Estimated survival for patients based on increasing risk score (R)
R = 0.535 × log [bilirubin (mg/dL)]
+ 0.486 × histologic stage
+ 0.041 × age (years)
+ 0.705 (if splenomegaly is present)

We have used these models to demonstrate that liver transplantation is indeed associated with prolonged survival in patients with end-stage disease

7   Complications

A   Complications related to liver failure and portal hypertension

1 The end stages of PSC are frequently associated with complications of portal hypertension:

- esophageal variceal bleeding
- peristomal variceal bleeding
- ascites
- spontaneous bacterial peritonitis
- portosystemic encephalopathy

2 Complications of portal hypertension are not specific to PSC, with the exception of bleeding from peristomal varices in patients who have undergone a proctocolectomy for underlying inflammatory bowel disease and who have an ileal stoma

3 Bleeding from peristomal varices can be controlled by a surgical portosystemic shunt or in some instances by a transjugular intrahepatic portosystemic shunt. Complications of peristomal variceal bleeding can be prevented by performing an ileoanal anastomotic surgical procedure in patients with PSC who need a proctocolectomy for chronic ulcerative colitis. With this procedure the formation of an ileal stoma is avoided

B   Complications of chronic cholestasis

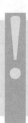

- fatigue
- pruritus
- steatorrhea
- fat-soluble vitamin deficiency (A, D, E, and K)
- metabolic bone disease

1 Fatigue and pruritus are the most common symptoms of PSC and can be quite debilitating and lead to a diminished quality of life

2 Steatorrhea associated with fat-soluble vitamin deficiency has also been described and is felt to be related to a decrease in the duodenal concentration of bile acids and thus a decrease in micellar formation

3 In patients with PSC, steatorrhea can be caused by concurrent conditions such as chronic pancreatitis and celiac disease

4 Fat-soluble vitamin deficiency, including deficiencies of vitamin A, D, E, and K, can be seen generally in patients who are jaundiced and have cirrhotic-stage disease

5 Metabolic bone disease, namely osteoporosis, occurs in approximately 50% of patients, who are at increased risk for nontraumatic fractures

6 Patients who have bone mineral densities below the fracture threshold frequently suffer compression fractures of trabecular bone

C   Complications specific to PSC

- bacterial cholangitis
- biliary stone disease
- dominant stricture
- cholangiocarcinoma

1 Bacterial cholangitis frequently occurs in patients who have had a previous biliary surgical procedure and who have an obstructing dominant stricture

2 Gallbladder and biliary stones are found in approximately 30% of patients with PSC sometime during the course of the disease

3 Approximately 20% of patients develop an obstructing dominant stricture of the biliary tree

4 The most common site for a dominant stricture is in the biliary hilum; however, strictures can occur in the common bile duct and common hepatic duct. In such cases, surgical reconstructive procedures should be avoided and balloon dilatation should be attempted either via an endoscopic or percutaneous route

5 Long-term follow-up studies have shown that cholangiocarcinoma may develop in up to 30% of patients with long-standing PSC. **We consider PSC a premalignant condition of the biliary tree just as chronic ulcerative colitis is a premalignant condition of the colon**

6 Bile duct carcinomas have been difficult to diagnose in patients with PSC since there are no serologic markers and biliary cytology has been insensitive for the early diagnosis of cholangiocarcinoma

7 Reports suggest that measuring serum CA 19-9 levels may be helpful in diagnosing cholangiocarcinoma in patients with PSC. Further studies to evaluate the specificity and sensitivity as a screening marker for cholangiocarcinoma are needed

8 Treatment

Management goals

- relieve symptoms
- prevent or treat complications
- halt progression of disease
- optimize timing of liver transplantation

A Management of symptoms related to chronic cholestasis (see also Ch. 14)

1 Pruritus occurs commonly in patients with PSC and can lead to a diminished quality of life. Therapeutic options for pruritus include:
- cholestyramine
- activated charcoal
- phenobarbital
- rifampin
- opiate antagonists (naloxone)
- plasmapheresis
- charcoal hemoperfusion

2 Patients with fat-soluble vitamin deficiency should be treated with replacement therapy

3 Osteoporosis – no effective therapy known; correct vitamin deficiency if it exists, administer supplemental calcium, and give estrogens to postmenopausal women

B Complications specific to PSC

1 Bacterial cholangitis – treat with broad-spectrum i.v. antibiotics. Prophylactic

therapy with ciprofloxacin, which achieves high biliary concentrations, is often effective

2 A dominant stricture which is associated with the recent onset of symptoms, including jaundice, pruritus, and bacterial cholangitis, should be treated endoscopically or radiologically with balloon dilatation. In all cases, biliary cytology and brush cytology should be obtained to attempt to exclude cholangiocarcinoma. Long-term stenting is often necessary

3 Cholangiocarcinoma carries a poor prognosis and responds poorly to chemotherapy or radiation therapy. Many liver transplant programs consider cholangiocarcinoma associated with PSC to be an absolute or relative contraindication to liver transplantation

C Management of complications of portal hypertension

1 Variceal bleeding is best treated with sclerotherapy or banding

2 A surgical shunt should be avoided in patients with Child's B or C cirrhosis. A transjugular intrahepatic portosystemic shunt (TIPS) should be considered in these patients as a bridge to liver transplantation

3 Management of ascites and encephalopathy are similar to that utilized for patients with other types of end-stage liver diseases (see Chs 9–13)

D Specific therapy aimed at retarding disease progression

A number of medical, radiologic, endoscopic, and surgical therapies have been utilized in an attempt to halt the progression of PSC:

1 **Medical**
   a Supportive
   b Possible definitive treatment
      • cupruretic
        – penicillamine
      • antifibrogenic
        – colchicine
      • immunosuppressive
        – prednisone
        – azathioprine
        – cyclosporine
        – methotrexate
        – choleretic
        – ursodeoxycholic acid

2 **Radiologic/endoscopic**
   • cholangioplasty

3 **Surgical**
   • reconstructive biliary tract

- procedures
- proctocolectomy
- liver transplantation

1 Overall medical therapy has been disappointing and controlled clinical trials evaluating D-penicillamine, cyclosporine, methotrexate, colchicine, and ursodeoxycholic acid have all failed to show a beneficial effect on disease progression on the basis of clinical, biochemical, radiological, histological, and survival parameters

2 While endoscopic and radiologic therapy have been demonstrated to improve jaundice and to relieve bacterial cholangitis, a long-term benefit of halting disease progression has never been demonstrated

3 Biliary reconstructive surgical procedures likewise have also been shown to relieve symptoms and have the advantage of excluding cholangiocarcinoma. However, a long-term impact on delaying disease progression has not been shown

4 Biliary reconstructive surgery has been associated with increased morbidity in liver transplantation

5 Proctocolectomy, while indicated for patients who have severe symptoms related to inflammatory bowel disease or who have colon cancer or dysplastic lesions, does not improve or prevent progression of PSC

6 Liver transplantation is currently the treatment of choice for patients with end-stage primary sclerosing cholangitis

7 Recent results of liver transplantation in PSC have shown patient survival rates of up to 90% at 1 year and 75% at 5 years

8 Recurrence of PSC most likely occurs in 15–20% of patients following liver transplantation. However, the diagnosis of recurrent PSC is difficult because of the lack of a gold standard diagnostic criterion. Indeed, there are a number of other factors, such as use of a Roux-en-Y bile duct anastomosis, chronic rejection, cytomegalovirus infection, and prolonged ischemia time, which have been implicated in bile duct stricturing after transplantation

References

1 Broome U, Lofberg R, Veress B, Eriksson LS. *Primary sclerosing cholangitis and ulcerative colitis: rvidence for increased neoplastic potential.* (Hepatology 1995) 22: 1404–8

2 Lee Y-M, Kaplan MM. *Primary sclerosing cholangitis.* (N Engl J Med 1995) 332: 924–37

3 Ramage JK, Donaghy A, Farrant JM, et al. *Serum tumor markers for the diagnosis of cholangiocarcinoma in primary sclerosing cholangitis.* (Gastroenterology 1995) 108: 805–9

4 Wiesner RH. *Primary sclerosing cholangitis.* In: Schiff L, Schiff ER (eds). *Diseases of the Liver*, 7th edn, Vol. 1. (Philadelphia: Lippincott, 1993) 411–26

5 Wiesner RH. *Current concepts in primary sclerosing cholangitis.* (Mayo Clin Proc 1994) 69: 969–82

6 Wiesner RH, Porayko MK, Hay JE, et al. *Liver transplantation for primary sclerosing cholangitis: impact of risk factors on outcome.* (Liver Transplant Surg 1996) 5 Suppl.: 99–108

Hemochromatosis

KRIS V. KOWDLEY, M.D., F.A.C.P.
ANTHONY S. TAVILL, M.D., F.R.C.P., F.A.C.P.

Key Points

1 Hereditary hemochromatosis is a common disorder, with a prevalence of up to 1/250–300 in persons of northern European descent

2 The disease is often unrecognized and diagnosed only in the setting of advanced disease

3 Patients detected early and treated with iron reduction therapy can have a normal life expectancy

4 Patients who have cirrhosis are at a significantly increased risk for hepatocellular carcinoma; patients undergoing liver transplantation for hereditary hemochromatosis have an increased risk of mortality due to cardiac and infectious complications

5 Screening for hemochromatosis is cost effective and relatively inexpensive; suspected cases should be confirmed with liver biopsy and measurement of liver iron concentration

1 Genetics

A Overview

1 There is an increased frequency of hereditary hemochromatosis (HHC) in persons with human leukocyte antigen **HLA A3** (75% in HHC patients versus 25% in the general population); the A3,B7 and A3,B14 haplotypes are the most commonly associated with HHC

2 HLA A and B haplotype linkage has been used to establish **autosomal recessive inheritance**

3 Siblings who share one HLA haplotype with the proband are putative heterozygotes

4 Siblings who share both HLA haplotypes are putative homozygotes (Fig. 16.1). Heterozygotes may have elevated indirect iron markers but not clinically significant iron overload

5 **Recently, a major histocompatibility complex class I-like gene which is mutated in patients with HHC has been identified. The mutation in homozygous form was present in ~85% of HHC patients (HFE gene)**

B Prevalence

1 **HHC is the most common genetic disease in white persons of northern European descent. The approximate prevalence of homozygotes is 1 : 300. The carrier rate is estimated at 1 in 10–12 of the white population**

2 The gene prevalence is estimated to be 0.05%

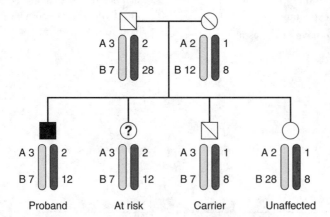

Fig. 16.1   HLA linkage for gene tracking in pedigrees with hemochromatosis. In this pedigree the hemochromatosis allele is carried on the HLA haplotypes A3,B7 and A2,B12; thus the sibling with an HLA type identical to the proband is also at risk of developing the disorder. The sibling sharing only one HLA haplotype with the proband is a putative carrier (Reproduced from Today's Life Science (1993) 5(1): 34–36, with permission)

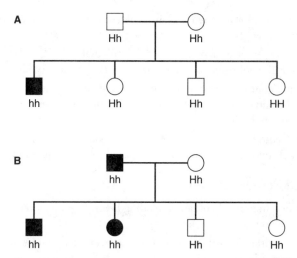

Fig. 16.2   Pattern of inheritance of hemochromatosis. H, normal allele; h, hemochromatosis allele; n, individuals with hemochromatosis. (a) Mendelian autosomal recessive mode of inheritance. (b) Apparent dominant mode of inheritance (Reproduced from Medicine International 84: 3496, by courtesy of The Medicine Group (Journals) Ltd)

3 Because of the high heterozygote prevalence, homozygote : heterozygote pairings may occur, leading to "pseudodominant" inheritance (Fig. 16.2)

4 The gene is present on the short arm of chromosome 6 telomeric to the HLA A3 locus

5 The major mutation of the HFE gene is the cys282tyr substitution

C   Relationship of genetic defect to metabolic abnormality

1 The basic defect leading to increased intestinal iron absorption in HHC is still unknown

2 It is unknown if the metabolic consequence of the gene defect is localized to the small bowel, although it is likely that the metabolic defect will have an impact on iron absorption and transport to the circulation (which normally occurs in the small bowel)

3 Ferritin function in small bowel and liver are apparently normal; however, ferritin synthesis is apparently defective in the enterocyte

4 There is some evidence that the carrier for nontransferrin bound iron may be abnormally delivered to its tissues

5 A primary hepatocyte defect is unlikely as the cause of iron overload in HHC.

6 Liver transplantation in HHC patients may help elucidate the site of the abnormality in iron overload; if hepatic iron overload does recur, then a primary intestinal mucosal defect is likely

2   Pathophysiology

A   Iron transport in HHC

1 Iron absorption is inappropriately high for dietary intake

2 The transferrin receptor in mucosa is upregulated and iron is transported across the intestinal mucosa into plasma at an increased rate

3 The transferrin receptor in hepatocytes is downregulated in HHC but is restored after iron removal, confirming that the alteration is a secondary phenomenon

4 Small bowel mucosal ferritin and ferritin mRNA levels are inappropriately decreased. This pattern is normally found in patients with iron deficiency and is corrected by iron repletion

5 In vivo kinetic studies indicate that increased transport of iron from the serosal side of intestinal cell into plasma drives the increased iron absorption in HHC

B   Parenchymal iron deposition in HHC

1 Iron is deposited in multiple organs including heart, liver, pancreas, joints, skin, gonads, and other endocrine organs

2 The major site of iron deposition in HHC is the liver, consistent with its role as the major storage organ for iron

3 Iron is deposited primarily in hepatocytes, with a decreasing gradient of iron deposition from periportal (zone 1) to pericentral (zone 3) hepatocytes

4 Late in the disease, iron may be deposited in Kupffer's cells and bile duct cells

5 Saturation of serum transferrin precedes hepatic iron accumulation and is responsible initially for increased iron delivery to the tissues

6 Later, nontransferrin-bound iron may play a role in iron delivery and toxicity

7 There is also a possible defect of iron storage in reticuloendothelial cells

Co-factors which may influence iron absorption and accumulation in HHC:

- vitamin C (ascorbic acid) intake
- amount of dietary iron
- bioavailability of dietary iron
- type of dietary iron (heme iron absorption > nonheme)
- gender: women have a lower degree of iron overload and express disease later than men because of menstrual blood loss, but they possess the abnormal genotype with equal frequency

C   Effect of alcohol intake in HHC

1 Earlier reports speculated that heavy alcohol intake alone could lead to hemochromatosis

2 Heavy alcohol intake alone is insufficient to lead to iron loading in the HHC range

3 Heterozygotes for HHC who drink heavily do not develop symptomatic iron overload, although serum iron markers (see below) are often elevated

4 Heavy alcohol intake may accelerate liver damage in homozygous HHC (damage occurs at an earlier age and at lower levels of hepatic iron)

D   Liver damage in HHC

1 Excess iron may mediate liver damage and/or promote liver fibrosis by a number of mechanisms:

- iron may catalyze the formation of free radicals that may damage cell organelles
- iron may directly damage DNA leading to mutations and carcinogenesis
- iron may directly lead to hepatic fibrosis by increasing collagen synthesis in response to lipid peroxidation

2 Liver disease in HHC is characterized by progressive fibrosis, but without significant inflammation

3 The presence of hepatitis (inflammatory changes) may suggest coexistent viral infection or alcoholic liver disease

4 Cirrhosis or hepatocellular carcinoma develops with long-standing iron overload

5 There is a correlation between elevated liver iron concentrations and fibrosis or cirrhosis

6 Fibrosis or cirrhosis is observed at >40 years in men and >50 years in women, and earlier if there is a significant pathogenetic co-factor (viral hepatitis or alcohol)

3   Clinical Features of HHC

1 The clinical presentation of patients with HHC has changed over the last several decades. Prior to 1960, patients were often seen with the classic presentation of "bronze diabetes," arthritis, liver disease, and cardiac failure. With increased awareness of the disease, patients are now frequently detected through laboratory testing while asymptomatic. Adams et al. (1991)[1] compared the presentation of patients seen between 1985 and 1995 with those seen between 1954 and 1985 and found the following differences:

- a greater proportion had no evidence of cirrhosis or diabetes
- fewer patients presented with liver disease
- more presented with arthritis, since joint involvement frequently is an early manifestation

2 The most common presenting symptoms in order of decreasing frequency:

- incidental diagnosis (unrelated to HHC) or serendipitous discovery of elevated serum iron markers
- chronic liver disease
- joint pains (arthritis)

3 The most common reasons that HHC is suspected:

- abnormal serum iron studies:
  - elevated serum transferrin iron saturation
  - elevated serum ferritin level
- hepatomegaly
- abnormal liver function tests (enzymes)
- iron studies and liver function tests ordered to evaluate abdominal pain

4 Symptoms

A Many patients are completely asymptomatic:

- 10% of males and 25% of females

B Common symptoms

- weakness and lassitude or fatigue
- joint symptoms (women > men)
- right upper quadrant pain, nonspecific in nature
- impotence (men)
- it is estimated that 43% of males and 28% of females may develop life-threatening symptoms

C Other symptoms and signs

- diabetes mellitus
- increased skin pigmentation
- shortness of breath
- amenorrhea (women)

D Liver disease

Progression of liver disease in HHC:

Fibrosis → cirrhosis → carcinoma

- increased frequencies of chronic viral hepatitis B and C have been reported in patients with HHC
- end-stage liver disease is a well-recognized complication
- increased mortality occurs in patients who also consume large quantities of alcohol
- HHC is associated with a 200-fold increased risk of hepatocellular carcinoma
- cirrhosis and hepatocellular carcinoma are associated with increased mortality and decreased life expectancy in HHC

E Cardiac disease

- restrictive cardiomyopathy has been described
- congestive heart failure and arrhythmias are common clinical manifestations
- endomyocardial biopsy may reveal evidence of iron overload
- major cause of morbidity associated with liver transplant action for HHC
- iron depletion prior to the development of dilated cardiomyopathy improves cardiac function

F   Diabetes mellitus

- probably due to iron deposition in the pancreas
- may often be associated with increased plasma insulin levels, suggesting peripheral insulin resistance

G   Joint disease

- chondrocalcinosis is associated with HHC joint disease
- degenerative arthritis and pseudogout are common manifestations
- a major cause of morbidity
- phlebotomy is unlikely to improve joint disease or clinical symptoms

H   Infections

Patients with HHC are reported to have an increased risk of bacterial and viral infections

1   Possibly increased risk of chronic hepatitis B and C
2   Uncommon bacterial infections associated with HHC:
- *Vibrio vulnifucus*
- *Yersinia enterocolitis*
- *Yersinia pseudotuberculosis*
- *Listeria monocytogenes*
3   Sepsis is a major cause of mortality after liver transplantation for HHC
4   Infections in HHC may be related to impaired phagocytosis and decreased free transferrin levels due to iron overload

5   Natural History and Prognosis

1   Liver disease in HHC is slowly progressive, but is usually mild when the hepatic iron concentration is < 200 µmol/g dry weight
2   Twenty-five percent of patients in early reports died of complications of liver disease
3   Significantly increased risk of hepatocellular carcinoma (200-fold increased risk) in patients with cirrhosis
4   Occasional cholangiocarcinomas may develop
5   Patients with cirrhosis at the time of diagnosis have a significantly decreased life expectancy
6   Patients without cirrhosis can expect a normal life expectancy if they are compliant with treatment
7   Liver transplantation for end-stage liver disease has had relatively disappointing results with only 50–60% 1-year survival rates

6   Diagnosis

A   Clinical suspicion and laboratory tests

1   suspect HHC in any individual with an unexplained elevation in serum ferritin levels or iron saturation

2 a transferrin saturation > 45 l warrants further evaluation for HHC

3 Consider HHC in patients with degenerative athropathy, type 2 diabetes, unexplained hepatomegaly or liver disease, or unexplained hypogonadism

B Liver biopsy

1 **Liver biopsy with determination of the hepatic iron concentration is the best method for establishing a definitive diagnosis**

2 Hepatic iron concentration can be measured in fresh, formalin-preserved, or paraffin-embedded tissue

3 A hepatic iron index > 1.9 is diagnostic (hepatic iron concentration in μmol/g ÷ age in years)

4 Hepatic iron stain is still important because sampling variability may yield a low hepatic iron index

5 Suggested strategy for diagnostic evaluation in liver tissue:

  a Perls' Prussian blue iron stain on half the core of tissue; if negative, iron overload is excluded

  b If positive, send remainder of tissue (fresh or preserved) for quantitative biochemical iron determination

6 Liver biopsy for staging disease:

- histopathology is the only reliable method of determining presence or absence of cirrhosis
- patients with cirrhosis have increased risk of mortality and hepatocellular carcinoma
- knowledge of the presence or absence of cirrhosis may influence management
- patients with cirrhosis need surveillance for hepatocellular carcinoma

C Genotyping

- After phenotypic confirmation of the diagnosis of HHC by liver biopsy, genotyping defines the homozygous mutation in the proband

7 Differential Diagnosis

Iron overload also can be the result of iron loading from increased red cell turnover, as in disorders of ineffective erythropoiesis, increased iron absorption (other than HHC), or a combination of increased red cell turnover and increased iron absorption. Secondary iron overload may also occur due to multiple repeated blood transfusions

A Other causes of iron overload due to increased iron absorption:

- a form of dietary iron overload due to consumption of beer brewed in steel drums has been described in South African blacks. Although this type of iron overload was initially felt to be due to increased iron consumption and absorption, recent studies indicate that these patients may have an inherited tendency towards iron loading

- homozygous beta thalassemia may be associated with increased iron loading due to blood transfusions and to increased iron absorption
- porphyria cutanea tarda (PCT) is a disorder of mild hepatic iron overload associated with defective uroporphyrinogen decarboxylase activity
- alcoholic liver disease is associated with mild hepatic iron overload
- post-shunt (portacaval) iron overload, or siderosis, may be observed. The mechanism for iron overload after portosystemic shunt surgery is unknown
- the amount of iron loading in PCT, alcoholic liver disease, and post-shunt siderosis is mild, with <5 g of storage iron

B   Hepatic iron index may be helpful in differentiating these disorders from HHC

However, measurement of hepatic iron concentration and hepatic iron index cannot distinguish HHC from transfusional iron overload

1   In early forms of secondary iron overload such as that due to blood transfusions, iron deposition is primarily noted in the Kupffer's cells and reticuloendothelial cells, with a paucity of iron in the hepatocytes. Furthermore, a periportal to pericentral "iron gradient" is not observed. Therefore, the hepatic iron stain can be helpful in distinguishing early forms of transfusional iron overload from hereditary hemochromatosis

2   Quantitative phlebotomy
- can be helpful when biopsy is not possible
- number of units of blood removed can estimate body iron stores
- each unit of 500 mL has approximately 250 mg of iron
- patients with HHC usually have >4 g of storage iron

C   Family members of HHC patients

1   25% prevalence of homozygosity in first-degree relatives of probands
2   Siblings who possess both HLA haplotypes identical to probands are presumed homozygotes. HFE gene can be determined to confirm homozygosity
3   Most homozygotes can be expected to express the disease and accumulate iron over their lifetimes; now defined as homozygosity for the HFE mutation

8   Treatment of Iron Overload in HHC

1   iron reduction by weekly phlebotomy achieves iron mobilization
2   phlebotomy is usually done weekly or biweekly until the serum ferritin is <50 ng/mL. The hematocrit should be checked at each session and the serum ferritin every 3 months
3   once iron stores have been mobilized, phlebotomy three to four times per year may be adequate
4   high doses of ascorbic acid should be avoided

5 moderate consumption of meats is permissible

6 alcohol should be avoided

7 chelation therapy is less effective, may have adverse side effects, and currently has to be administered parenterally

9 Family Screening

1 All first-degree relatives of homozygous HHC patients above age 20 years should be screened

2 Initial screening should include (fasting) serum iron (Fe), total iron binding capacity (TIBC) and serum ferritin

3 Homozygous men over 30 and women over 40 may demonstrate significantly increased body iron stores

4 The transferrin saturation may be increased at an early age, before the serum ferritin is elevated

5 Genotyping of a proband and family members may also be performed for family screening. Those who are identical to proband are (presumed) homozygotes

6 Liver biopsy should be strongly considered in such patients for diagnostic confirmation and to assess fibrosis

10 Population Screening

1 Several studies have demonstrated that screening is cost effective

- initial indirect screening should be performed with serum iron, TIBC, or unsaturated iron binding capacity (UIBC), a new inexpensive test of iron status
- serum Fe and TIBC should be repeated (fasting) along with serum ferritin, if initially elevated
- liver biopsy with iron staining and measurement of hepatic iron concentration and calculation of hepatic iron index should be performed when serum tests are suggestive of HHC to confirm diagnosis and to stage the disease. This is particularly relevant when the age of the individual makes target organ damage likely

2 Serum iron studies are unreliable in patients with evidence of liver disease

3 Hepatic iron measurement and calculation of the hepatic iron index is specific for HHC in patients with liver disease

4 The cost effectiveness of genotypic screening has not been evaluated; questionable since cys282tyr homozygotes do not invariably have phenotypic expression

References

1 Adams PC, Kertesz AE, Valberg LS. *Clinical presentation of hemochromatosis: a changing scene.* (Am J Med 1991) 90: 445–9

2 Adams PC, Valberg LS. *Evolving expression of hereditary hemochromatosis.* (Semin Liver Dis 1996) 16: 47–54

3 Bassett ML, Halliday JW, Ferris RA, Powell LW. *Diagnosis of hemochromatosis in young subjects: predictive accuracy of biochemical screening tests.* (Gastroenterology 1984) 87: 628–33

4 Bassett ML, Halliday JW, Powell LW. *Value of hepatic iron measurements in early hemochromatosis and determination of the critical iron level associated with fibrosis.* (Hepatology 1986) 6: 24–9

5 Deugnier YM, Guyader D, Crantock L, et al. *Primary liver cancer in genetic hemochromatosis: a clinical, pathological, and pathogenetic study of 54 cases.* (Gastroenterology 1993) 104: 228–34

6 Fargion S, Mandelli C, Piperno A, et al. *Survival and prognostic factors in 212 Italian patients with genetic hemochromatosis.* (Hepatology 1992) 15: 655–9

7 Niederau C, Fischer R, Sonnenberg A, Stremmel W, Trampisch HJ, Strohmeyer G. *Survival and causes of death in cirrhotic and in noncirrhotic patients with primary hemochromatosis.* (N Engl J Med 1985) 313: 1256–62

8 Niederau C, Stremmel W, Strohmeyer GWW. *Clinical spectrum and management of haemochromatosis.* (Baillìere's Clin Haematol 1994) 7: 881–901

9 Feder FN, Gnirke A, Thomas W, et al. *A novel MHC class-l-like gene is mutated in patients with hereditary hemochromatosis.* (Nature Genetics 1996) 14: 399–408

Wilson's disease and related disorders

WISAM F. ZAKKO, M.D.
JOHN L. GOLLAN, M.D., Ph.D.

▼

Key Points

1 The Wilson's disease (WD) gene is located on chromosome 13 and encodes a copper-transporting P-type ATPase protein.

2 Deficiency of the WD gene product is likely to be responsible for the lack of copper incorporation into ceruloplasmin and the defective biliary excretion of copper in WD.

3 The majority of symptomatic WD patients present with hepatic or neuropsychiatric features; the principal hepatic manifestations include fulminant hepatic failure, chronic hepatitis, and cirrhosis.

4 In patients with a low serum ceruloplasmin, diagnosis of WD in the absence of Kayser–Fleischer rings requires determination of hepatic copper concentration. Serum detection of radiocopper incorporation into ceruloplasmin may be a useful alternative test when liver biopsy is contraindicated

5 The use of DNA marker studies is limited largely to genetic screening of young family members or difficult diagnostic situations, using the index patient's DNA as a reference

▶

6 The drug of choice for treating WD patients is D-penicillamine, but alternatives under selected circumstances include trientine, zinc, or tetrathiomolybdate

7 Liver transplantation is indicated for patients with fulminant hepatitis or decompensated cirrhosis unresponsive to therapy

1 Copper Metabolism (see Figs. 17.1 and 17.2)

- dietary copper (1–2 mg/day) is actively transported into the proximal small intestinal epithelial cells
- a fraction (25–60%) is absorbed and transferred into the portal circulation bound to serum albumin. The remaining intraepithelial copper is bound to metallothioneins and is subsequently excreted when intestinal epithelial cells are sloughed
- it is likely that the Menke's gene (ATP7A) product plays an important role in copper absorption. Deficiency of the Menke's gene product in intestinal epithelial cells is believed to be the cause of the copper deficiency state responsible for the manifestations of Menke's disease

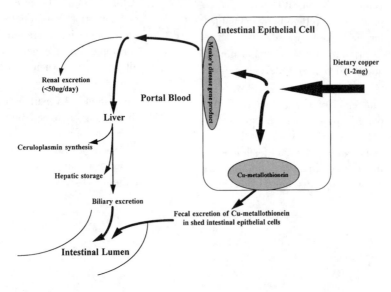

Fig. 17.1   Copper absorption and excretion. Dietary copper (1–2 mg/day) is transported into the intestinal epithelial cell, with the Menke's gene product regulating absorption (25–60%). The remaining intraepithelial copper is bound to metallothionein and is subsequently excreted in feces as the intestinal epithelial cells are sloughed. A small amount of the absorbed copper is excreted in urine, the majority is taken up by the hepatocyte and is either excreted in bile, synthesized into ceruloplasmin, or stored in the liver

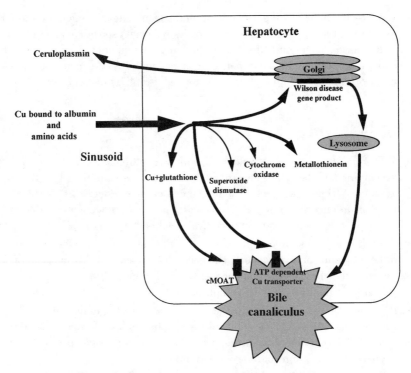

Fig. 17.2. Hepatocellular copper metabolism. Copper is taken up by hepatocytes, where it interacts with metallothionein and glutathione. A portion of the intracellular copper is incorporated into metalloenzymes, and some is transported into the Golgi apparatus by the WD gene product (ATP7B protein), where it is incorporated into ceruloplasmin. It is postulated that copper is also routed from the trans-Golgi apparatus to lysosomes for subsequent excretion in bile. Copper bound to glutathione is also excreted via the canalicular organic anion transporter (cMOAT), or by direct interaction with a postulated ATP-dependent copper transporter (adapted from Schilsky 1996[9])

- only a small fraction (<50 μg/24 h) of serum albumin-bound (nonceruloplasmin) copper is normally excreted by the kidney. The majority is taken up by hepatocytes via an undefined mechanism
- in the hepatocyte, copper is complexed with metallothioneins or glutathione and is utilized as a co-factor for specific cellular enzymes, incorporated into ceruloplasmin, or excreted in the bile. Metallothioneins and glutathione act as intracellular antioxidants and play an important role in copper detoxification
- present evidence based on the study of the Long–Evans Cinnamon rat, a rodent model of WD, suggests that the site of copper incorporation into ceruloplasmin may be the Golgi apparatus. It is speculated that the WD gene (ATP7B) product, which exhibits a subcellular localization to the trans-Golgi apparatus of liver cells, is responsible for copper transport in this compartment and subsequent incorporation into ceruloplasmin
- biliary excretion of copper occurs partly via a vesicular pathway involving lysosomes. Another, perhaps less important route of excretion, is as

copper–glutathione by the canalicular multispecific organic anion transporter (cMOAT). A third potential excretory pathway is via a specific copper transporter in the plasma membrane; the ATP7B protein is absent at the plasma membrane and the bile canaliculus, but there is evidence for an ATP-dependent copper-transporting system in the plasma membrane of rat liver distinct from cMOAT

2 Genetics

- WD is an autosomal recessive disease with a gene frequency of 0.3–0.7%, accounting for a heterozygote carrier rate of slightly greater than 1 in 100. In 1985 the WD gene was linked to the red cell enzyme, esterase D, establishing a location on **chromosome 13**. Using multipoint linkage techniques, the abnormal gene locus was more specifically defined as 13q14–q21
- the WD gene was subsequently isolated in 1993 using positional cloning by three different groups of investigators. The gene, designated ATP7B, spans an 80 kb region of the chromosome and encodes a 7.5 kb transcript that is expressed primarily in the liver, kidney, and placenta
- the gene product is a 1411 amino acid protein, a member of the cation-transporting P-type ATPase subfamily, and is highly homologous to the Menke's gene (ATP7A) product and the copper-transporting ATPase (cop A) found in copper-resistant strains of *Enterococcus hirae*
- over 40 mutations of the WD gene have been identified to date. The variety of mutations in the WD gene may affect copper transport to varying degrees and may explain the clinical diversity of the disease. Thus, patients with early-onset liver disease appear to be more likely to have mutations which would lead to absence of or a severely defective protein.
- while one normal allele is adequate to prevent clinical disease, heterozygotes for the WD gene may demonstrate subclinical abnormalities in copper metabolism.

3 Pathogenesis

- copper toxicity plays a primary role in the pathogenesis of this disorder. Affected organs invariably exhibit elevated copper levels, and reduction in the copper content results in improvement
- maintenance of normal copper homeostasis depends on the balance between gastrointestinal absorption and biliary excretion. Intestinal copper absorption in WD patients does not differ from that of normal or cirrhotic subjects
- **biliary excretion of copper is reduced in WD**. Studies in the Long–Evans Cinnamon (LEC) rat indicates a possible defect in the entry of copper into lysosomes, but with normal delivery of lysosomal copper to bile. It is suggested that copper transport into the trans-Golgi apparatus by the WD gene product may be essential for its routing and excretion via the lysosomal pathway
- **deficiency of the plasma copper protein ceruloplasmin is unlikely to have a role in the pathogenesis of WD**. Studies with LEC rats have demonstrated normal transcription and translation of ceruloplasmin RNA. It is

now believed that the low serum ceruloplasmin level is the result of a lack of incorporation of copper into apoceruloplasmin, which has a shorter half-life than the copper-bound ceruloplasmin.

- excess copper appears to exert toxic effects by the generation of free radicals, which result in lipid peroxidation, depletion of antioxidants, and polymerization of Cu-thionein. In favor of the role of copper as a pro-oxidant is the reduced hepatic content of antioxidants like glutathione and vitamin E, the rise in circulating levels of lipid peroxides, and decreased plasma levels of vitamin E in patients with untreated WD. Oxidant damage to the mitochondria, DNA, lysosomes and various enzymes and proteins takes place and may be accompanied by abnormal respiration of mitochondria and reduced activity of cytochrome oxidase. Morphologic changes have been identified, particularly in mitochondria

- pathologic copper deposition in the brain, particularly in the caudate nucleus and the putamen, results in the neurologic and psychiatric manifestations of the disease, while excessive deposition in Descemet's membrane of the cornea gives rise to Kayser–Fleischer rings.

4   Clinical Manifestations

Clinical symptoms are rarely observed before age 5 years. WD patients may be asymptomatic, although the majority present with hepatic or neurologic manifestations. In one large series the initial clinical manifestations were hepatic in 42%, neurologic in 34%, psychiatric in 10%, and hematologic in 12%. Less commonly, patients present with renal, skeletal, cardiac, ophthalmologic, endocrinologic, or dermatologic symptoms

A   Hepatic

Clinical hepatic manifestations tend to occur at a younger age (mean, 8–12 years) than neurologic manifestations. Three major patterns may occur: cirrhosis, chronic hepatitis or fulminant hepatic failure

1 Cirrhosis
- early in the course, there may be minimal or no symptoms with near normal liver function tests
- later there is an insidious but relentless progression to cirrhosis, which may be associated with fatigue, anorexia, jaundice, ascites, and variceal bleeding

2 Chronic hepatitis
- it is estimated that less than 5% of patients with chronic hepatitis under age 35 years have WD as the underlying cause, and an estimated 5–30% of patients with WD present with the features of chronic hepatitis
- modest elevation of serum aminotransferase levels in the presence of severe hepatocellular necrosis and inflammation is a distinctive feature of Wilsonian chronic hepatitis
- the diagnosis may be difficult, because almost 50% of these patients have no evidence of Kayser–Fleischer rings and lack neurologic manifestations of the

disease; moreover, patients with severe hepatic inflammation may have normal serum ceruloplasmin levels.

- the prognosis for treated patients is good even if they have cirrhosis

3 Fulminant hepatic failure

- Patients tend to be young, and the clinical picture may be indistinguishable from that of viral-induced massive hepatic necrosis
- characteristic clinical features include intravascular hemolysis, splenomegaly, Kayser–Fleischer rings, and a fulminant course; patients rarely survive longer than days to weeks unless liver transplantation is performed
- Serum aminotransferases are mildly to moderately elevated, with marked elevation of the serum bilirubin, a low serum alkaline phosphatase level, and evidence of hemolytic anemia. Serum ceruloplasmin may be in the normal range; however, 24-hour urinary copper and free serum copper levels are usually elevated
- liver biopsy, if performed, will document an elevated hepatic copper content and usually coexistent cirrhosis

B Neurologic

- tends to occur in the second to third decades of life
- Kayser–Fleischer rings are almost invariably present on ophthalmologic examination
- common early symptoms are dysarthria, clumsiness, tremor, drooling, gait disturbance, and mask-like facies
- rigidity with overt parkinsonian features, flexion contractures, grand mal seizures, and spasticity are seen less often and in the later stages of the disease
- cognitive ability usually remains normal despite severe neurologic impairment
- neurologic symptoms may improve markedly with treatment, although residual deficits are common despite adequate chelation therapy
- three subgroups have been defined by clinical and magnetic resonance imaging (MRI) findings:

1 MRI shows dilatation of the third ventricle in a subgroup of patients with bradykinesia, rigidity, and cognitive impairment
2 A second group is characterized by ataxia, tremor, and reduced functional capacity; MRI reveals focal thalamic lesions
3 A third subgroup exhibits dyskinesia, dysarthria, and an organic personality syndrome; MRI shows focal lesions in the putamen and globus pallidus

C Psychiatric

- one third of all WD patients may present with psychiatric symptoms. Patients may be mistakenly diagnosed with a progressive psychiatric illness and institutionalized prior to the diagnosis of WD

- psychiatric symptoms are present in virtually all neurologically affected patients; the severity tends to parallel that of the neurologic abnormalities
- early symptoms may be limited to subtle behavioral changes and deterioration of academic and work performance
- later, patients present with personality changes, lability of mood, emotionalism, impulsive and antisocial behavior, depression that may lead to suicidal ideation, and increased sexual preoccupation
- schizophreniform psychosis, anxiety, other psychotic disturbances and cognitive impairment occur rarely in WD patients
- psychiatric symptoms usually resolve with chelation therapy

D Ophthalmologic

1 Kayser–Fleischer rings

- a golden brown or greenish discoloration in the limbic area, evident initially at the superior and inferior corneal poles and eventually becoming circumferential
- consist of electron-dense granules rich in copper and sulfur, suggesting that the copper is bound to metallothionein
- presence or absence should be confirmed by an ophthalmologist with slit-lamp examination

- occurs in most symptomatic WD patients and 90–100% of those with neurologic manifestations. Generally absent in asymptomatic cases and in more than 40% of patients with hepatic disease, particularly those who present with chronic hepatitis

- not pathognomonic of WD, since they also are seen in patients with long standing cholestasis, such as intrahepatic cholestasis of childhood, primary biliary cirrhosis, and partial biliary atresia
- the rings resolve in 80% of patients with chelation therapy over 3–5 years

2 Sunflower cataracts

- typically found with Kayser–Fleischer rings but less frequently
- vision is unimpaired
- resolve more quickly than Kayser–Fleischer rings with treatment

E Renal

- proximal renal tubular acidosis or features of Fanconi's syndrome with aminoaciduria, glucosuria, uricosuria, hyperphosphaturia, and hypercalciuria.
- distal renal tubular acidosis also may occur and is a likely factor in the increased incidence of renal calculi in WD
- hematuria, mostly microscopic, may be due to nephrolithiasis or glomerular disease
- proteinuria has been noted as a manifestation of WD, although nephrotic syndrome and Goodpasture's syndrome are more likely to be a side effect of D-penicillamine therapy (see below)
- chelation therapy results in marked improvement in renal function

F Skeletal

- over half the patients exhibit osteopenia on radiologic examination, due to osteomalacia, osteoporosis, or both
- symptomatic arthropathy occurs in 25–50% of patients. Radiographically it is a degenerative joint disease that resembles premature osteoarthritis and involves the spine and large joints
- osteochondritis dissecans, chondromalacia patellae, and chondrocalcinosis have also been described

G Miscellaneous

- acute intravascular hemolysis may be the presenting manifestation in up to 15% of patients; it is transient and self-limited but often associated with fulminant hepatic failure or chronic hepatitis
- cardiac involvement has been underestimated in the past. EKG abnormalities are detected in one third of cases; findings include left ventricular or biventricular hypertrophy, ST–T changes, arrythmias, and conduction disturbances
- azure lunulae (blue discoloration of the bases of finger nails) is an unusual but characteristic finding
- there is an increased incidence of pigment and cholesterol gallstones
- delayed puberty, gynecomastia, and amenorrhea have been noted

5 Diagnosis

A When to look for Wilson's disease?

Individuals between ages 3 and 40 years with:

- unexplained serum aminotransferase elevations, fulminant hepatic failure, chronic hepatitis, or cirrhosis
- neurologic features of unexplained etiology (abnormal behavior, incoordination, tremor, dyskinesia)
- a psychiatric disorder with signs of hepatic or neurologic disease, or patients who are refractory to therapy
- Kayser–Fleischer rings detected on routine eye examination
- unexplained, acquired Coombs-negative hemolytic anemia
- a sibling or a parent carrying the diagnosis of WD

B Diagnostic modalities

1 Ceruloplasmin

- normal serum concentration is 20–40 mg/dL
- 90% of all patients and 65–85% of patients presenting with hepatic manifestations have levels below the normal range
- normal levels are found in ≥15% of WD patients with liver involvement, as part

of an acute-phase response to hepatic injury, and in patients with elevated serum estrogen levels secondary to pregnancy or exogenous administration

- a decreased level is not pathognomonic of WD. The following non-Wilsonian causes should also be considered:

  - diminished synthetic function as a consequence of severe liver diseases
  - nephrotic syndrome, protein-losing enteropathy, and malabsorption
  - 10–20% of asymptomatic heterozygote carriers of the WD gene (approximately 1 in 2000 in the general population)
  - children up to age 2 years
  - hereditary aceruloplasminemia associated with iron overload, unrelated to WD

2 Urinary copper excretion

- normal urinary copper excretion is less than 40 µg/24 hours. **Most patients with symptomatic WD have a urinary copper excretion greater than 100 µg/24 hours, and patients with fulminant hepatic failure often have levels that exceed 1000 µg/24 hours**
- asymptomatic WD patients may have normal urinary copper excretion
- elevated levels may be seen in other hepatic disorders such as primary biliary cirrhosis, and chronic hepatitis, and in severe proteinuria due to ceruloplasmin loss in urine
- the test is useful in confirming the diagnosis of WD and in monitoring compliance and response to chelation therapy
- D-penicillamine administered in a dose of 0.5 g prior to 24-hour urine collection has been shown to increase urinary copper excretion, but does not reliably distinguish WD from other liver diseases

3 Nonceruloplasmin serum copper

- the mean free (nonceruloplasmin) serum copper concentration can be calculated by subtracting the amount of ceruloplasmin copper (0.047 µmol copper per mg of ceruloplasmin) from the total serum copper concentration
- patients with WD have elevated concentrations of copper bound to serum albumin, amino acids, or transcuprein (nonceruloplasmin copper). However, total serum copper, generally remains below 80 µg/dL
- the test is useful in monitoring the adequacy of chelation therapy during maintenance treatment

4 Liver biopsy

- changes on light microscopy are nonspecific. Early features include glycogen deposition in the nuclei of periportal hepatocytes and moderate fatty infiltration. The fatty changes progressively increase and in some cases may resemble steatosis induced by ethanol
- in more advanced cases, cirrhosis is present. In fulminant hepatitis and chronic hepatitis, submassive necrosis with Mallory bodies are seen with cirrhosis

- histochemical staining of liver biopsy specimens for copper using rhodanine or rubeanic acid is of little value, unless positive, since during the initial stages of copper accumulation the metal is distributed diffusely in the cytosol
- **a hepatic copper concentration >250 µg/g dry liver (normal 15–55 µg/g) accompanied by a low serum ceruloplasmin establishes the diagnosis of Wilson disease.** There are **two caveats:**
  - the biopsy needle and the specimen container should be free from copper. It is recommended that a disposable needle made from steel, or a Klatskin or Menghini needle, washed in 0.1M EDTA and rinsed with demineralized water, be used
  - the finding of a normal hepatic copper concentration excludes the diagnosis, but an elevated level alone may also be found in other liver diseases.

a **Cholestatic disorders**
  - primary biliary cirrhosis
  - primary sclerosing cholangitis
  - intrahepatic cholestasis of childhood
  - biliary atresia
b **Indian childhood cirrhosis**
c **Idiopathic copper toxicosis**

5 Incorporation of orally administered radiocopper into ceruloplasmin

- serum radioactivity (mainly as radiocopper-containing ceruloplasmin) is measured after oral administration of radiolabeled copper (^{64}Cu or ^{67}Cu) at 1, 2, 4, and 48 hours. Normally there is prompt appearance of radiolabeled copper in serum, followed by disappearance (as circulating copper is cleared by the liver for incorporation into newly synthesized ceruloplasmin), and then reappearance of copper in ceruloplasmin
- in WD the radioactivity does not reappear in serum. Heterozygotes exhibit a slower and lower level of reappearance than normal subjects
- this test may be useful in diagnostic dilemmas, when a liver biopsy is contraindicated, and in other hepatic disorders which exhibit an elevated hepatic copper concentration and/or Kayser–Fleischer rings

6 Genetic diagnosis

- in family studies linkage analysis has been used for carrier detection with less than 1–2% error. Use of DNA marker studies in the diagnosis of WD, however, has several limitations:
  - currently the technique is relatively expensive and labor intensive
  - WD is caused by a wide variety of mutations in a single gene
  - DNA marker studies can be performed only within families in which the diagnosis is already established in one family member using the index patient DNA as a reference
- The application of this technique is likely to be applied to genetic screening of young family members particularly when standard biochemical methods do not provide a definitive answer

C   Diagnostic approach

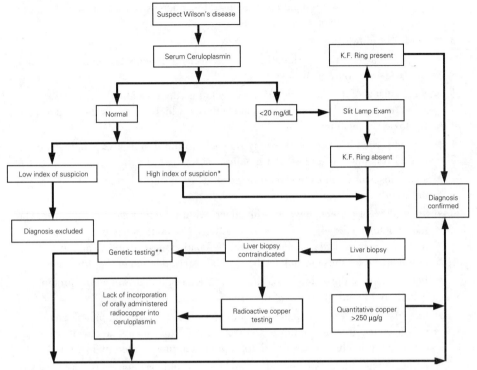

Fig. 17.3.   Wilson's disease diagnostic algorithm. *Example: presence of Kayser–Fleischer (K.F.) ring, high urinary copper excretion, and neuropsychiatric symptoms with liver involvement. **Genetic testing is performed within families where the diagnosis is already established in one family member using the index patient DNA as a reference

6   Treatment

A   Diet

- A low-copper diet is rarely prescribed or necessary
- tips to decrease dietary copper intake include:
  - avoid foods with a high copper content, e.g., liver, chocolate, nuts, mushrooms, legumes, and shellfish
  - use deionized or distilled water if the drinking water copper content is >0.2 ppm
  - avoid use of domestic water softeners and untested well water

B   Pharmacotherapy

1   BAL (British Anti-Lewisite)

- the first effective copper chelating agent

- abandoned because it requires painful intramuscular injection
- the only occasional situation in which BAL may be useful is in combination with D-penicillamine, when a patient demonstrates progressive neurological deterioration while on penicillamine

2 D-Penicillamine

- an amino acid derivative identified in the urine of patients taking penicillin and the **first-line drug** in WD
- mechanisms of action include copper chelation, detoxification, and possibly induction of cellular metallothionein synthesis, which enhances the proportion of nontoxic Cu-metallothionein
- best absorbed if taken on an empty stomach. Initial dose is 1–2 g daily, with a standard maintenance dose of 1 g daily.
- small doses of pyridoxine should be given daily, because of the weak antipyridoxine effect of D-penicillamine.
- about 20% of patients develop side effects within the first month of therapy. The most common side effect is a hypersensitivity reaction, consisting of fever, malaise, rash, and occasionally lymphadenopathy; most patients can be desensitized for these symptoms by gradual reintroduction of the drug
- bone marrow suppression or significant (>1 g/24 hours) or worsening proteinuria usually requires withdrawal of the drug
- may also precipitate autoimmune features such as myasthenia, pemphigus, polymyositis, or systemic lupus erythematosus. When such side effects occur, the drug should be discontinued and appropriate alternative therapy instituted
- dermatologic side effects include pemphigus, acanthosis nigricans, and elastosis perforans serpiginosa. The last of these, which also may occur with trientine, may respond to isotretinoin

3 Trientine

- introduced in 1969 as an alternative chelating agent to D-penicillamine
- mechanisms of action include copper chelation and detoxification
- daily dosage is similar to penicillamine: 1–2 g administered orally in three divided doses, taken on an empty stomach
- sideroblastic anemia is the only major side effect of this agent; other reported side effects include skin rash, gastrointestinal distress, and rhabdomyolysis
- most of the side effects of D-penicillamine, with the exception of elastosis perforans serpiginosa, subside when the patient is converted to trientine
- because it is a less potent copper chelator than D-penicillamine and because of limited experience in its use, trientine should remain as second-line therapy

4 Zinc

- the rationale for use of zinc is its ability to induce intestinal and hepatic metallothionein synthesis
- zinc decreases copper absorption by increasing the formation of Cu-metallothionein in intestinal epithelial cells; copper is not absorbed in this form but is excreted when the intestinal epithelial cells are shed
- in the hepatocyte, the increase in metallothionein synthesis appears to be protective, since the Cu-metallothionein complex is nontoxic

- zinc is relatively safe; common side effects include gastrointestinal upset and headache
- the dose is 150 mg daily of zinc acetate or sulfate, divided in two to three doses between meals
- experience with zinc in WD is limited. Its role in therapy is mainly in presymptomatic patients who have been previously decoppered and possibly as a temporary measure during pregnancy

5 Ammonium tetrathiomolybdate

- decreases intestinal copper absorption by forming complexes with intraluminal copper
- following absorption, the drug forms nontoxic complexes with serum copper, preventing its uptake by tissues
- because its affinity for copper is higher than that of metallothionein, the drug can remove copper bound to metallothionein, potentially making it a more potent chelator than D-penicillamine and trientine
- the drug appears to be useful in removing redistributed copper during initial treatment with D-penicillamine or trientine when there is neurologic deterioration
- the potential side effects of bone marrow suppression and skeletal abnormalities (in animals) limit its usefulness and warrant further testing before FDA approval and routine use can be recommended

C   Treatment regimens

1 Initial therapy

- a baseline 24-hour urinary copper should be obtained
- treatment is initiated with D-penicillamine
- starting dose is 250–500 mg gradually increasing to 1.0–1.5 g, which is usually required to achieve the desired level of copper excretion (rarely a dose of >2.0 g is required)
- because of the potential for bone marrow suppression and nephrotic syndrome (rarely Goodpasture's syndrome), a complete blood count and routine urinalysis should be performed every 2 weeks during the first 2 months of therapy
- patients intolerant of D-penicillamine may be treated with trientine. Zinc or tetrathiomolybdate may be utilized when side effects caused by D-penicillamine are also known to be associated with trientine
- clinical signs of improvement may be delayed until at least 6–12 months of uninterrupted therapy
- patients with severe hepatic insufficiency unresponsive to pharmacotherapy should be considered for liver transplantation (see below)

2 Maintenance therapy

- maintenance doses of D-penicillamine are usually 0.75–1.25 g/day
- patients maintained on an adequate therapeutic regimen exhibit a progressive fall in urinary excretion of copper to 0.5–1 mg/24 hours, and of the free serum copper level to less than 0.1 mg/L

- yearly slit-lamp examination will document fading of Kayser–Fleischer rings, if the patient is adequately decoppered
- alternative therapeutic agents, such as zinc and trientine, may be used, but experience with D-penicillamine is more extensive
- treatment of asymptomatic WD patients, diagnosed by screening of family members, may be started at age 3 years
- **lifelong therapy, without interruption, is essential in all patients with WD. Cessation of therapy may result in rapid and irreversible hepatic and neurologic deterioration**

3 Pregnancy

- **therapy for WD patients should be continued throughout pregnancy**
- D-penicillamine, as well as trientine and zinc, appear to be safe during pregnancy in humans
- **it is recommended that the daily dose of D-penicillamine should not exceed 1.0 g during pregnancy**, and if cesarean section is anticipated the dose should be reduced to 0.5 g/day 6 weeks prior to delivery and until wound healing is complete

4 Patients with neurologic disease

- about 10–20% (up to 50% in one series) of patients presenting with neurologic disease have worsening of neurologic symptoms during initial treatment with D-penicillamine
- this phenomenon is most likely caused by the mobilization and redistribution of copper during initial treatment, resulting in higher levels of copper in certain areas in the brain
- treatment with D-penicillamine should be continued in these patients, with gradual adjustment of the dose to increase urinary copper excretion
- if neurologic manifestations continue to worsen, alternative approaches may include:
  - the addition of BAL, which has the advantage of crossing the blood–brain barrier
  - substituting tetrathiomolybdate for penicillamine (this approach remains experimental)
- differential diagnosis of neurologic deterioration during initial treatment with D-penicillamine also includes progression of the disease due to subtherapeutic dosage or, rarely, a side effect of D-penicillamine, such as a lupus-like central nervous systems vasculitis and cerebritis

D Liver transplantation

- results in complete reversal of the metabolic defect in copper metabolism, marked cuperiuresis, and improvement in hepatic and neurologic manifestations
- in 55 patients with WD undergoing liver transplantation, the indications were fulminant hepatitis in 38%, hepatic insufficiency unresponsive to medical therapy in 58%, neurologic disease in one patient, and recurrent gastrointestinal bleeding in another

- in the absence of severe hepatic disease, liver transplantation for refractory neurological manifestations should be considered as experimental; however, there are several reports of improvement in these patients after liver transplantation
- in fulminant hepatic failure, the selection of patients is facilitated by determination of the prognostic index (Table 17.1); the outcome of liver transplantation in these selected patients is good, with 90% survival in one series.

Score[a]	0	1	2	3	4
Bilirubin (nl, 3–20 mol/L)	<100	100–150	151–200	201–300	>300
AST (nl, 7–40 U/L)	<100	100–150	151–200	201–300	>300
Prolongation of PT (s)	<4	4–8	9–12	13–20	>30

Adapted from Nazer et al. 1986[1]
[a]Patients with a prognostic index (score) of 7 or greater should be considered for liver transplantation

(Table 17.1: Prognostic index in Wilsonian fulminant hepatitis)

7 Other Copper-related Hepatic Disorders

A Indian childhood cirrhosis

- rapidly progressive cirrhosis presenting at 6 months to 5 years of age, generally restricted to the Indian subcontinent
- grossly increased hepatic, urinary, and serum copper concentrations
- environmental ingestion of excessive amounts of copper, due to use of copper and brass vessels, is the likely cause of copper overload in this disorder, although a genetic predisposition may also coexist in some patients
- this entity was one of the most common causes of chronic liver disease in India, but is rarely seen now due to health education and avoidance of use of brass vessels

B Idiopathic copper toxicosis

- rare disorder with only 20 reported cases
- severe, progressive cirrhosis, with clinical onset usually by age 2 years.
- liver biopsy reveals cirrhosis with Mallory bodies and a hepatic copper concentration >400 µg/g dry weight
- serum ceruloplasmin is normal
- may be caused by an unidentified genetic defect or excessive environmental copper exposure (e.g., contaminated spring water)

C Menke's disease

- X-linked recessive disorder characterized by altered absorption and distribution of copper leading to a severe copper deficiency state

- symptoms usually appear before the age of 3 months
- characterized by growth retardation, hypothermia, skin and hair depigmentation, osteoporosis, tortuosity and dilatation of major arteries, varicosities of veins, and profound central nervous system damage
- Generally results in death by age 5 or 6 years

References

1   Nazer H, Ede RJ, Mowat AP, Williams R. *Wilson's disease: clinical presentation and use of prognostic index.* (Gut 1986) 27: 1377–81

2   Akil M, Brewer GJ. *Psychiatric and behavioral abnormalities in Wilson's disease.* (Adv Neuro 1995); 65: 171–8

3   Cuthbert JA. *Wilson's disease: a new gene and an animal model for an old disease.* (J Invest Med 1995); 43: 323–36

4   Linder M, Hazegh-Azam M. *Copper biochemistry and molecular biology.* (Am J Clin Nutr 1996); 63: 797S–811S

5   Pandit A, Bhave S. *Present interpretation of the role of copper in Indian childhood cirrhosis.* (Am J Clin Nutr 1996); 63: 830S–835S

6   Sallie R, Katsiyiannakis L, Baldwin D, et al. *Failure of simple biochemical indexes to reliably differentiate fulminant Wilson's disease from other causes of fulminant liver failure.* (Hepatology 1992); 16: 1206–11

7   Scheinberg IH, Sternlieb I. *Wilson disease and idiopathic copper toxicosis.* (Am J Clin Nutr 1996); 63: 842S–845S

8   Schilsky ML, Scheinberg IH, Sternlieb I. *Liver transplantation of Wilson's disease: indications and outcome.* (Hepatology 1994); 19: 583–7

9   Schilsky ML, Scheinberg IH, Sternlieb I. *Prognosis of Wilsonian chronic active hepatitis.* (Gastroenterology 1991); 100: 762–7

10 Schilsky ML. *Wilson disease: genetic basis of copper toxicity and natural history.* (Semin Liver Dis 1996); 16: 83–95

11 Zucker SD, Gollan JL. *Wilson's disease and hepatic copper toxicosis.* In: Zakim D, Boyer TD (eds). *Hepatology: A Text book of Liver Disease.* (Philadelphia: Saunders 1996) 1405–39

Alpha-1 antitrypsin deficiency and other metabolic liver diseases

HUGO R. ROSEN, M.D.

▼

Key Points

1 Alpha-1 antitrypsin deficiency (α-1ATD) should be considered in the differential diagnosis in any adult who presents with chronic hepatitis or cirrhosis of unknown etiology, although α-1ATD does not invariably lead to chronic liver disease

2 Hereditary tyrosinemia is associated with high serum alpha fetoprotein levels and regenerative macronodules, making screening for hepatocellular carcinoma problematic

3 Considerable variation in the severity of liver disease exists in patients with Gaucher's disease; bone marrow transplantation and orthotopic liver transplantation have successfully treated the disease

4 Cystic fibrosis, the most common autosomal recessive childhood disorder among whites, is frequently manifested by hepatobiliary complications, particularly as more patients live into adulthood

5 Liver transplantation may be indicated for hepatic-based metabolic disorders not associated with any overt liver disease (e.g., primary hyperoxaluria, familial homozygous hypercholesterolemia)

6 Gene therapy, although tremendously promising for clinical application to metabolic liver diseases, is still in its embryonic stages

▲

1 Pathogenesis and Treatment of Metabolic Liver Disease: Overview

A General principles

1 Inherited disorders have been increasingly recognized as a cause of acute and chronic liver diseases

2 Establishing the diagnosis is not difficult in most cases; the liver is often the sole organ clinically affected by the metabolic disease

3 Some of the diseases are relatively common

4 Collectively, genetic/metabolic liver diseases account for approximately 30% of children who undergo liver transplantation each year

5 In general, liver transplantation should be considered in any child with metabolic liver disease and growth failure or complications secondary to progressive liver disease (e.g., ascites, variceal hemorrhage) (see Ch. 31)

6 Psychological consequences of screening for metabolic disorders can be adverse

B Insight into pathogenesis derived from basic science research

Our understanding of the inborn errors of metabolism has been greatly enhanced by advances in cellular and molecular biological principles and techniques (see Table 18.1)

Disease	Technique
Alpha-1 antitrypsin deficiency	Analysis of an abnormally folded protein within the vacuolar secretory pathway resulted in identification of liver disease related defect in quality control
Hereditary tyrosinemia	Characterization of tyrosine degradation permitted development of a compound preventing accumulation of hepatotoxic intermediate
Gaucher's disease	Use of the receptor-mediated pathway for endocytosis and delivery of ligands to lysosome allowed targeted enzyme replacement therapy

Reproduced with permission from Teckman & Perlmutter (1995)[1]

(Table 18.1: Application of scientific techniques to disease)

2 Alpha-1 antitrypsin deficiency (α-1ATD)

A Genetics and function

1 Alpha-1 antitrypsin is encoded by a gene on the long arm of chromosome 14; and the phenotype is transmitted by autosomal co-dominance inheritance

2 Alpha-1 antitrypsin functions to protect tissues from proteases such as neutrophil elastase.

3 The phenotype PiMM (Pi = protease inhibitor), which is present in 95% of the

population, is associated with normal serum levels of α-1AT. There are about 75 different α-1AT alleles

4 A single nucleotide substitution (glu to lys) leads to Z α-1AT protein. In northern European descendants, the PiZ gene frequency is 1–2% with a homozygote prevalence of one in 2000 births

5 The PiZZ phenotype is accompanied by severe deficiency, whereas the PiMZ phenotype (heterozygote) leads to intermediate deficiency

B Symptoms and signs

1 α-1ATD predisposes children to liver disease and adults to emphysema and liver disease

- Deficiency of α-1AT in serum leads to lung disease.
- in contrast, the liver disease relates to the presence of the abnormal Z protein in the liver, not to the serum level of α-1AT
- liver disease can occur not only in persons deficient in α-1AT (PiZZ) but also in persons heterozygous for the Z allele (PiMZ) who do not have α-1AT deficiency in the serum

2 liver involvement is often first identified in the newborn period because of persistent jaundice; in fact, most infants with α-1ATD are indistinguishable from those with idiopathic neonatal hepatitis

- 10% of this population develop moderate to severe clinical liver disease with ascites, coagulopathy, and poor growth during the first few years of life
- a large 18-year-long Swedish study has demonstrated that both clinical and laboratory signs of liver disease improve with time[2] (see Table 18.2)

All patients with PiZZ or PiSZ	Infancy (1–4 months)	At 18 years of age
Abnormal serum alanine aminotransferase	48%	10%
Abnormal serum gamma glutamyltranspeptidase	60%	8%
Clinical signs of liver disease	17%	0%

(Table 18.2: Improvement of signs of liver disease with time, as found by Sveger & Eriksson (1995)[2])

3 The incidence of liver disease in adolescents with α-1ATD is 2% by age 20–40 years, 5% by age 40–50 years, and 15% thereafter, with a slight male predominance

4 α-1ATD should be considered in the differential diagnosis in any adult who presents with chronic hepatitis, cirrhosis, portal hypertension, or hepatocellular carcinoma of unknown etiology

C Pathogenesis and diagnosis

1 The pathogenesis of chronic liver disease associated with α-1ATD is still a matter of controversy

- the "accumulation" theory, in which liver damage is caused by accumulation of the mutant α-1AT molecule in the endoplasmic reticulum (ER) of liver cells, is the most widely accepted and substantiated by studies in transgenic mice expressing the human α-1AT Z variant.

- other researchers have postulated that additional inherited traits (e.g., lag in degradation of abnormally folded polypeptide) or environmental factors (e.g., viral hepatitis) may exaggerate the intracellular accumulation of mutant α-1AT.
- liver damage does not appear to be a consequence of a "proteolytic attack" mechanism, which probably underlies the destructive lung disease

2 The number of patients seen with liver or lung disease associated with α-1ATD is far fewer than would be expected from projections based on population genetic estimates

- numerous studies have demonstrated a disproportionately high prevalence of hepatitis B and C markers in α-1AT-deficient patients, underscoring that α-1ATD may only predispose to the development of chronic liver disease[3]

3 Diagnosis is established by a serum α-1AT phenotype determination (Pi typing)

- serum α-1AT concentrations may be misleading; the host response to inflammation may lead to false elevations (even in homozygous ZZ individuals)
- the distinctive histological feature of α-1ATD is the aggregation of eosinophilic, periodic acid–Schiff-positive, diastase-resistant globules in the ER of periportal hepatocytes (see Fig. 18.1, plate section)

D Treatment and screening

1 The most important treatment for α-1ATD is avoidance of cigarette smoking, which markedly accelerates the destructive lung disease. Infusions of α-1AT derived from pooled plasma or obtained by recombinant DNA methods are under investigation for treatment of pulmonary disease

2 Orthotopic liver transplantation (OLT)

- α-1ATD is the most common metabolic deficiency and the second most common

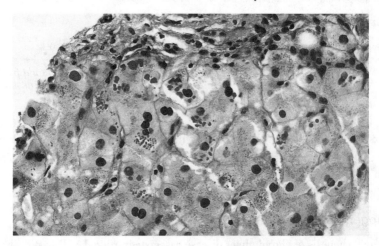

Fig. 18.1   Alpha-1 antitrypsin deficiency: periportal hepatocytes contain numerous eosinophilic, periodic acid–Schiff-positive, diastase-resistant globules (×110). See page xxi.

childhood liver disease (after biliary atresia) for which OLT is performed (see Chs 23 and 31)

- the recipient assumes the Pi phenotype of the donor
- long-term survival post OLT is excellent, especially for children. OLT should be performed before advancing lung disease complicates or precludes transplantation

3 Somatic gene therapy

- potentially less expensive than replacement therapy with purified α-1AT protein
- would be useful only in ameliorating pulmonary disease, because liver disease is associated with mutant Z protein in hepatocytes, not deficient serum or tissue levels of α-1AT
- strategies may eventually focus on delivering peptides to ER to prevent polymerization of α-1AT or manipulating the degradative system in the subpopulation of PiZZ individuals predisposed to liver injury
- currently limited by low and nonsustained levels of transferred gene product

4 Screening

- phenotype determination of relatives of patients with α-1ATD to distinguish between ZZ and heterozygous allotypes is important for genetic counseling
- patients and afflicted family members should be informed of the great variability in clinical course
- newborn screening in Sweden for α-1ATD was associated with severe negative psychological effects in more than half of the families that was still evident 5–7 years later
- concern has been raised about potential repercussions of positive genetic information, particularly the possibility of their discriminatory use by employers and insurance carriers

3 Hereditary Tyrosinemia

A General features

1 Molecular defects

- defects in the fumarylacetoacetate hydrolase (FAH) gene; the enzyme product catalyzes the last step in tyrosine degradation
- autosomal recessive defect most prevalent in French Canadian descendants in Quebec

2 Clinical features

- characterized by progressive liver failure, renal tubular dysfunction, and hypophosphatemic rickets
- patients with acute form usually referred for poor growth, irritability, and vomiting. Hepatomegaly, coagulopathy, ascites, and death from liver failure by 1 year of age not uncommon.
- patients may develop neurologic crises that resemble acute intermittent porphyria, presumably resulting from competitive inhibition of δ-aminolevulinic

acid dehydratase by succinylacetone, an accumulated metabolite of tyrosine degradation

- increased susceptibility to hepatocellular carcinoma even within the first 1–5 years of life

3 Laboratory and pathologic evaluation

- markedly prolonged prothrombin time despite only mild elevation of liver enzymes and bilirubin levels
- elevated urine succinylacetone and plasma tyrosine, methionine, and alpha fetoprotein levels
- urinary abnormalities consistent with proximal renal tubular acidosis
- liver biopsy notable for hepatocellular inflammation and necrosis, fatty infiltration, and marked nodular regeneration

B Treatment

1 Nutritional and pharmacological

- dietary restriction of phenylalanine, tyrosine, and methionine with regular estimation of serum amino acids to ensure that they remain in normal range
- vitamin D and phosphate supplements to prevent rickets
- treatment with a novel drug, 2-(2-nitro-4-trifluoromethylbenzoyl)-1,3-cyclohexanedione (NTBC), has been shown to prevent the accumulation of toxic derivatives of tyrosine and lead to improvement in prothrombin time, and biochemical parameters and reduction in serum alpha fetoprotein and hepatic nodularity, as assessed by computed tomography
- these measures may improve well-being and promote growth, but it remains to be shown whether they delay the onset of liver failure

2 Orthotopic liver transplantation

- should be performed as soon as growth arrest occurs or liver function deteriorates
- appears to have a beneficial effect on the renal disease
- It has been suggested OLT be performed electively between ages 2 and 3, particularly because high serum alpha fetoprotein levels and the emergence of regenerative macronodules make it virtually impossible to identify the development of malignant transformation

4 Gaucher's Disease

- most common of the lysosomal storage diseases, caused by a deficiency of the enzyme glucocerebrosidase, leading to accumulation of the enzyme substrate (glucosylceramide) in reticuloendothelial cells throughout the body
- inherited in an autosomal recessive fashion

A Types

1 Type I is most common phenotype: **1** incidence in Ashkenazi Jews of approximately one homozygote per 1000; **2** usually presents with painless splenomegaly, anemia,

hepatomegaly, and elevated serum aminotransferase levels, although liver failure is rare; **3** most frequent serious complications are skeletal, specifically osteoporosis-related fractures

2 Types II and III are dominated by neurologic manifestations; Type III can be associated with hepatic dysfunction, but usually to a lesser extent than Type I

B Diagnosis

- Gaucher's disease should be considered in children or adults with unexplained liver dysfunction, splenomegaly, bleeding, or skeletal abnormalities
- histopathologically, the disorder is characterized by the Gaucher cell: lipid-laden histiocytic cells abundant in the spleen, hepatic sinusoids, bone marrow, and lymph nodes (see Fig. 18.2, plate section)
- considerable variation in the severity of liver disease exists in patients with Gaucher's disease. In general, the degree of liver involvement correlates with the severity of extrahepatic manifestations: **1** location of storage cells is predominantly centrizonal in the majority of cases; **2** patients can develop cirrhosis with portal hypertensive bleeding from gastroesophageal varices
- the definitive diagnostic test for homozygotes is glucocerebrosidase activity in blood leukocytes or urine
- prenatal diagnosis is possible with amniotic or chorionic villus sampling

C Treatment and screening

- In the past, patients often underwent splenectomy when bleeding or mechanical complications of splenomegaly developed
- effective enzyme replacement with alglucerase (Ceredase), "the world's most expensive medicine," represents a major breakthrough in the treatment of this disorder. **1** Based on the ability of the macrophage mannose receptor to deliver

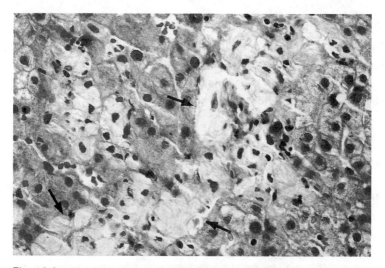

Fig. 18.2 Gaucher's disease: lipid-laden histiocytic cells (arrows) in the hepatic sinusoids (H&E, ×110). See page xxi.

partially deglycosylated glucocerebrosidase to its natural site of action, the lysosome of macrophages. **2** Shown to induce considerable decreases in the size of the liver and spleen over relatively short time intervals
- the occurrence of cell migration after liver transplantation (microchimerism) may explain why patients with lysosomal storage diseases experience more benefit from liver replacement than simply improved hepatic function
- Gaucher's disease is a disorder of the hematopoietic stem cell and is cured by bone marrow transplantation.
- it is possible to screen the Jewish population for the carrier state. Prenatal diagnosis can be offered to couples when both are carriers. Unlike Tay–Sachs disease, which usually leads to early death, the clinical course of Gaucher's disease is often benign

5 Glycogen Storage Diseases (GSD)

A Features

- characterized by abnormal accumulation of glycogen in tissues, including liver, heart, skeletal muscle, kidney, and brain
- children often present with nonspecific gastrointestinal symptoms and failure to thrive. Without intervention progresses to hepatosplenomegaly, portal hypertension, ascites, liver failure, and death between 2 and 4 years of age from liver disease
- cardiac, neurologic, and myopathic symptoms may predominate
- inherited in an autosomal recessive fashion, except for one variant of Type III
- Types I, III, and IV are associated with liver disease: **1** Hepatocellular adenomas occur in up to 50% of children with Type I who survive beyond the first decade. **2** Type IV (Andersen's disease) is characterized by cirrhosis with or without evidence of cardiac or brain involvement. Death usually occurs by age 5 years.

B Treatment

- a key objective of treatment is to maintain the blood sugar within the normal range, utilizing frequent feeds and/or administration of glucose polymers
- OLT has been successfully performed for GSD, with subsequent resorption of abnormal amylopectin-like polysaccharide as confirmed by endomyocardial biopsy specimens

6 Cystic Fibrosis (CF)

A General features

- CF, an autosomal recessive inherited disease of epithelial cell ion transport, is the most common potentially lethal genetic defect of the white population, affecting about one in 2000 newborns
- the gene responsible for CF is on the long arm of chromosome 7 and encodes for the cystic fibrosis transmembrane regulator (CFTR)

- more than 200 different mutations of the CFTR gene responsible for CF have been identified
- epithelial cells in different organs are affected by the CF defect, accounting for the protean manifestations of this multisystemic disease. **1** Sweat glands, pancreas, and lungs are the most commonly affected organs. **2** With improved life expectancy of CF patients, now approaching a median of 30 years, there has been increased appreciation of hepatobiliary complications.

B Hepatobiliary features

- a rise in prevalence and severity of liver involvement is observed with increasing age
- biochemical abnormalities may be intermittent and often do not correlate with the presence or severity of liver disease.
- the sweat test is recommended as part of the diagnostic workup in infants with neonatal cholestasis
- the pathognomonic lesion of CF-associated liver disease is focal biliary cirrhosis **1** The patchy distribution of cirrhotic transformation (predominantly portal tracts) spares many areas of hepatic tissue, preserving the general architecture of the liver. Therefore, liver biopsy has a limited diagnostic role because sampling error can occur. **2** Probably explains the typically mild and insidious course of liver disease in patients with CF
- biliary tree abnormalities are not infrequent. **1** Prevalence of gallstones ranges from 12% to 27%. **2** Nearly one-third of patients show morphologic and functional abnormalities of the gallbladder (i.e., microgallbladder). **3** Sclerosing cholangitis has also been reported in adult patients with CF-associated liver disease
- cirrhosis and portal hypertension affect only 1.5% of the total CF population but account for about 10% of all complications reported by the American Cystic Fibrosis Patient Registry[4]

C Treatment

- in patients with massive hepatic steatosis, correction of pancreatic insufficiency with enzyme replacement and improvement of nutritional status with hypercaloric diet has been advocated
- a recent double-blind multicenter trial of ursodeoxycholic acid (UDCA, 15 mg/kg/day) demonstrated improvement in serum gamma glutamyltranspeptidase levels and decreased deterioration of overall clinical status as compared with placebo controls[5]
- taurine supplementation is advisable in CF patients with severe pancreatic insufficiency and poor nutritional status during chronic administration of UDCA
- OLT is an effective treatment for CF patients with end-stage liver disease and mild pulmonary involvement. Combined liver/lung transplant has been performed. Cyclosporine dosing may be problematic secondary to intestinal malabsorption and altered drug metabolism
- experimental studies in the rat indicate that somatic gene transfer into the biliary tract with correction of the CF defect is feasible.[6] Pilot human studies have not yet been initiated

7 Inborn Errors of Metabolism Leading to Hyperammonemia or Damage to Other Vital Organs

A Hyperammonemic syndromes

- may be caused by any of a number of deficiencies, including urea cycle enzyme deficiencies (e.g., ornithine transcarbamylase), transport defects of urea cycle intermediates, organic acidemias, fatty acid oxidation disorders, and disorders of pyruvate metabolism
- symptoms tend to vary with the age of patient. 1 Neonates with hyperammonemia have poor suck, lethargy, and even seizures or coma. 2 Older children present more insidiously with failure to thrive and persistent vomiting or irritability. These episodes may be precipitated by processes causing endogenous protein catabolism (e.g., excessive protein intake or infections)
- should be considered in any child with a family history of sudden infant death, Reye's syndrome, cyclic vomiting, ataxia, or unexplained failure to thrive
- measurement of serum ammonia, acid–base balance, glucose, lactate, pyruvate, ketones, plasma amino acids, and urine organic and orotic acid excretion is essential in making the diagnosis and excluding other inborn errors of metabolism[7]
- treatment: 1 Facilitate ammonia removal (dialysis, divert nitrogen from urea to other waste products with sodium benzoate) 2 Decrease ammonia production (antibiotics) 3 OLT appears to correct the metabolic abnormalities completely 4 Gene therapy for urea cycle defects appears to be a future therapeutic possibility

B Specific disorders causing irreversible damage to other vital organs (see also Ch. 23)

1 Crigler–Najjar Type II

- heterogeneous deficiency of hepatic microsomal UDP-glucuronyltransferases → complete failure of bilirubin glucuronide formation in the liver
- enzymatic activity cannot be induced by phenobarbital
- all patients must be considered at risk for irreversible brain damage if they survive the neonatal period
- exchange transfusion and phototherapy may reduce plasma bilirubin levels
- cholestyramine (in an attempt to interrupt the enterohepatic circulation of unconjugated bilirubin) has not been useful
- to date, no therapy short of OLT has proven effective for the long-term mananagement of this disorder

2 Primary hyperoxaluria (Type I oxalosis)

- autosomal recessive disorder with both genetic and phenotypic heterogeneity
- medical management includes large fluid intake, low intake of calcium and oxalate, and supplementation with pyridoxine and phosphate or magnesium oxide
- initially, renal transplantation was attempted, but early graft failure resulted from calcium oxalate deposition

- OLT is now advocated prior to the development of renal dysfunction. It is essential to maintain a high urinary output immediately post OLT when the renal oxalate load is greatly elevated

3 Primary hypercholesterolemia

- homozygous deficiency of low-density lipoprotein receptors
- associated with myocardial ischemia and death within first three decades of life
- recent trend to perform OLT to normalize metabolic defect before development of atherosclerosis
- combined liver–heart transplantation has been performed for this disorder

References

1   Teckman J, Perlmutter DH. *Conceptual advances in the pathogenesis and treatment of childhood metabolic liver disease.* (Gastroenterology 1995) 108: 1263–78

2   Sveger T, Eriksson S. *The liver in adolescents with alpha-1 antitrypsin deficiency.* (Hepatology 1995) 22: 514–17

3   Propst T, Propst A, Dietze O, Judmaier G, Braunsfeiner H, Vogel W. *High prevalence of viral infection in adults with homozygous or heterozygous alpha-1 antitrypsin deficiency and chronic liver disease.* (Am Intern Med 1992) 117: 641–7

4   Annual Data Report (American Cystic Fibrosis Registry 1992)

5   Colombo C, Battezzati PM, Podda M, Bettinardi N, Giunta A and the Italian Group for the study of ursodeoxycholic acid in cystic fibrosis. (Hepatology 1996) 23: 1484–90

6   Yang Y, Raper SE, Cohn JA, Engelhardt JF, Wilson JM. *An approach for treating the hepatobiliary disease of cystic fibrosis by somatic gene transfer.* (Proc Natl Acad Sci USA 1993) 90: 4601–5

7   Treem WR. *Inherited and acquired syndromes of hyperammonemia and encephalophathy in children.* (Semin Liver Dis 1994) 14: 236–58

8   Kumar A, Riely CA. *Inherited liver disease in adults.* (West J Med 1995) 163: 382–6

9   Lavine JE, Jonas MM. *Pediatric liver disease.* (Semin Liver Dis 1994) 14: 213–317

10 Mowat AP. *Orthotopic liver transplantation in liver-based metabolic disorders.* (Eur J Pediatr 1992) 151: S32–S38

11 Sharp HL. *Wherefore art thou liver disease associated with alpha-1 antitrypsin deficiency?* (Hepatology 1995) 22: 667–9

12 Starzl TE, Demetris AJ, Trucco M, Ricordi C, et al. *Chimerism after liver transplantation for type IV glycogen storage disease and type 1 Gaucher's disease.* (N Engl J Med 1993) 328: 745–9

Budd–Chiari syndrome and other vascular disorders

MACK C. MITCHELL Jr, M.D., F.A.C.P., F.A.C.G.

▼

Key Points

1 Hepatic vein occlusion, or Budd–Chiari syndrome, is an uncommon disorder characterized by hepatomegaly, ascites and abdominal pain. The disorder most often occurs in patients with underlying thrombotic diathesis including myeloproliferative disorders such as polycythemia vera and paroxysmal nocturnal hemoglobinuria pregnancy, tumors, chronic inflammatory diseases, clotting disorders and infections

2 Diagnosis is confirmed by visualization of thrombus or absent flow in hepatic veins on Doppler ultrasound or magnetic resonance imaging. Hepatic venography and liver biopsy provide definitive confirmation of Budd–Chiari syndrome

3 Budd–Chiari syndrome is often fatal. Medical therapy with diuretics and conventional anticoagulation provides only short-term symptomatic relief. Most patients require portosystemic decompression or liver transplantation for long-term relief of symptoms and correction of the underlying pathophysiology

4 Transjugular intrahepatic portal shunts and hepatic venous stents are promising options to replace or delay the need for surgery

5 Veno-occlusive disease of the liver is an occlusive disease of the small hepatic venules that mimics Budd–Chiari syndrome and develops primarily in patients following

▶

allogeneic or autologous bone marrow transplantation. It is probably the result of toxic injury to the endothelial cells

due to cytoreductive therapy. Treatment is largely supportive

1 Budd–Chiari Syndrome (BCS)

BCS results from obstruction to hepatic venous outflow, due to either thrombotic or nonthrombotic occlusion to flow

A Classification and etiology

1 Classified according to:
  a The duration of symptoms and signs of liver disease:
  - acute
  - subacute
  - chronic
  b The site of obstruction:
  - small hepatic veins, excluding terminal venules
  - large hepatic veins
  - hepatic inferior vena cava (IVC)
  c Cause of obstruction
  - membranous webs
  - direct infiltration by tumor or metastasis along veins
  - thrombosis

2 The majority of patients with BCS present within 3 months of the onset of symptoms. Most have subacute or chronic disease at the time of presentation, suggesting that thrombosis of intrahepatic veins leads subsequently to occlusion of large collecting veins

3 Membranous occlusion of the hepatic veins (MOHV) is the most common cause of BCS worldwide. However, this condition is rarely seen in the USA. The pathogenesis is the subject of controversy; many investigators have assumed that webs are congenital, but the onset of symptoms in the fourth decade of life and the pathological features are more suggestive of a post-thrombotic event

4 The majority of patients with BCS have an underlying thrombotic diathesis. In less than 30% of cases is the disorder idiopathic. Disorders associated with BCS include the following:

a Hematological disorders
  - polycythemia rubra vera

- paroxysmal nocturnal hemoglobinuria
- unspecified myeloproliferative disorder
- antiphospholopid antibody syndrome

b Inherited thrombotic diathesis
- protein C deficiency
- protein S deficiency
- antithrombin III deficiency
- factor V Leiden mutation

c Pregnancy or high-dose estrogen use (oral contraceptives)

d Chronic infections
- aspergillosis
- amebic abscess
- hydatid cysts
- tuberculosis

e Tumors
- hepatocellular carcinoma
- renal cell carcinoma
- leiomyosarcoma

f Chronic inflammatory diseases
- Behçet's disease
- inflammatory bowel disease
- sarcoidosis

B   Clinical manifestations and routine laboratory tests

1 The **classic triad of hepatomegaly, ascites, and abdominal pain** is seen in the vast majority of patients, but is nonspecific.
- splenomegaly may develop in almost half of patients
- peripheral edema suggests the possibility of thrombosis or compression of the inferior vena cava
- jaundice is rare

2 The natural history of untreated patients is progression of symptoms often resulting in death due to complications of portal hypertension. In the presurgical era, death was almost invariable except in some patients with membranous webs, in whom symptoms developed slowly

3 Routine biochemical and hematological parameters
- little value in differential diagnosis
- abnormal but nonspecific
- no obvious pattern of abnormalities

4 Ascitic fluid characteristics are useful clues to diagnosis
- high protein concentration (>2.0 g/dL)
- white cell count is usually <500
- serum-ascites albumin gradient is usually >1.1

5 Differential diagnosis includes:
   - right-sided congestive heart failure
   - constrictive pericarditis
   - metastatic disease involving the liver
   - alcoholic liver disease
   - granulomatous liver disease

C   Diagnosis

1 A high index of suspicion is necessary for diagnosis because clinical manifestations and laboratory results are nonspecific

2 Imaging techniques for visualizing hepatic veins
   a Ultrasound
      - color flow Doppler ultrasound is better than duplex ultrasound which is superior to real-time ultrasound
      - provides cost-effective confirmation of low or absent hepatic venous blood flow
      - occasionally can visualize thrombus within hepatic veins
      - sensitivity for color flow Doppler is 85–90% with similar specificity
   b Magnetic resonance imaging (MRI) scanning with pulsed sequencing
      - can visualize thrombus and detect absence of hepatic venous blood flow
      - higher cost is seldom justifiable if Doppler ultrasound is available
      - sensitivity and specificity are approximately 90%
   c Computed tomographic (CT) scanning less sensitive and less specific than Doppler ultrasound and MRI
   d Nuclear scintiscanning shows central hotspot due to hypertrophy of caudate lobe; has largely been replaced by above tests

3 Hepatic venography
   - thrombus within hepatic veins
   - "spider-web" pattern of collaterals
   - inability to cannulate the hepatic vein orifices

4 Pathological findings on liver biopsy
   - evidence of high-grade venous congestion
   - centrilobular liver cell atrophy
   - thrombi within terminal hepatic venules occasionally seen
   - heterogeneous involvement of liver is occasionally problematic

5 The diagnostic approach to a patient suspected of having hepatic vein occlusion should begin with color Doppler ultrasound. If positive or suspicious for BCS, then hepatic venography with inferior vena cavography should be performed to confirm the diagnosis and guide surgical treatment. Liver biopsy is valuable in identifying the extent of fibrosis, which can also guide therapeutic decisions

D   Therapy

1 **Medical therapy** provides only short-term, symptomatic benefit

- the 2-year mortality rate with supportive medical therapy alone is approximately 85–90%
- diuretics are useful for relieving ascites but do not alter the long-term outcome
- anticoagulation with heparin or warfarin may be useful in preventing repeat thromboses but has not been beneficial in relieving symptoms or preventing long-term morbidity and mortality
- thrombolytic therapy has been used successfully in a few reported cases, although the long-term benefit is unclear

2 Portosystemic shunting

a Rationale
   - hepatocellular injury results from microvascular ischemia due to congestion as blood flows into, but not out of, the liver
   - portosystemic shunting provides a low-pressure path for the egress of blood from the congested liver

b Options include:
   - side-to-side portacaval shunt
   - mesocaval shunt
   - mesoatrial shunt
   - side-to-side portacaval with cavoatrial shunt

c Success of portosystemic shunting[1] depends on the following:
   - experience of the surgeon with particular shunts
   - the underlying disease
   - host factors including the extent of fibrosis and/or presence of cirrhosis
   - overall hepatic function at the time of operation

d Patency rates of 65–95%[2] depend on:
   - duration of disease: longer duration, lower patency
   - presence of fibrosis or cirrhosis lowers patency rates
   - the type of shunt: rates for mesoatrial shunts slightly lower than those for mesocaval shunts
   - continued thrombotic diathesis from underlying disease

e Survival rates of 38–87% at 5 years[1–3] depend on:
   - continued patency of graft
   - degree of fibrosis
   - type of shunt

3 Liver transplantation[3,4]

- in theory, transplantation corrects some underlying clotting disorders and restores hepatocellular function
- actuarial 5-year survival rates are approximately 70%; slightly lower than rates for patients with other chronic liver diseases
- some surgeons advocate orthotopic liver transplantation for all patients with BCS
- other surgeons recommend liver transplantation in selected patients with liver failure, cirrhosis, extensive fibrosis, or partial thrombosis of the portal vein

4 **Transcardiac membranotomy** has been used to relieve membranous obstruction of the IVC and rarely the hepatic veins. Other surgical procedures have been used in small numbers of patients with BCS from other causes. The results have been variable and are subject to the bias of reporting successes more often than failures. Approaches include the following:

- hepatopneumopexy
- splenopneumopexy
- Senning operation
- dorsal resection of the liver

5 **Peritoneovenous shunts** have been used to relieve refractory ascites in patients who were not candidates for other surgical procedures. This operation provides only palliation.

6 **Interventional radiologic techniques** have been used to relieve portal hypertension and/or hepatic vein occlusion, nonoperatively.

- angioplasty has been used successfully to relieve hepatic and IVC webs. For other lesions, relief of obstruction is temporary and repeated treatment is required for long-term management
- placement of metal stents in the hepatic veins following angioplasty of short-segment stenoses has been used to improve long-term patency
- placement of stents in the vena cava provides relief of compression from an enlarged caudate lobe and can be followed by side-to-side portacaval or mesocaval shunts, if necessary[5]

7 **Transjugular intrahepatic portal shunts** (TIPS) have been used successfully to correct portal hypertension for up to 3 years in some patients.

- mortality following TIPS occurred in 3 of 12 patients, with one additional patient requiring liver transplantation in a recently published series[6]
- several patients required stent revision after 6–12 months
- of all the interventional techniques, this one holds the most promise both as a temporizing measure to improve hepatic function in patients with BCS prior to definitive surgical treatment and as a potential method for avoiding shunt surgery or transplantation altogether

E   Algorithm for evaluation and management of BCS

1 **The diagnosis of BCS should be suspected in any patient with ascites and hepatomegaly, particularly if there is evidence of a thrombotic diathesis.** A high ascitic protein content or serum-ascites albumin gradient is a clue to the diagnosis

2 Color Doppler or duplex ultrasound should be used to visualize hepatic veins and determine patency of the IVC. If there is doubt, hepatic venography is indicated

3 If there is evidence of hepatic vein outflow obstruction, liver biopsy should be performed unless ascites or coagulopathy cannot be corrected. **The finding of cirrhosis or extensive fibrosis warrants consideration of liver transplantation**

4 **If cirrhosis is absent, options include TIPS or portosystemic shunting.** Hepatic venography and vena cavography are required to determine the need for a

mesoatrial versus a mesocaval shunting. Mesoatrial shunts are preferable in patients with a high pressure gradient across the hepatic cava, provided the surgeon is experienced in this operation. If the IVC is patent, mesocaval shunting with or without placement of an IVC stent is possible. An IVC stent can be placed to relieve compression temporarily by an enlarged caudate lobe. **All patients should undergo early portosystemic decompression**

5 **If cirrhosis or hepatic decompensation is present, liver transplantation is indicated.** Early portosystemic decompression with TIPS is desirable until a donor organ is available

2 Hepatic Veno-occlusive Disease (VOD)

A Definition and etiology

1 Originally described by Chiari in 1899; further described as hepatic vein endophlebitis by Bras in 1954. Histologic features include:
   - subendothelial sclerosis of terminal hepatic venules
   - thrombosis secondary to sclerosis
   - perivenular and sinusoidal fibrosis, particularly in later stages and with chronic injury
   - centrilobular hepatocyte necrosis (may be a primary event)

2 VOD is most often seen
   - in an **acute form** following bone marrow transplantation; thought to be due to toxicity from the preparative regimen of high-dose cytoreductive therapy with or without hepatic irradiation
   - as a **chronic, more indolent form** following toxicity of pyrrolizidine alkaloids from plants of the *Crotalaria*, *Senecio*, and *Heliotropium* genera. The alkaloids are ingested in the form of herbal teas, hence the term Jamaican bush tea disease.

3 Using a definition of VOD based on clinical manifestations (see below), there is no single histologic feature that is pathognomonic. There is a correlation between the number of histologic abnormalities and the clinical severity of VOD[7]

B Clinical manifestations

1 VOD following bone marrow transplantation has been defined as the occurrence of two or more of the following characteristics appearing within 20 days after transplantation:[8]
   - painful hepatomegaly
   - sudden weight gain > 2% of baseline body weight
   - total serum bilirubin > 2.0 mg/dL (34.2 µmol/L)

2 The occurrence of VOD is significantly correlated with subsequent development of renal insufficiency, pleural effusions, cardiac failure, pulmonary infiltrates, and bleeding requiring blood transfusions

3 Using clinical definitions, approximately 50% of bone marrow transplant patients develop VOD. The mortality rate for all patients with clinical evidence of VOD is approximately 40%

4 A more chronic form of VOD develops in those who ingest pyrrolizidine alkaloids.

Clinical features of this condition are similar to those of hepatic vein occlusion, and include tender hepatomegaly, abdominal pain, ascites, and fatigue. The absence of specific features and the lack of noninvasive methods for detecting this condition make diagnosis difficult. Liver biopsy usually shows sinusoidal and perivenular fibrosis as well as subendothelial sclerosis. Poisoning is most often inadvertent and can be due to contamination of foodstuffs with pyrrolizidine-containing plants

C   Risk factors for acute VOD following bone marrow transplantation

1   Risk factors for VOD occurring after bone marrow transplantation[8] include:
   - pretransplant elevation in serum alanine aminotransferase (AST) or alanine aminotransferase (ALT) levels
   - past history of viral or drug-induced hepatitis
   - past history of abdominal radiation
   - fever before cytoreductive therapy not responsive to broad-spectrum antibiotics
   - fever occurring after cytoreductive therapy and before transplantation

2   Cytoreductive regimens associated with an increased incidence of VOD:
   - radiation dose > 12 Gy
   - cyclophosphamide plus busulfan
   - cyclophosphamide, BCNU, and etoposide

D   Pathogenesis

1   Cytoreductive therapy is toxic primarily to endothelial cells, both sinusoidal and vascular. These cells are more susceptible to glutathione depletion in response to a variety of agents, including dacarbazine, azathioprine, and monocrotaline[9]

2   Various cytokines including tumor necrosis factor α (TNF-α) are released in response to cytoreductive therapy. Patients with hepatic and multi-organ failure syndrome have been shown to have high circulating levels of TNF-α and other cytokines. TNF in particular exerts procoagulant effects on protein C and may be involved in the pathogenesis of thrombosis in VOD. However, much of the pathophysiology is speculative at present

E   Treatment

1   Treatment of VOD following bone marrow transplantation is largely supportive.
   - attention should be paid to the patient's fluid status, avoiding excess fluid administration which results in worsening of cardiac and pulmonary function
   - support with platelets and red blood cell transfusions is often necessary because of the profound cytopenias that accompany marrow transplantation
   - use of dopamine and other pressors is often necessary to maintain renal perfusion, particularly in the presence of a capillary leak syndrome.
   - broad-spectrum antibiotics are used to treat presumptive infection, pending identification of a specific causative organism
   - there is interest in the use of drugs such as pentoxifylline that inhibit release of TNF-α, but this approach is still experimental

2   Treatment of chronic VOD associated with ingestion of pyrrolizidine alkaloids often

requires liver transplantation because of the extensive fibrosis that is usually present at the time of diagnosis. Early cases may be managed with portosystemic shunts

References

1 Klein A, Sitzmann J, Coleman J, Herlong F, Cameron J. *Current management of the Budd–Chiari syndrome.* (Ann Surg 1990) 212: 144–9

2 Panis Y, Belghiti J, Valla D, Berthamou J, Fekete F. *Portosystemic shunt in Budd–Chiari syndrome: long-term survival and factors affecting shunt patency in 25 patients in western countries.* (Surgery 1994) 115: 276–81

3 Hemming A, Langer B, Greig P, Taylor B, Adams R, Heathcote J. *Treatment of Budd–Chiari syndrome with portosystemic shunt of liver transplantation.* (Am J Surg 1996) 171: 176–81

4 Ringe B, Lang H, Oldhafer KJ, et al. *Which is best surgery for Budd–Chiari Syndrome: venous decompression or liver transplantation? A single-center experience with 50 patients.* (Hepatology 1995) 21: 1337–1344

5 Venbrux AC, Mitchell SE, Savader SJ et al. *Long-term results with the use of metallic stents in the inferior vena cava for treatment of Budd–Chiari syndrome.* (J Vasc Interv Radiol 1994) 5: 411–16

6 Blum U, Rossle M, Haag K, et al. *Budd–Chiari syndrome: technical, hemodynamic and clinical results of treatment with transjugular intrahepatic portosystemic shunt.* (Radiology 1995) 197: 805–11

7 Shulman HM, Fisher LB, Schoch HG, Henne KW, McDonald GB. *Venoocclusive disease of the liver after marrow transplantation: Histological correlates of clinical signs and symptoms.* (Hepatology 1994) 19: 1171–81

8 McDonald G, Hinds M, Fisher L, et al. *Veno-occlusive disease of the liver and multiorgan failure after bone marrow transplantation: a cohort study of 355 patients.* (Ann Intern Med 1993) 118: 255–67

9 DeLeve LD, Wang X, Kuhlenkamp JF, Kaplowitz N. *Toxicity of azathioprine and monocrotaline in murine sinusoidal endothelial cells and hepatocytes: the roles of glutathione and relevance to hepatic venoocclusive disease.* (Hepatology 1996) 23: 589–99

10 Dilawari J, Bambery P, Chawla Y, et al. *Hepatic outflow obstruction (Budd–Chiari syndrome): experience with 177 patients and a review of the literature.* (Medicine 1994) 73: 21–36

11 Ludwig J, Hashimoto E, McGill D, Heerden J. *Classification of hepatic venous outflow obstruction: ambiguous terminology of the Budd–Chiari syndrome.* (Mayo Clin Proc 1990) 65: 51–5

12 Mitchell M, Boitnott J, Kaufman S, Cameron J, Maddrey J. *Budd–Chiari syndrome: etiology, diagnosis and management.* (Medicine 1982) 61: 199–218

13 Valla D, Casadevell N, Lancombe C, et al. *Primary myeloproliferative disorders and hepatic vein thrombosis: a prospective study of erythroid colony formation in vitro in 20 patients with Budd–Chiari syndrome.* (Ann Intern Med 1985) 103: 329–334

The liver in heart failure

FLORENCE WONG, M.D., F.R.A.C.P.
SUSAN GREENBLOOM, M.D., F.R.C.P.(C.)
LAURENCE M. BLENDIS, M.D., F.R.C.P.(C.)

▼

Key Points

1 Liver involvement in either forward or backward cardiac failure is frequent

2 Backward cardiac failure will cause congestion of the liver with hepatomegaly and nonspecific liver function test abnormalities

3 Forward cardiac failure will cause ischemic damage to the liver if the circulatory failure is severe and prolonged. The pattern of a very rapid rise and fall in aminotransferase levels is characteristic

4 Beware of alternative diagnoses if liver abnormalities are unusually high when not in an acute setting, in particular, if the alkaline phosphatase level is more than twice normal or if the ALT is much higher than the AST

5 The frequency and severity of liver involvement depend on the severity of cardiac failure

6 There is no specific treatment for the liver dysfunction. Improvement in cardiac function will result in return of liver tests to normal, unless cardiac cirrhosis is already present

7 The severity of the cardiac, not the hepatic, dysfunction will determine prognosis, unless cardiac cirrhosis is already present

▲

1 Introduction

1 Liver dysfunction has long been recognized as a complication of both severe acute and chronic congestive heart failure

2 Heart failure is usually due to pump failure leading to decreased cardiac output, venous congestion and retention of extracellular fluid

3 An understanding of the hepatic circulation and normal liver architecture is important to appreciate how the hemodynamic changes of heart failure affect the liver, leading to the associated clinical, biochemical, and histologic features

2 The Hepatic Circulation

A Hepatic blood supply

1 The liver has a dual blood supply:
- The portal vein supplies approximately 66–83% of the blood flow to the liver, bringing nutrient-rich but relatively less well-oxygenated venous blood from the stomach, intestine, and spleen
- The hepatic artery, a branch of the celiac axis, provides the remaining 17–34% of its blood supply with arterial blood and supplies approximately 50% of hepatic oxygen

2 A reduction in portal inflow or sinusoidal pressure results in a reflex increase in hepatic arterial blood flow, thereby ensuring a constant sinusoidal pressure

3 Primary changes in hepatic arterial blood are not associated with changes in portal venous blood flow

4 A decrease in cardiac output usually results in decreased hepatic blood flow. The percentage of cardiac output received by the liver, however, remains relatively stable

5 Decreased perfusion is usually compensated by increased oxygen extraction

6 Hypercapnia, if present, will cause generalized vasodilation, increasing blood flow to the liver further

B Hepatic venous drainage

1 The liver is drained by the hepatic vein, which is formed by the right, middle, and left hepatic veins

2 The hepatic vein in turn drains into the inferior vena cava and then into the right side of the heart

C The hepatic microcirculation

1 The portal vein and the hepatic artery divide into branches to the right and left lobes of the liver. These further subdivide five to six times until their terminal branches reach the portal triad

2 The portal vein tributaries open directly into sinusoids. The hepatic artery branches open into some but not all sinusoids. The sinusoids anastomose freely at all levels between the portal vein tributaries and the terminal hepatic venules.

3 Hepatic sinusoids:
  • form a rich vascular network that converges towards the terminal hepatic venule
  • are lined by both endothelial cells and specialized macrophages called Kupffer's cells. There is no basement membrane underlying the endothelial cells
  • the porous nature of the sinusoids allows for a low hydrostatic pressure and free flow between the sinusoids and the interstitial space – the space of Disse
  • the diameter of the sinusoid is less than that of the erythrocytes, which therefore have to squeeze through the lumen
4 Narrowing of the sinusoidal lumen has serious consequences for the oxygenation of the hepatocytes

3   Liver Architecture

1 The histologic unit of the liver is the lobule (Fig. 20.1A):
  • its boundaries are surrounded by connective tissue stroma and the portal triads
  • the center of the lobule is the terminal hepatic vein
2 The functional unit of the liver is the acinus (Fig. 20.1B)
  • liver parenchymal cells are grouped into concentric zones centered around the portal triad – zone 1 is nearest, while zones 2 and 3 are more distal to the afferent blood vessels
  • the oxygen tension and nutrient level of the blood decrease from zone 1 to zone 3
  • zone 1 hepatocytes are first to receive oxygenated blood and last to undergo necrosis
  • zones 2 and 3 receive blood of considerably less oxygen and nutrient content and are more vulnerable to hepatotoxins and hypoxic injuries

4   Pathophysiology

1 Forward failure of the heart leads to decreased cardiac output and hepatic blood flow
2 Backward failure with venous engorgement causes hepatic congestion

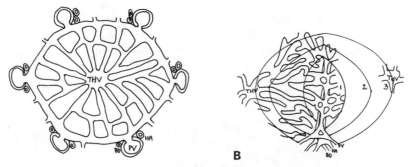

Fig. 20.1   **A** The histologic unit of the liver – the lobule. **B** the functional unit of the liver – the acinus. THV, terminal hepatic vein; HA, hepatic artery; PV, portal vein; BD, bile duct; 1,2,3, zone 1, zone 2, zone 3 of Rappaport

3 Both forward and backward failures lead to cellular hypoxia and liver damage

4 Decreased arterial oxygen saturation also contributes to the liver damage (Fig. 20.2)

A Chronic passive congestion

1 In congestive heart failure with low cardiac output, total hepatic blood flow falls by about one-third

2 The increased systemic venous pressure is reflected as hepatic venous hypertension, which can cause hepatic cell atrophy via sinusoidal congestion and expansion

3 The accompanying perisinusoidal edema can result in decreased diffusion of oxygen and other metabolites to hepatocytes

4 Collagenosis of Disse's space from chronic congestion may play a minor role in impairing oxygen diffusion

5 Low cardiac output and the consequent circulatory changes in the intestinal wall may allow an increased diffusion of endotoxin into the portal blood and augment damage to the liver.[1] The role of endotoxemia in liver damage associated with cardiac failure is still to be confirmed

B Decreased hepatic blood flow

1 Increased oxygen extraction by the liver in situations of low hepatic flow ensures a constant oxygen consumption within wide limits of hepatic flow. The liver therefore does not suffer from hypoxia as a result of decrease in hepatic flow under basal conditions

2 A reduction in hepatic flow of greater than 70% results in decreased oxygen uptake, galactose elimination capacity, and adenosine triphosphate concentrations and increased lactate/pyruvate ratio (an index of tissue hypoxia)

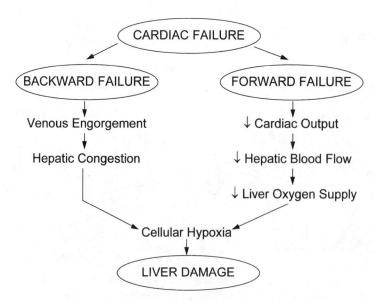

Fig. 20.2 The pathophysiology of liver dysfunction in cardiac failure

3 Hepatic arterial vasoconstriction and intense selective splanchnic vasoconstriction in significant hypoperfusion and shock causes hypoxic damage to the liver

4 Hypoxic damage characteristically occurs in the area adjacent to the terminal hepatic vein (zone 3 of the acinus) – the area that is furthest away from the oxygen-carrying blood supply

5 High aminotransferase levels (aspartate aminotransferase (AST) and alanine aminotransferase (ALT) greater than 20 times upper limit of normal) are the typical hallmark of zone 3 necrosis

6 Insufficient substrates and accumulation of metabolites both contribute to hypoxic damage

7 Loss of mitochrondrial oxidative phosphorylation as a result of hypoxia leads to impaired membrane function, disrupted intracellular ion homeostasis, and reduced protein synthesis

8 In acute cardiac failure, both a reduction of hepatic blood flow and increased central venous pressure contribute to the development of hypoxic hepatitis[2]

5 Pathology

A Macroscopic

1 The liver is enlarged and purplish with rounded edges (Fig. 20.3, see plate section)

2 Nodularity is inconspicuous, but if nodular regenerative hyperplasia (see below) or cardiac cirrhosis is present, nodules may be seen

3 The cut surface shows prominent hepatic veins which may be thickened

4 There is a "nutmeg" appearance from the contrasting combination of hemorrhagic

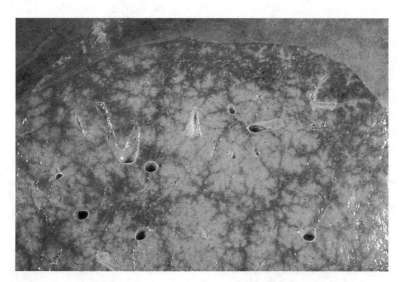

Fig. 20.3   Macroscopic appearance of the liver in congestive cardiac failure. See page xxii.

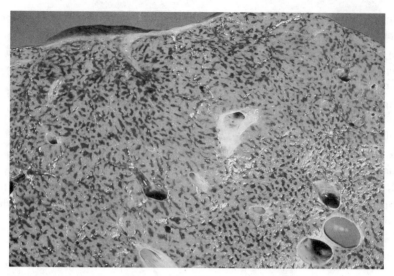

Fig. 20.4   Cut surface of the liver in congestive cardiac failure showing the "nutmeg appearance". See page xxii.

central areas of the lobules and the normal yellow portal and periportal areas (Fig. 20.4, see plate section)

5 A more yellow than usual appearing portal area may be due to increase in portal fat

B   Microscopic

1 The hepatic histology generally correlates with the clinical or biochemical severity of cardiac failure and with cardiac weight and chamber size

2 Early in congestive cardiac failure, the terminal hepatic veins become engorged and dilated. Sinusoids adjacent to the terminal hepatic veins are also dilated and filled with erythrocytes for a variable extent towards the portal areas

3 There is also compression and variable atrophy of the liver cell plates and an apparent increase in the amount of lipofuscin in the cytoplasm of liver cells

4 Moderately severe congestive cardiac failure can result in zone 3 liver cell necrosis. Cellular infiltrate is inconspicuous

5 In acute severe hypotension and shock, mid-zone necrosis can also occur

6 The necrotic hepatocytes are often packed with a brownish pigment which probably is related to bilirubin degradation

7 Liver cell necrosis progresses from zone 3 to the portal areas as the heart disease progresses.[3] In the most severe form of liver congestion from cardiac failure, only a small area of normal-appearing hepatocytes remains in the periportal area

8 The reticulin network condenses and may collapse around the terminal hepatic vein following loss of liver cells (Fig. 20.5, see plate section)

   • bridging can be seen extending from and joining adjacent terminal hepatic veins

   • ultimately, the unaffected portal areas are surrounded by rings of fibrous tissue, resulting in reverse lobulation

9 True cardiac cirrhosis is rare. When present, it is associated with intimal fibrosis

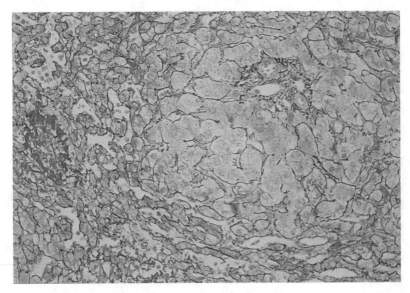

Fig. 20.5   Collapse of reticulin network around terminal hepatic veins and nodular transformation in congestive cardiac failure. See page xxiii.

and thrombosis of small and medium-sized hepatic veins. The resultant ischemia is responsible for hepatocellular necrosis, and the stasis augments fibroblast activation and collagen deposition[4]

10   Regeneration of hepatocytes around the periportal area can occur, leading to liver cell plates many cells thick. These can reorganize into rounded periportal masses abutting on compressed central hepatocytes and congested and dilated sinusoids. Such changes are best described as nodular regenerative hyperplasia[5] (Fig. 20.6, see plate section)

11   The wall of the terminal hepatic vein can undergo varying degrees of fibrous thickening called phlebosclerosis (Fig. 20.7, see plate section)

12   Liver damage associated with congestive cardiac failure is reversible once the cardiac failure is treated. Hepatocytes regenerate, fibrous bands become narrower and acellular, and near-normal hepatic architecture is restored[6]

6   Etiology (see Table 20.1)

1   Left and right ventricular failure often coexist, resulting in hepatic congestion

2   Acute myocardial infarction with arrhythmia and cardiogenic shock can complicate coronary artery disease, resulting in ischemic hepatitis, superimposed on the chronic hepatic congestion

3   Rheumatic heart disease, with mitral stenosis and tricuspid regurgitation, appears to produce the most severe hepatic congestion

4   The abrupt onset of atrial fibrillation or the development of bacterial endocarditis can decrease left ventricular output and aggravate hypoxic liver damage

5   Children with hypoplastic left heart syndrome and coarctation of the aorta are

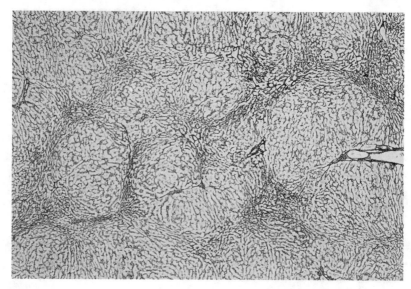

Fig. 20.6 Nodular regenerative hyperplasia associated with congestive cardiac failure. See page xxiii.

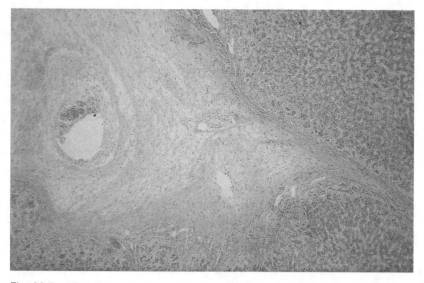

Fig. 20.7 Phlebosclerosis observed in the wall of the terminal hepatic vein in congestive cardiac failure. See page xxiv.

particularly prone to hepatic necrosis. This may be due to the combination of reduced systemic blood flow, a left-to-right shunt, and markedly elevated right ventricular pressure

7 Prevalence

1 Liver involvement is common in severe cardiac failure

	% of total
Coronary artery disease	33
Hypertension	22
Rheumatic valve disease	32
Cor pulmonale	6
Constrictive pericarditis	4
Congenital heart disease	2
Miscellaneous	<1

Reprinted by permission of the publisher from 'Alterations in indices of liver function in congestive heart failure with particular reference to serum enzymes' by S.M. Richman, A. Delman and D. Grob, *American Journal of Medicine* 30: 217–25. Copyright 1961 by Excerpta Medica Inc.

(Table 20.1: Common causes of cardiac failure leading to liver congestion[7])

2 As the incidence of rheumatic valve disease declines, coronary artery disease and the associated congestive cardiomyopathy is becoming an important cause of liver congestion

3 The overall prevalence of liver congestion in congestive cardiac failure depends on patient selection and the criteria used for defining liver involvement (clinical, biochemical, or histologic)

4 In patients with a cardiac index above 2 L/min/m^2, only 20–30% of patients have minor elevations of liver enzymes. In contrast, up to 80% of patients with a cardiac index below 1.5 L/min/m^2 have some major biochemical abnormalities[8]

8 Clinical Features

1 The clinical picture is dominated by signs and symptoms of right-sided cardiac failure rather than those of liver disease, in the majority of patients (see Table 20.2)

2 Stigmata of chronic liver disease, such as palmar erythema, spider telangiectases, and caput medusa are rare

3 Right-upper-quadrant pain is due to stretching of the liver capsule and mediated via the phrenic nerve

4 The liver can return to normal size as fibrosis develops during the course of severe hepatic congestion, but it is never reduced in size

5 Hyperbilirubinemia and jaundice:
  • mild jaundice is common, but deep icterus is rare
  • jaundice increases with prolonged and repeated bouts of congestive cardiac failure
  • part of the hyperbilirubinemia may be unconjugated, related to infarcts of tissues, especially pulmonary infarcts. The jaundice may then be prolonged due to inability of the hypoxic liver to handle the bilirubin load

Symptom/sign	Patients showing symptom/sign (%)
Right-upper-quadrant discomfort	30
Hepatomegaly	95–99
Marked hepatomegaly (>5 cm below the right costal margin)	50
Jaundice	10–20
Peripheral edema	75
Ascites	25
Pleural effusion	20
Splenomegaly	20

Reprinted by permission of the publisher from 'Alterations in indices of liver function in congestive heart failure with particular reference to serum enzymes' by S.M. Richman, A. Delman and D. Grob, *American Journal of Medicine* 30: 217–25. Copyright 1961 by Excerpta Medica Inc.

(Table 20.2: Common signs and symptoms of liver congestion[7])

6 With tricuspid regurgitation, a palpable systolic pulsation over the liver, related to the transmission of right atrial pressure to the hepatic vein, is present

7 Splenomegaly is frequent, but other features of portal hypertension are usually absent, except in severe cardiac cirrhosis associated with constrictive pericarditis

8 The presence of ascites is most likely related to increased sinusoidal pressure and permeability, and increased leakage of lymph, rather than a manifestation of cirrhosis. This accounts for the **high ascitic protein** content (with a high serum-ascites albumin gradient) found in these patients

9 The presence of peripheral edema and pleural effusion probably reflects the cardiac disease rather than the concomitant hepatic congestion

10 **Ischemic hepatitis** as a result of low cardiac output may not be clinically obvious. Hypotension is not always documented and the left-sided cardiac failure may be subtle. Diagnosis is often based on the abnormal biochemical tests and a high index of suspicion

11 Fulminant hepatic failure with asterixis and coma as a complication of circulatory failure is rare. It usually develops 2–3 days after the circulatory failure. Serum aminotransferases can rise to over 1000 U/L. Prognosis is poor, with half of the patients dying from the underlying cardiac disease

9 Laboratory Abnormalities

1 The frequency of abnormal liver function tests in patients with cardiac failure varies widely in the published literature. This is most likely due to the heterogeneity of the patients described

2 There is no absolute correlation between the clinical severity of the cardiac failure and the abnormalities of liver function tests. In general, however, patients with higher right atrial pressures and the more profound clinical manifestations of cardiac failure tend to have more abnormal liver function tests

A Bromsulphalein (BSP) retention test

- this is the most sensitive test of hepatic dysfunction in congestive cardiac failure and may be the only abnormal liver function test
- abnormal in over 80% of patients and correlates well with central venous pressure elevation
- however, the test is no longer widely available and is rarely used

B Bilirubin

- increased bilirubin reported in 25–75% of patients with congestive cardiac failure. Jaundice is usually mild in congestive cardiac failure, with serum bilirubin generally less than 80 mmol/L (4.5 mg/dL)
- markedly elevated serum bilirubin levels are usually seen in acute right-sided heart failure. The hyperbilirubinemia appears to be related to hepatocellular dysfunction per se
- about 50–60% of the serum bilirubin is unconjugated, due to a combination of mild hemolysis, reduced uptake, and decreased conjugation by hepatocytes
- serum bilirubin levels may fall rapidly after improvement of the congestion, resulting in normal levels in 3–7 days
- in patients with prolonged congestive cardiac failure, serum bilirubin levels may not return to normal for many months after the relief of the congestion. This may be due to covalent bonding of conjugated bilirubin with albumin to form delta bilirubin, with a prolonged half-life of 21 days

C Aminotransferases

- in stable congestive cardiac failure without decompensation, the aminotransferases are only elevated in 5–30% of patients. Levels are usually two to four times the upper limit of normal.
- markedly elevated levels (more than 10 times the upper limit of normal) are seen in patients with acute worsening of severe chronic congestive cardiac failure, hypotension or shock[9]
- AST tends to be higher than ALT, due to the AST-rich cardiac myocytes; the increase in AST generally appears earlier than the increase in ALT
- very high levels of AST can also be found in patients with drug-induced or viral hepatitis, but ALT levels are usually higher in the latter (see Ch. 1)
- if the elevation in AST is due to cardiac failure, the level can be expected to fall within a few days of circulatory improvement. In contrast, high levels of AST usually persist in cases of viral or drug-induced hepatitis and are independent of improvement in circulatory status

- moderate increases in AST can also be due to myocardial infarction, a not uncommon scenario. The consequent myocardial dysfunction and congestive cardiac failure can make the interpretation of the AST level difficult. Simultaneous measurements of other enzymes, such as the MB fraction of creatine kinase, are helpful in diagnosing myocardial injury
- there is a significant, albeit weak, correlation between the aminotransferase levels and the height of the right atrial pressure and the cardiac index. Improvement of cardiac function will result in return of aminotransferase levels towards normal in 3–7 days.

D   Alkaline phosphatase

- elevated alkaline phosphatase levels are uncommon in congestive cardiac failure. When present, the elevation is mild, usually not exceeding twice the upper limit of normal
- the exact mechanism leading to increased alkaline phosphatase in liver congestion is unknown. Both pressure-induced intrahepatic biliary obstruction and hepatic dysfunction may both play a role
- when nodular regenerative hyperplasia complicates congestive cardiac failure, the only abnormal liver function test is an elevated alkaline phosphatase

E   Prothrombin time

- increased prothrombin time is observed in over 80% of patients with congestive cardiac failure
- prolongation of the prothrombin time is more common with acute than chronic congestion. In acute congestion, the prothrombin time may rapidly increase to twice normal, is not responsive to vitamin K administration, and may return to normal rapidly with successful treatment of the congestion
- these patients are therefore very sensitive to the effects of warfarin
- with successful treatment of chronic congestive cardiac failure, prothrombin time takes 2–3 weeks to return to normal

F   Serum albumin

- the serum albumin is moderately decreased in 30–50% of patients with congestive cardiac failure. Lower albumin levels are seen in patients with ascites and edema
- the low serum albumin level may be due in part to decreased hepatic synthesis and in part to a dilutional effect secondary to fluid retention
- in general, the serum albumin does not correlate with either the duration of congestive cardiac failure or the extent of hepatic damage
- the serum albumin level may require more than a month to improve following resolution of congestive cardiac failure

G   Ischemic hepatitis

- Changes in biochemical tests in ischemic hepatitis are characteristic, and the diagnosis can be made by observing the evolution of these changes:
  - marked increases in aminotransferase levels with AST greater than ALT (up to 100 times normal) within 24–48 hours of the acute circulatory failure
  - a rapid return of the aminotransferase levels to normal in 3–11 days after treatment of acute circulatory failure
  - a similar rise and fall of serum lactic dehydrogenase (LDH)
  - serum bilirubin may rise but is rarely greater than four times the upper limit of normal
  - alkaline phosphatase levels generally remain normal
  - the prothrombin time is only mildly prolonged by 1 or 2 seconds

H   Cardiac cirrhosis

- there is no biochemical test that distinguishes a congested noncirrhotic liver from one with cardiac cirrhosis. Therefore, cardiac cirrhosis is a clinical diagnosis

- suspect cardiac cirrhosis in a patient with well-documented tricuspid regurgitation and absent hepatic pulsation
- Cardiac cirrhosis should also be considered in:
  - severe mitral stenosis
  - constrictive pericarditis
  - prolonged or recurrent severe congestive cardiac failure
  - clinically severe passive congestion of the liver, with a small liver, splenomegaly, and ascites

10   Radiological Changes

Suggestive findings on contrast-enhanced computed tomographic (CT) scan

1. Lobulated, patchy, and inhomogeneous pattern in a large liver
2. Irregular perivascular enhancement or delayed parenchymal enhancement
3. Distended inferior vena cava and early reflux of contrast medium into the inferior vena cava and hepatic veins

11   Treatment

1. Treatment of liver congestion should be directed towards the primary problem, that is, cardiac failure

2 Clinical improvement in cardiac function can be dramatic following definitive treatment of cardiac failure such as valve replacement, pericardiectomy for constrictive pericarditis, or correction of a congenital anomaly

3 However, the presence of cardiac cirrhosis with or without hepatic failure results in a significant rise in perioperative mortality rate and may therefore be a contraindication to surgery (see Ch. 30)

4 Improvement of liver function tests usually follows clinical improvement unless cardiac cirrhosis is already present

12 Prognosis

1 The prognosis is that of the underlying cardiac disease
2 In chronic congestive cardiac failure, if the condition is treated and the congestion resolves, the outcome will be positive
3 In ischemic hepatitis, the prognosis is often poor. Prolonged jaundice, especially if severe, is a bad prognostic sign
4 Death in ischemic hepatitis is usually due to circulatory failure. The hepatic disorder usually has little or no influence on the eventual outcome

References

1 Shibayama Y. *The role of hepatic venous congestion and endotoxaemia in the production of fulminant hepatic failure secondary to congestive heart failure.* (J Pathol 1986) 151: 133–8

2 Henrion J, Descamps O, Luwaert R, et al. *Hypoxic hepatitis in patients with cardiac failure: incidence in a coronary care unit and measurement of hepatic blood flow.* (J Hepatol 1994) 21: 696–703

3 Kanel GC, Ucci AA, Kaplan MM, et al. *A distinctive perivenular hepatic lesion associated with heart failure.* (Am J Clin Pathol 1980) 73: 235–39

4 Wanless IR, Liu JJ, Butany J. *Role of thrombosis in the pathogenesis of congestive hepatic fibrosis (cardiac cirrhosis).* (Hepatology 1995) 21: 1232–7

5 Lefkowitch JH, Mendez L. *Morphologic features of hepatic injury in cardiac disease and shock.* (J Hepatol 1986) 2: 313–27

6 Arcidi JM, Moore GW, Hutchins GM. *Hepatic morphology in cardiac dysfunction: a clinicopathologic study of 1000 subjects at autopsy.* (Am J Pathol 1981) 104: 159–66

7 Richman SM, Delman A, Grob D. *Alterations in indices of liver function in congestive heart failure with particular reference to serum enzymes.* (Am J Med 1961) 30: 211–25

8 Kubo SH, Walter BA, John DHA, et al. *Liver function abnormalities in chronic heart failure: influence of systemic hemodynamics.* (Arch Intern Med 1987) 147: 1227–30

9 Bynum TE, Boitnott JK, Maddrey WC. *Ischaemic hepatitis.* (Dig Dis Sci 1979) 24: 129–35

The liver in pregnancy

JACQUELINE L. WOLF, M.D.

▼

Key Points

1 Liver diseases in pregnancy include those present at the time of pregnancy, those that occur coincidentally with pregnancy and those that occur exclusively in pregnancy

2 The time of gestation when abnormal liver function tests develop, the occurrence of multiple births, a history of past pregnancies, and the family history provide clues to the etiology of pregnancy-associated liver disease

3 Symptoms and physical findings such as pruritus, hypertension, edema, and abdominal pain are particularly important to note

4 Diagnostic tests with particular importance to diagnosing liver disease in pregnancy are proteinuria, hyperuricemia, elevated serum bile acids, thrombocytopenia, and anemia. Abdominal ultrasound and/or limited abdominal computed tomography may be helpful. Liver biopsy is rarely done but may be diagnostic for acute fatty liver of pregnancy

5 Diagnosis guides treatment. Delivery is the treatment of choice for severe preeclampsia, eclampsia, acute fatty liver of pregnancy, and severe HELLP syndrome. Immunization of infants born to mothers with hepatitis B is critical

▲

---

1   The Liver in Pregnancy

A   Overview

1 **Liver diseases in pregnancy consist of:**
   - **those present at the time of pregnancy**
   - **those that occur coincidentally with pregnancy**
   - **those that occur exclusively during pregnancy**

2 De novo liver function test abnormalities occur in up to 5% of pregnancies in the USA

3 Liver function tests may differ in the gravid and nongravid state (see Table 21.1)

4 Chronic hepatitis B infection is present in 5–15 per 1000 pregnancies in the USA

5 The frequency of chronic hepatitis C infection is as high as 2.3% in an indigent population

Test	Effect	Trimester of maximum change
Albumin	↓ 10–60%	Second
Gamma globulin	nl to sl ↓	
Fibrinogen	↑ 50%	Second
Transferrin	↑	Third
Bilirubin	nl	
Alkaline phosphatase	↑ 2 to 4-fold	Third
AST/SGOT	nl	
ALT/SGPT	nl	
Cholesterol	↑ 2-fold	Third

nl, normal; sl, slight; ↑, increase; ↓, decrease; AST, aspartate aminotransferase; ALT, alanine aminotransferase
Reprinted with permission from Olans & Wolf (1995)[1]

(Table 21.1: Changes in Liver function test results in normal pregnancy)

2   Approach to the Pregnant Patient

A   History

1 **Relation to time of gestation** (see Table 21.2)

2 **Pruritus**
   - characteristic of intrahepatic cholestasis of pregnancy
   - affects palms of hands and soles of feet initially, then elsewhere

3 **Nausea and vomiting**
   - occurs in 50–90% of all pregnancies

Trimester of pregnancy	Differential diagnosis
First	Hyperemesis gravidarum Gallstones Viral hepatitis Drug-induced hepatitis Intrahepatic cholestasis of pregnancy[a]
Second	Intrahepatic cholestasis of pregnancy Gallstones Viral hepatitis Drug-induced hepatitis Pre-eclampsia/eclampsia[a] HELLP syndrome[a]
Third	Intrahepatic cholestasis of pregnancy Pre-eclampsia/eclampsia HELLP syndrome Acute fatty liver of pregnancy Hepatic rupture Gallstones Viral hepatitis Drug-induced hepatitis

[a]Uncommon in this trimester
HELLP hemolytic anemia, elevated liver function tests, low platelets
Reprinted with permission from Olans & Wolf (1995)[1]

(Table 21.2: Differential diagnosis of elevated serum aminotransferase levels and/or jaundice in pregnancy)

- key features of hyperemesis gravidarum
- when associated with headache and peripheral edema may indicate pre-eclampsia
- when associated in late pregnancy with abdominal pain and with or without hypotension, may indicate hepatic rupture

4 Abdominal pain
- note location, character, duration, and factors that induce or relieve pain
- right-upper-quadrant or mid-abdominal pain in late pregnancy may have ominous implications. Consider cholelithiasis, acute fatty liver of pregnancy, hepatic rupture, pre-eclampsia

5 Jaundice
- note relation to onset of other symptoms
- follows pruritus in intrahepatic cholestasis of pregnancy

6 Systemic symptoms
- headache, peripheral edema, foamy urine, oliguria, and neurological symptoms may occur in pre-eclampsia
- fever, malaise, change in stools may indicate infection such as hepatitis
- easy bruisability may occur in HELLP syndrome
- weight loss or gain or dizziness may occur with liver disease in pregnancy

7 History of past pregnancy and birth control use (see Table 21.3)

- note time of onset of symptoms in previous pregnancies
- note outcome of previous pregnancies
- jaundice may occur with birth control use in patients who have had intrahepatic cholestasis of pregnancy

Intrahepatic cholestasis of pregnancy	Frequently
HELLP	2–43%
Acute fatty liver of pregnancy	Occasionally
Pre-eclampsia	4–27%

(Table 21.3: Rates of recurrence of pregnancy-associated liver disease)

8 Relevant pregnancy-related factors

- multiple verus single gestation
- primiparous verus multiparous
- medications

B Physical examination

- spider telangiectases and palmar erythema occur in normal pregnancy
- abnormal findings occurring with liver disease in pregnancy are jaundice, hepatomegaly, hepatic tenderness, friction rub or bruit, splenomegaly, Murphy's sign, diffuse excoriations
- systemic findings that may occur with liver disease in pregnancy are hypertension, orthostatic hypotension, peripheral edema, asterixis, hyperreflexia or other neurologic findings, ecchymoses, and petechiae

C Diagnostic tests

- only major restriction compared to nongravid state is limitation on radiation exposure
- routine blood chemistries and blood count helpful. Uric acid level often elevated in acute fatty liver of pregnancy and may be elevated in pre-eclampsia
- low platelet counts and hemolysis in HELLP syndrome. Disseminated intravascular coagulation with low fibrinogen, increased fibrin split products, and elevated partial thromboplastin time may also occur in HELLP
- elevations in serum bile acid levels occur before or concurrent with onset of intrahepatic cholestasis of pregnancy
- check amylase and lipase if abdominal pain
- in suspected viral hepatitis, check serologic tests for hepatitis A (IgM and IgG antibodies); hepatitis B (surface antigen (HBsAg) and antibody, core antibody, and, if surface antigen positive, "e" antigen and antibody); hepatitis C, (antibody and possibly hepatitis C viral RNA). If foreign travel to endemic area, consider testing for hepatitis E (see Ch. 3)

- endoscopy, including endoscopic retrograde cannulation of pancreatic and biliary ducts, is safe in pregnancy so long as radiation exposure is limited
- abdominal ultrasound is safe and useful
- abdominal computed tomography (CT), limiting exposure to one or two views, may be preferable for defecting acute fatty liver of pregnancy or hepatic rupture
- angiography is rarely needed for hepatic rupture
- magnetic resonance imaging (MRI) is probably safe, though not conclusively proven

3   Liver Disorders Unique to Pregnancy

See Table 21.4 for the laboratory findings associated with these disorders.

	Amino-transferases	Bile acids	Bilirubin	Alkaline phosphatase	Uric acid	Platelets	PT/PTT	Urine protein
Hyperemesis gravidarum	1–2×	nl	<5 mg/dL	1–2×	nl	nl	nl	nl
Intrahepatic cholestasis of pregnancy	1–4×	30–100×	<5 mg/dL	1–2×	nl	nl	nl	nl
Acute fatty liver of pregnancy	1–5×	nl	<10 mg/dL	1–2×	↑	±↓	±↑	±↑
Pre-eclampsia/ eclampsia	1–100×	nl	<5 mg/dL	1–2×	↑	±↓	±↑	↑
HELLP	1–100×	nl	<5 mg/dL	1–2×	↑	↓	±↑	±↑
Hepatic rupture	2–100×	nl	±↑	↑	nl	±↓	±↑	nl

PT, prothrombin time; PTT, partial thromboplastin time

(Table 21.4: Results of laboratory tests in pregnancy-associated liver disease)

A   Hyperemesis gravidarum

1 **Definition:** Intractable vomiting in pregnancy that leads to dehydration, electrolyte disturbances, or nutritional deficiencies.

2 **Epidemiology**
- most common in first trimester
- occurs more frequently in women under age 25 years who are overweight, multiparous, and with multiple births
- incidence of 0.2–6.0 per 1000 deliveries in USA

3 **Clinical and laboratory findings**
- liver function test abnormalities in 50% of patients

- ALT elevation generally one- to three-fold but may reach 20 times the upper limit of normal
- occasional alkaline phosphatase and bilirubin elevations
- concomitant hyperthyroidism in 50%

4 **Treatment**: symptomatic with rehydration and antiemetics

5 **Outcome**: carriage to term actually better than in normal population

B Intrahepatic cholestasis of pregnancy (IHCP)

1 **Definition**: cholestatic disorder characterized by pruritus which typically resolves within 2 days of delivery

2 **Epidemiology**
- incidence in USA unknown but reported to be 0.1% in Canada
- highest incidence (12–22%) in Chilean Araucanian Indians
- increased frequency in those with past medical or family history of IHCP and in women with history of intrahepatic cholestasis due to oral contraceptive or estrogen ingestion

3 **Etiology**: theories include inherited sensitivity to estrogens; alteration of sodium–potassium–adenosine triphosphatase activity in hepatocyte membranes; decreased membrane fluidity due to increased cholesterol uptake; and production of cholestatic metabolites

4 **Clinical and laboratory findings** (see Table 21.5)

Drug	Mechanism of action	Dose
Cholestyramine	Binds bile acids	4 g q.d to q.i.d.
Ursodeoxycholic acid (Ursodiol)	Modifies bile acid pool Inhibits absorption of more hydrophobic bile acids Modifies the expression of major histocompatibility antigens on hepatocyte membrane	300 mg t.i.d. to q.i.d.
Dexamethasone	Unknown (efficacy controversial)	12 mg/day

(Table 21.5: Management of IHCP)

- most common in third trimester but can occur in any trimester
- jaundice occurs in 25% and follows onset of pruritus
- aminotransferase levels increased up to four-fold. Serum cholesterol and triglyceride levels may be increased. Serum bile acid levels elevated 30–100×.
- liver biopsy (not usually indicated) reveals cholestasis with minimal hepatocellular necrosis

5 **Outcome**
- mother does well

- increased risk of prematurity (3×), perinatal deaths, fetal distress, and meconium staining of amniotic fluid (1.5×)

C Acute fatty liver of pregnancy (AFLP)

1 Epidemiology
- occurs in last trimester but as early as 26 weeks
- incidence of 1 in 13,000 deliveries
- more common during first pregnancy, with multiple gestations, and with male fetuses

2 Etiology
- as many as 70% of cases are due to homozygous long-chain 3-hydroxyacyl coenzyme dehydrogenase (LCHAD) deficiency in fetus with a heterozygous mother
- nutritional factors, alterations in lipoprotein synthesis, and enzyme deficiencies in the mitochondrial urea cycle also proposed

3 Clinical and laboratory findings
- symptoms include headache, fatigue, malaise, nausea, vomiting, and abdominal pain in right upper quadrant, epigastrium, or diffusely
- jaundice may follow prodrome
- progressive liver failure may occur with coagulopathy, encephalopathy, and/or renal failure
- pre-eclampsia occurs in 20–40%
- aminotransferase levels almost always elevated but usually less than 500 U/L
- alkaline phosphatase and bilirubin levels mildly to moderately elevated
- hyperuricemia in 80%

4 Diagnosis
- ultrasound imaging shows increased echogenicity of liver
- abdominal CT shows decreased attenuation of signal in liver and is more sensitive than ultrasound, but risks radiation exposure to infant
- microvesicular fatty infiltrate of liver detectable by oil-red-O stain of frozen liver biopsy section

5 Treatment: rapid delivery of mother is critical. Most women improve but fulminant hepatic failure may occur and treatment with orthotopic liver transplantation has been reported.

6 Outcome
- maternal mortality rate of 8–18%
- fetal mortality rate of 18–23%

D Pre-eclampsia/eclampsia

1 Definition
- multisystem disease characterized by renal, hematologic, hepatic, central nervous system, and fetal–placental involvement
- also characterized by hypertension, proteinuria, and edema

2 Epidemiology
- usually occurs after 20 weeks of pregnancy. May occur postpartum

- pre-eclampsia occurs in 5–7% of pregnancies, eclampsia in 0.1–0.2%
- most common in primigravidas
- increased incidence associated with diabetes mellitus, hypertension, extremes of age (less than age 20 or greater than 45 years), a family history of pre-eclampsia/eclampsia, plural gestations, hydatidiform mole, fetal hydrops, polyhydramnios, and inadequate prenatal care

3 **Etiology**: unknown. Proposed mechanisms include vasospasm, abnormal endothelial reactivity, activation of coagulation, and decreased nitric oxide synthesis

4 **Clinical and laboratory findings**
- in mild pre-eclampsia blood pressure is ≥140/90 mmHg but <160/110 mmHg
- in severe pre-eclampsia blood pressure is ≥160/110 mmHg
- eclampsia includes signs and symptoms of pre-eclampsia plus convulsions or coma
- in severe disease headaches, visual changes, abdominal pain, congestive heart failure, respiratory distress, or oliguria may occur

5 **Diagnosis**
- clinical diagnosis
- elevated serum AST/ALT levels in 84%/90% with eclampsia, 50%/24% with severe pre-eclampsia, and 24%/20% with mild pre-eclampsia.
- aminotransferase level elevations 5–100× with modest increase in bilirubin (≤5 mg/dL)
- there may be thrombocytopenia and microangiopathic hemolytic anemia
- liver biopsy, if done, may demonstrate periportal deposition of fibrin and fibrinogen associated with hemorrhage with or without necrosis

6 **Outcome**
- morbidity and mortality rates correlate with severity
- most common cause of death cerebral involvement
- increased risk of hepatic rupture
- risks to fetus include prematurity, fetal growth retardation, abruptio placentae, and low birthweight
- increased perinatal morbidity and mortality in mother and fetus correlate with severity of pre-eclampsia, preterm delivery, multiple gestations, and pre-existing maternal medical conditions
- post-delivery liver function test abnormalities generally resolve

7 **Treatment**
- treatment of eclampsia and near-term pre-eclampsia is delivery of infant. Management remote from term is controversial
- prevention with low-dose aspirin may be beneficial

E HELLP syndrome

1 **Definition**: hemolytic anemia, elevated liver function tests, and low platelets

2 Epidemiology
- occurs in 0.2–0.6% of pregnancies
- occurs in 4–12% of women with pre-eclampsia/eclampsia
- may occur in AFLP or de novo
- increased risk in white multiparous women and those, older than age 25 years
- two-third of cases antepartum usually at or after 32 weeks but as early as 25 weeks
- one-third of cases occur postpartum, the majority within 2 days of delivery sometimes later

3 Etiology: unknown but may include abnormal vascular tone, vasospasm, coagulation, or LCHAD deficiency in the infant

4 Clinical and laboratory findings
- proteinuria, microangiopathic hemolytic anemia with increased serum lactic dehydrogenase and indirect bilirubin levels and decreased haptoglobin levels
- decreased platelets (may be <10,000/mm^3)
- positive D-dimer test may help predict development of HELLP in pre-eclamptic patients
- postpartum resolution of:
  - abnormal platelets – usually within first 5 days,
  - hypertension or proteinuria if present – up to 3 months
- see Table 21.6 for symptoms in HELLP

	Percentage of cases
Epigastric pain	65
Nausea or vomiting	30
Headache	31
Hypertension	85
Other: visual changes, weight gain, edema	

(Table 21.6: Symptoms in HELLP syndrome)

5 Outcome
- maternal and fetal outcomes are independent of liver involvement
- increased risk of maternal disseminated intravascular coagulation, abruptio placentae and renal, cardiopulmonary, or hepatic failure
- infant mortality rate 10–60%
- increased risk of infant prematurity, intrauterine growth retardation, disseminated intravascular coagulation, and thrombocytopenia

6 Treatment
- delivery of infant indicated if there is maternal or fetal distress
- treatment with glucocorticoids may be beneficial antepartum and glucocorticoids or plasma exchange postpartum

7 Recurrence
- recurrence rate of HELLP in future pregnancies 4–22%
- risk of recurrent pre-eclampsia is 2–43%

F Hepatic rupture

1 Epidemiology
- occurs in one to 77 per 100,000 deliveries
- 80% of cases are associated with pre-eclampsia or eclampsia
- also occurs with AFLP, HELLP, hepatocellular carcinoma, adenoma, hemangioma, and hepatic abscess
- recurrence is rare

2 Etiology: unknown

3 Clinical and laboratory findings
- usually occurs in last trimester or occasionally within 24 hours of delivery
- typical symptoms: sudden onset of abdominal pain, nausea, and vomiting followed by abdominal distention and hypovolemic shock
- usually involves right lobe of liver but may occur in either or both lobes
- liver function test results increased 2–100× and associated with anemia and consumptive thrombocytopenia with or without disseminated intravascular coagulation

4 Diagnosis
- abdominal ultrasound, CT, MRI, and angiography are useful

5 Outcome
- maternal mortality rates of 50–75%
- maternal mortality is caused by hemorrhage
- fetal mortality rate of about 60%
- fetal mortality correlates directly with prematurity

6 Treatment
- early recognition with prompt delivery and surgical or radiologic intervention
- surgical therapies include application of direct pressure, evacuation, packing or hemostatic wrapping, topical hemostatic agents, oversewing lacerations, hepatic artery ligation, partial hepatectomy, and transplantation
- angiographic embolization is an alternative option

4 Pregnancy in Patients with Chronic Liver Disease

A Overview
- patients have more difficulty conceiving
- pregnancy has no adverse effect on the progression of liver disease

B Cirrhosis
- incidence of bleeding esophageal varices may be increased or unchanged

- bleeding is more common if varices are present at conception; risk increases from 20–27% to 52–78%[2]
- bleeding is more common in second or third trimester
- treatment is the same as in nongravid patient and includes sclerotherapy, band ligation, and, if necessary, transjugular intrahepatic portosystemic shunt placement or portosystem shunt surgery
- maternal mortality rate is 20%
- fetal mortality depends on health and nutrition of mother
- fetal stillbirths in 13% and neonatal mortality rate of 4.8%[2]

5   Viral Hepatitis in Pregnancy

A   Overview

- of all viral hepatitides, only the course of hepatitis E is affected by pregnancy
- may occur throughout pregnancy

B   Hepatitis A

- occurs in as many as one in 1000 pregnancies
- course and management unaffected by pregnancy
- perinatal transmission is rare
- prevention with immune globulin is safe for mother and fetus
- for infants of mothers infectious at or soon after delivery, the dose of immune globulin is 0.02 mL/kg i.m.

C   Hepatitis B

1 Epidemiology
- acute disease occurs in two of 1000 pregnancies
- chronic disease occurs in 5–15 per 1000 pregnancies

2 Transmission to infant without immunoprophylaxis[3]
- when mother is HBsAg positive, the rate is 10–20%
- when mother is HBsAg and hepatitis B e antigen positive, the rate is 90%
- following infection in first trimester, 10% of neonates become HBsAg positive
- following infection in third trimester, 80–90% of neonates become HBsAg positive
- transmission to neonate usually occurs at birth

3 Treatment

Combination active and passive immunotherapy is 85–95% effective in preventing transmission to neonate (see Table 21.7)

D   Hepatitis C

- does not adversely affect pregnancy

Treatment	Hepatitis B surface antigen in mothers		
	+	Unknown	−
Hepatitis B immune globulin (0.5 ml i.m.)	≤12 hours	≤12 hours	No
Hepatitis B vaccine	≤12 hours	≤12 hours	≤1 week
Recombivax HB 5 μg (0.5 ml)	1 month	1–2 months	1–2 months
Engerix-B 10 μg (0.5 ml)	6 months	6 months	6–18 months

Table modified from ACOG Technical Bulletin (1993)

(Table 21.7: Treatment of neonates born to mothers with hepatitis B infection)

- risk of infection to neonate correlates with titer of HCV RNA in mother[4]
- risk of transmission to neonate is 10% or less
- no effective prevention is available for infants

E   Hepatitis D

- rare instances of vertical transmission
- control hepatitis B infection to prevent spread

F   Hepatitis E

- jaundice is nine times more common in pregnant than nonpregnant women
- disease in third trimester is more severe than at often times, with 20% mortality rate compared to 0.5–4% mortality rate in nonpregnant patients
- 12% risk of abortion and intrauterine death
- vertical transmission occurs
- no known therapy

6   Budd–Chiari Syndrome (see also Ch. 19)

A   Definition: Occlusion of one or more of the three hepatic veins

B   Epidemiology

- 20% of cases associated with pregnancy and contraception therapy
- postpartum onset is rare and associated with a poor prognosis

C   Etiology

- hypercoagulable state
- may be associated with anti-phospholipid antibodies, pre-eclampsia, and ingestion of herbal teas

D   Clinical and laboratory findings

- symptoms are usually acute in pregnancy
- abdominal pain, hepatomegaly, ascites

E   Diagnosis

- MRI, real-time ultrasound, liver biopsy
- if possible, avoid venography or angiography until after pregnancy

F   Outcome

- maternal mortality rate as high as 70% with acute onset in pregnancy

G   Treatment

- same as in nonpregnant patients

7   Cholelithiasis and Cholecystitis in Pregnancy (see also Ch. 33)

A   Epidemiology/prevalence

- the frequency of cholelithiasis varies from 2.5% in 20–29-year-old women to 25% in 60–64-year-olds
- relative risk of developing gallstones increases to 3.3 after four pregnancies in women less than age 50 years
- incidence rates of new biliary sludge and gallstones in pregnancy are 14% and 2%, respectively, at end of second trimester and 31% and 2% 2–4 weeks post partum[5]
- sludge disappears in 61% at 3 months and in 96% at 12 months after delivery, while gallbladder stones disappear in 13–28% of women by 1 year

B   Etiology

- increased lithogenicity of bile in second and third trimesters
- progressive decrease of chenodeoxycholic and deoxycholic acid concentrations in bile and increase in cholic acid during pregnancy
- fractional turnover rate of each primary bile acid decreases
- number of enteropathic cycles per hour of bile acid pool is also decreased
- increase in gallbladder volume in second and third trimesters

C   Clinical and laboratory findings[5]

- vomiting 32%, dyspepsia 28%, pruritus 10%
- biliary pain in 29% with stones, 4.7% with sludge, respectively, but does not generally occur in patients with new sludge or stones

D   Treatment

- whether to treat medically or surgically is controversial
- surgical management in second trimester is safe
- questionable increase in spontaneous abortions when surgery is performed in first trimester
- surgery in third trimester is associated with premature labor in 40% of cases
- laparoscopic cholecystectomy is an option

References

1　Olans LB, Wolf JL *Liver disease in pregnancy*. In: Carlson KJ, Eisenstat SA (eds). *The Primary Care of Women*. (St. Louis: Mosby–Yearbook, 1995) 79–86

2　Homburg R, Bayer I, Lurie B. *Bleeding esophageal varices in pregnancy: a report of two cases*. (J Reprod Med 1988) 33: 784–6

3　American College of Obstetricians and Gynecologists Technical Bulletin (Hepatitis in Pregnancy 1993)

4　Ohto H, Terazawa S, Sasaki N, et al. Transmission of hepatitis C virus from mothers to infants. (N Engl J Med 1994) 330: 744–50

5　Maringhini A, Ciambra M, Baccelliere P, et al. *Biliary sludge and gallstones in pregnancy: incidence, risk factors, and natural history*. (Ann Intern Med 1993) 119: 116–20

6　Barron WM. *The syndrome of preeclampsia*. (Gastroenterol Clin North Am 1992) 21: 851–72

7　Khuroo MS, Datta DV. *Budd–Chiari syndrome following pregnancy: report of 16 cases, with roentgenologic, hemodynamic and histologic studies of the hepatic outflow tract*. (Am J Med 1980) 68: 113–121

8　McKellar DP, Anderson CT, Boynton CJ. *Cholecystectomy during pregnancy without fetal loss*. (Surg Gynecol Obstet 1992) 174: 465–8

9　Reyes H, Simon FR *Intrahepatic cholestasis of pregnancy*: an estrogen-related disease. (Semin Liver Dis 1993) 13: 289–301

10　Sibai BM, Ramadan MK, Chari RS, Friedman SA. *Pregnancies complicated by HELLP syndrome (hemolysis, elevated liver enzymes, and low platelets): subsequent pregnancy outcome and long-term prognosis*. (Am J Obstet Gynecol 1995) 172: 125–9

11　Singer AJ, Brandt LS. *Pathophysiology of the gastrointestinal tract during pregnancy*. (Am J Gastroenterol 1991) 86: 1695–712

12　Treem WR, Rinaldo P, Hale DE. *Acute fatty liver of pregnancy and long-chain 3-hydroxyacyl-coenzyme A dehydrogenase deficiency*. (Hepatology 1994) 19: 339–45

13　Wolf JL. *Liver disease in pregnancy*. Med Clin North Am 1996) 80: 1167–87

14　Mishra L, Seeff LB 1992 Viral hepatitis, A through E, complicating pregnancy. Gastroenterol Clin North Am 21: 873–87

15　Barbara L, Sama C, Labate AMM. *A population study on the prevalence of gallstone disease: the Sirmione Study*. (Hepatology 1987) 7: 913–7

16　Rioseco AJ, Ivankovic MB, Manzur A, Hamed F, Kato SR, Parer JJ, Germain AM. *Intrahepatic cholestasis of pregnancy: A retrospective case-control study of perinatal outcome*. (American Journal of Obstetrics and Gynecology 1994) 170: 890–5

17　Schorr-Lesnick B, Dworkin B, Rosenthal WS. *Hemolysis, elevated liver enzymes, and low platelets in pregnancy (HELLP syndrome): A case report and literature review*. (Digestive Diseases and Science 1991) 36: 1649–52

18　Schorr-Lesnick B, Lebovics E, Dworkin B, Rosenthal WS. Liver diseases unique to pregnancy. (American Journal of Gastroenterology 1991) 86: 659–70

19　Sullivan CA, Magann EF, Perry KG Jr, Roberts WE, Blake PG, Martin JN Jr. *The recurrence risk of the syndrome of hemolysis, elevated liver enzymes, and low platelets (HELLP) in subsequent gestations*. (American Journal of Obstetrics and Gynecology 1994) 171: 940–3

20　Treem W, Shoup M, Hale D. *Acute fatty liver of pregnancy (AFLP) and defects in fatty acid oxidation (FAO)*. (Gastroenterology 1994) 106 Abstract 1000

The liver in systemic disease

JAMES H. GRENDELL, M.D.

▼

Key Points

1 The liver is frequently involved as an incidental target organ in a wide variety of systemic conditions, in part because it is the body's largest parenchymal organ. However, in some systemic diseases, the liver can be so severely compromised as to threaten survival

2 In evaluating patients with systemic disease and liver dysfunction, the challenge for the clinician is to distinguish among hepatic manifestations of the systemic disease, liver toxicity from drugs being used to treat that disease, and coexisting primary liver disorders

▲

1 Amyloidosis

A Classification

1 Amyloid is an amorphous protein which produces damage when it is deposited in various tissues including the liver. In a number of published series, the liver has been involved in from 20% to nearly 100% of patients with systemic amyloidosis

2 Although a variety of types of amyloids have been described, the two major types, designated AL (primary amyloid) and AA (secondary amyloid), account for about 90% of cases

3 In patients with **primary amyloidosis** (about 80% of all cases), the amyloid consists of kappa or lambda immunoglobulin light chains produced by a monoclonal population of plasma cells. Bence-Jones proteinuria may also be present, and about one third of patients with primary amyloidosis meet the diagnostic criteria for multiple myeloma

4 In **secondary amyloidosis**, the amyloid is derived from serum amyloid A, a protein secreted by the liver as an acute phase reactant in response to chronic infections or inflammatory processes such as tuberculosis, lepromatous leprosy, osteomyelitis, rheumatoid arthritis, and lymphoma, as well as in amyloidosis associated with familial Mediterranean fever

B Pathology

1 The liver in amyloidosis is large, firm and has a yellow-to-light brown, waxy appearance. Hepatomegaly may be in part the result of chronic passive congestion due to heart failure secondary to cardiac deposition of amyloid

2 Microscopically, amyloid appears as a pink, amorphous material with hematoxylin and eosin staining. Following staining with Congo red, examination under a polarizing microscope demonstrates the amyloid as green birefringent material deposited throughout the hepatic lobule in the space of Disse, in periportal areas, and within the walls of blood vessels

C Clinical presentation

1 Symptoms of patients with hepatic amyloidosis are usually nonspecific, such as fatigue and weakness, weight loss, edema, and exertional dyspnea. Hepatomegaly is found in about 60% and splenomegaly in about 20%

2 Patients may present with symptoms related to involvement of other organs with amyloidosis: congestive heart failure, nephrotic syndrome, malabsorption, peripheral or autonomic neuropathy or carpal tunnel syndrome

D Laboratory tests

1 Abnormalities of liver tests do not correlate with the degree of hepatic involvement. Most patients will have an elevation in alkaline phosphatase, usually 2–4 times the upper limit of normal. The alanine aminotransferase (ALT) and aspartate amino-transferase (AST) levels are generally normal or elevated to less than twice normal, and jaundice is found in only about 5% of patients

2 About one third of patients with hepatic amyloidosis have proteinuria in the

nephrotic range; an acquired factor X deficiency may produce a prolonged prothrombin time

E Diagnosis

1 Hepatic amyloidosis should be suspected in patients with hepatomegaly in the setting of a chronic infectious or inflammatory process, particularly if associated with proteinuria or a monoclonal gammopathy.

2 Generally the diagnosis can be confirmed by Congo red staining of a biopsy of subcutaneous fat, gingiva, small intestine, or rectum

3 As there appears to be a small increased risk of bleeding following liver biopsy in patients with systemic amyloidosis, liver biopsy should be reserved for those patients in whom the diagnosis cannot be confirmed in other ways

F Treatment

1 The prognosis for patients with systemic amyloidosis is generally poor, with a median survival of less than 2 years. However, mortality is usually due to cardiac or renal disease and only very rarely to hepatic involvement

2 Specific treatment of underlying chronic infectious or inflammatory disorders, as well as treatment of familial Mediterranean fever with colchicine, may be beneficial in patients with amyloidosis. Some patients have been reported to benefit from therapy with melphalan and prednisone, although the results of chemotherapy have generally been disappointing

2 Cardiac Disease (see also Chapter 20)

A Congestive heart failure[2]

1 Hepatic congestion due to right heart failure (sometimes called congestive hepatopathy) is common in both congenital and acquired cardiac diseases

2 The liver is enlarged and purplish in color. The cut surface demonstrates a "nutmeg" appearance of alternating areas of pale, less involved areas and congested centrilobular regions. Microscopically, the central veins and centrilobular sinusoids are dilated and engorged with blood, but inflammation is not observed. Long-standing hepatic congestion can result in "cardiac cirrhosis" with development of extensive fibrosis

3 Symptoms in patients with hepatic congestion are those of heart failure rather than liver disease, except for a usually mild, aching discomfort in the right upper quadrant

4 On physical examination, signs of congestive heart failure are typically prominent, including jugular venous distension, hepatojugular reflux, and peripheral edema. Almost all patients will have hepatomegaly, and in about 50% of patients, it will be marked. Splenomegaly and ascites are observed in 10–20% of patients (Table 22.1)

5 Approximately 75% of patients with hepatic congestion have a prolonged prothrombin time and 20–40% of patients have elevated serum bilirubin levels, usually <3 mg/dL and predominantly unconjugated. The alkaline phosphatase level

	% in patients with acute heart failure	% in patients with chronic heart failure
Any hepatomegaly (> 11 cm)	99	95
Marked hepatomegaly (> 5 cm below right costal margin)	57	49
Peripheral edema	77	71
Pleural effusion	25	17
Splenomegaly	20	22
Ascites	7	20

Adapted from Richman (1961)[2]

(Table 22.1: Symptoms and signs of hepatic congestion in 175 patients with right-sided heart failure)

is typically normal. AST and ALT levels are generally normal or only mildly elevated, except in decompensated heart failure in which greater elevations may represent an element of left-sided failure

6 The signs and biochemical abnormalities of congestive hepatopathy usually improve with improvement in right heart function

B   Left heart failure

1 Acute left ventricular failure may result in centrilobular necrosis of the liver without inflammation, frequently termed "shock liver" or "ischemic hepatitis." This usually occurs in the setting of an acute myocardial infarction or cardiogenic shock but can result from an abrupt, severe decrease in cardiac output from any cause or as an effect of vasoactive drugs (e.g., cocaine, ergotamine overdosage)

2 The hepatic manifestations of left heart failure are biochemical. Elevated levels of AST, ALT, and lactate dehydrogenase (LDH) (predominantly hepatic fraction) to 25 or more times the upper limits are common, with values peaking within 1–3 days of the inciting event and rapidly returning to near normal, usually within 7–10 days. Generally serum bilirubin and alkaline phosphatase levels are normal or only mildly elevated

3 Mortality rates in patients with ischemic hepatitis are high (40–50% in some series) but do not correlate with the degree of liver function test abnormalities. The cause of death in these patients is related to the cause of the ischemic injury to the liver, not to liver failure. Treatment should be directed to correcting the underlying disease process

3   Nephrogenic Liver Dysfunction[3]

1 Nephrogenic hepatic dysfunction (Stauffer's syndrome) is a syndrome of abnormal liver function tests in association with renal cell carcinoma without liver metastases

2 Fever and weight loss are observed in >85% of patients, hepatomegaly in about 70% and splenomegaly in about 50%. A variety of laboratory abnormalities have been observed (Table 22.2), in particular, an elevated alkaline phosphatase level and prolonged prothrombin time, and decreased hematocrit and serum albumin levels

	No. of patients with/ No. of patients tested	%
Hematocrit < 35%	11/15	73
WBC >10,000	8/21	38
Platelets >350K	13/21	62
BUN >25 mg/dL	5/15	33
Bilirubin >1 mg/dL	2/20	10
AST >40 U/L	3/14	21
Elevated alkaline phosphates	24/27	90
Prolonged prothrombin time	18/23	77
Albumin <3.5 g/dL	18/22	82

From Strickland & Schenker (1977)[3]

(Table 22.2: Laboratory tests in nephrogenic hepatic dysfunction in 29 patients)

3 Liver biopsy demonstrates only nonspecific changes (scattered focal hepatocyte necrosis, steatosis, portal inflammation with lymphocytes, Kupffer's cell hyperplasia without cholestasis)

4 Resection of the renal cell carcinoma usually results in resolution of both clinical and biochemical abnormalities within 1–2 months. However, these abnormalities may recur with recurrence of the primary tumor

4   Collagen Vascular Disease

A   Systemic lupus erythematosus[4]

1 Although liver function test abnormalities are common in lupus, clinically significant liver disease is uncommon

2 About 20% of patients have elevations of serum aminotransferase or alkaline phosphatase levels, usually less than four times the upper limit of normal. Jaundice is observed in about 5% of patients

3 Liver biopsy or autopsy reveals a variety of findings, with steatosis the most common. Other findings include nonspecific portal inflammation, chronic hepatitis, nodular regenerative hyperplasia, arteritis, and cirrhosis. However, it is difficult to determine which of these findings may be directly related to lupus and which may be related to medications (e.g., salicylates, prednisone) or co-morbid conditions (e.g. hepatitis C)

4 Salicylates should be withdrawn from patients with collagen vascular diseases and symptoms, signs or laboratory evidence of hepatitis, to identify those patients in whom the salicylate is responsible for liver dysfunction

B Rheumatoid arthritis[5]

1 Liver disease is most commonly seen in patients who have Felty's syndrome (splenomegaly and neutropenia in the setting of rheumatoid arthritis). These patients frequently also have hepatomegaly, and about 25% will have elevations of serum aminotransferase and alkaline phosphatase levels. Biopsy findings are usually nonspecific, with infiltration of portal areas with lymphocytes and plasma cells and mild portal fibrosis

2 Some patients develop nodular regenerative hyperplasia with atrophy and formation of regenerative nodules, which may result in portal hypertension, ascites, and variceal hemorrhage. The pathogenesis of nodular regenerative hyperplasia has been proposed to be drug-induced or immune complex-induced obliteration of the portal venules

3 Hepatic toxicity can be produced in patients with rheumatoid arthritis due to treatment with salicylates, gold, and methotrexate

C Sjögren's syndrome[5]

1 About 5–10% of patients with Sjögren's syndrome and about 40% with Sjögren's syndrome and rheumatoid arthritis have an antimitochondrial antibody, and most of these patients also have an elevated serum alkaline phosphatase level

2 Liver biopsy in these patients frequently demonstrates changes of stage 1 primary biliary cirrhosis, even in the absence of liver function test abnormalities

3 At present the risk that these patients will develop clinical primary biliary cirrhosis is uncertain. Whether any early therapeutic intervention is of value is also unclear

D Scleroderma

1 About 25% of patients with scleroderma have an antimitochondrial antibody and these patients frequently have evidence of primary biliary cirrhosis on liver biopsy

2 Almost 5% of patients with primary biliary cirrhosis have symptoms of the CREST syndrome (calcinosis, Raynaud's phenomenon, esophageal dysmotility, sclerodactyly, and telangiectases), which may antedate the diagnosis of primary biliary cirrhosis by many years

E Polymyalgia rheumatica

1 Elevation of alkaline phosphatase or serum aminotransferase levels may be observed in patients with polymyalgia rheumatica

2 Liver biopsy demonstrates focal hepatocellular necrosis, portal inflammation, and scattered small epithelioid granulomas

3 Clinically important liver disease does not appear to result due to polymyalgia rheumatica.

5   Hematologic Diseases

A   Sickle cell anemia[6]

1 Although liver function test abnormalities are common in patients with sickle cell anemia, they are frequently due to other factors, such as chronic viral hepatitis or congestive heart failure

2 Hepatic crisis usually occurs in the setting of sickle cell crisis and is marked by right upper quadrant pain, jaundice, and tender hepatomegaly. Serum bilirubin levels are frequently as high as 10–15 mg/dL and may be as high as 40–50 mg/dL. AST and ALT levels are also elevated, usually 10 times normal. The LDH level may be markedly increased, reflecting both liver dysfunction and hemolysis. Liver biopsy demonstrates sinusoidal distension, erythrocyte sickling, and phagocytosis of erythrocytes by Kupffer's cells. Differential diagnosis includes acute cholecystitis and cholangitis. Care is supportive and usually results in clinical improvement in a few days, although fatal liver failure has been described

3 Pigment gallstones have been reported in 40–80% of patients with sickle cell anemia, and choledocholithiasis has been described in about 20–65% of patients at the time of cholecystectomy. Abdominal ultrasound or computed tomography (CT) and biliary scintigraphy may be helpful in establishing the diagnosis of cholecystitis, and endoscopic retrograde cholangiopancreatography (ERCP) may be necessary to identify and treat stones in the common bile duct

B   Lymphoma[7]

1 The liver is involved in up to 50% of patients with Hodgkin's lymphoma at the time of autopsy. In addition, nonspecific inflammatory infiltrates or noncaseating granulomas are seen in the absence of direct hepatic involvement with lymphomas. An elevated alkaline phosphatase level of 1.5–2.0 times the upper limits is common even in the absence of direct liver involvement. Jaundice is uncommon in Hodgkin's lymphoma and usually reflects hepatic infiltration with the lymphoma rather than extrahepatic biliary obstruction

2 Hepatic involvement is observed in 25% to nearly 50% of patients with non-Hodgkin's lymphoma; and, rarely, the liver may be the primary site. Typically, the lymphoma produces a nodular infiltrate of the portal areas. The clinical and laboratory presentation is similar to that of non-Hodgkin's lymphoma except that extrahepatic obstruction, usually at the level of the porta hepatis, is much more common

6   Obesity and Jejunoileal Bypass

A   Obesity[8] (see also Ch. 7)

1 Fatty infiltration is commonly present in morbidly obese individuals and can result in hepatomegaly and elevations in the AST, ALT and alkaline phosphatase levels, usually to 3–4 times upper limits

2 Abdominal ultrasound demonstrates an enlarged, diffusely echogenic liver. CT shows the liver to be of homogenously decreased density as compared to the spleen. Liver

biopsy demonstrates steatosis. Additionally, in <5% of patients, inflammation and fibrosis may be observed. In these latter patients, alcohol abuse must be excluded as a cause of these histologic findings. Unlike in alcoholic liver disease, in obese patients the elevated AST level generally does not exceed the ALT level, and the gamma glutamyltranspeptidase (GGTP) level is typically not elevated

3 Weight loss will usually result in improvement in steatosis, inflammation, and, in some patients, fibrosis

B Jejunoileal bypass[9]

1 Following jejunoileal bypass surgery for morbid obesity (rarely performed nowadays), patients may develop steatosis, fibrosis, and even cirrhosis and progressive liver failure. Liver disease may occur within the first few months following surgery or 10 or more years later

2 Liver tests are often normal or only mildly elevated until advanced liver disease is present and do not reflect the degree of liver injury. Liver biopsy shows steatosis and portal infiltration with lymphocytes. Mallory's hyaline and polymorphonuclear leukocytes may be found in the hepatic lobule as in alcoholic liver disease. In some patients, perivenular fibrosis may develop and progress to cirrhosis

3 Reversal of the bypass may be beneficial in patients with progressive liver disease. Patients with endstage liver disease may require transplantation and should have subsequent elective reversal of the bypass

7 Inflammatory Bowel Disease[10]

A Liver abnormalities

1 Mild elevations of serum aminotransferase and alkaline phosphatase levels are common in patients with inflammatory bowel disease, as are abnormalities on liver biopsy

2 Steatosis is the most commonly observed abnormality. Additionally, chronic hepatitis characterized by either portal or lobular infiltrates of mononuclear inflammatory cells may be found. However, it is not clear whether the hepatitis is a direct consequence of inflammatory bowel disease or a manifestation of sclerosing cholangitis or another cause of liver disease, such as hepatitis C or drugs

3 Patients with Crohn's disease infrequently develop hepatic granulomas or amyloidosis

E Biliary abnormalities

1 Primary sclerosing cholangitis is the most important hepatobiliary complication of inflammatory bowel disease, occurring in about 5–10% of patients with ulcerative colitis but in fewer than 1% of patients with Crohn's disease (see Ch. 15)

2 Patients may present with jaundice or pruritus, or the diagnosis may be suspected based on an elevated serum alkaline phosphatase level

3 Although progression may be insidious, most patients will develop biliary cirrhosis with increasing levels of serum bilirubin and alkaline phosphatase and portal

hypertension with ascites and variceal bleeding. Bacterial cholangitis may also be observed, particularly in patients who have undergone surgical or endoscopic manipulation of the bile ducts

4 About 10% of patients with primary sclerosing cholangitis develop cholangiocarcinoma

5 Diagnosis of sclerosing cholangitis is made by visualization of the biliary tree by ERCP. The typical pattern is one of multiple bile duct strictures with areas of beaded dilatation. Differentiation between benign strictures and cholangiocarcinoma by radiographic criteria is often uncertain. Brush cytology obtained at ERCP may be helpful

6 Neither medical nor surgical treatment of the underlying inflammatory bowel disease alters the course of primary sclerosing cholangitis. Treatment with ursodeoxycholic acid may result in some improvement in symptoms and liver function tests. Patients with advanced liver disease secondary to primary sclerosing cholangitis may be candidates for liver transplantation if they have not already developed cholangiocarcinoma

References

1 Gertz MA, Kyle RA. *Hepatic amyloidosis: clinical appraisal in 77 patients.* (Hepatology 1997) 25: 118–21

2 Richman SM, Delman AJ, Grob D. *Alterations in indices of liver function in congestive heart failure with particular reference to serum enzymes.* (Am J Med 1961) 30: 211–25

3 Strickland RC, Schenker S. *The nephrogenic hepatic dysfunction syndrome: a review.* (Am J Dig Dis 1977) 22: 49–55

4 Runyon BA, LaBrecque DR, Anuras S. *The spectrum of liver disease in systemic lupus erythematosus.* (Am J Med 1980) 69: 187–94

5 Webb J, Whaley K, MacSween RNM, Nuki G, Dick WC, Buchanan WW. *Liver disease in rheumatoid arthritis and Sjogren's syndrome.* (Ann Rheum Dis 1975) 34: 70–81

6 Charlotte F, Bachir D, Nenert M, Mavier P, Galacteros F, Dhumeaux D, Zafrani ES. *Vascular lesions of the liver in sickle cell disease. A clinicopathological study in 26 living patients.* (Arch Pathol Lab Med 1995) 119: 46–52

7 Harris AC, Ben-Ezra JM, Contos MJ, Kornstein MJ. *Malignant lymphoma can present as hepatobiliary disease.* (Cancer 1996) 78: 2011–9

8 Diehl AM, Goodman Z, Ishak KG. *Alcohollike liver disease in nonalcoholics.* (Gastroenterology 1988) 95: 1056–62

9 Peters RL, Gay T, Reynolds TB. *Post-jejunoileal bypass hepatic disease.* (Am J Clin Pathol 1975) 63: 318–31

10 Harmatz A. *Hepatobiliary complications of inflammatory bowel disease.* (Med Clin N Am 1994) 78: 1387–98

CHAPTER 23

Pediatric liver disease

MICHELLE S. KENNEDY, M.D.
WILLIAM F. BALISTRERI, M.D.

▼

Key Points

1 Acquired liver diseases seen in adults are rare in children. More commonly encountered are congenital or metabolic disorders

2 There is physiologic immaturity of the liver during the perinatal period, and significant maturational changes in hepatic metabolic processes occur during childhood; these affect the presentation of and reaction to viral and toxin exposure

3 Liver disease may present as hyperbilirubinemia, hepatomegaly, liver cell failure, cirrhosis, cystic disease of the liver, portal hypertension, or systemic disease due to to secondary effects of liver disease

4 The secondary effects of liver disease may be life threatening:
- metabolic derangement such as hypoglycemia
- coagulopathy secondary to low levels of vitamin K-dependent clotting factors resulting in intracranial hemorrhage in the infant
- persistent "toxin" exposure, as may be seen in diseases such as galactosemia or fructosemia
- sepsis as a cause of liver disease or as a result of secondary immunodeficiency due to malnutrition
- portal hypertension with potential gastrointestinal bleeding

▲

1   Physiologic Immaturity of the Liver

1   Altered metabolism and clearance of potentially toxic endogenous and exogenous potentially toxic compounds

- hepatic concentrations of cytochrome P-450 are low in infants. Similarly, activities of aminopyrine N-demethylase and aniline p-hydroxylase are low. Hepatic processes such as clearance of certain drugs or bilirubin which depend on these systems will be inefficient. Therefore, potentially toxic serum levels of such compounds may be reached more rapidly in the infant
- clearance of drugs which depend on cytochrome P-450 is more rapid in older children than adults. By puberty, an adult pattern of metabolism is established
- lower levels of glutathione peroxidase and glutathione S-transferase are present in infants, making the infant liver potentially more prone to oxidant injury

2   Alterations in the bile acid pool size and composition exist. It is unclear whether this is beneficial (some of the bile acids present may be more readily excreted in urine) or harmful (atypical bile acids formed may exacerbate cholestasis)

3   **Physiologic jaundice**: up to one third of newborns develop jaundice within the first week of life. Breast-fed infants have a higher risk of developing jaundice than formula-fed infants. This is most often referred to as "physiologic jaundice" and resolves spontaneously with no complications. Physiologic jaundice reflects the transition from clearance and metabolism of unconjugated bilirubin by the maternal system to that of the infant. This is likely multifactorial:

- increased production of bilirubin; the newborn has a large red cell mass and these cells have a shorter half-life than adult red blood cells.
- inefficient serum protein binding of bilirubin, which affects hepatocellular uptake
- immature intracellular conjugation within the liver; however, this remains unproven and is unlikely to be the sole cause

4   Warning signs of pathologic jaundice
- elevated bilirubin occurring before 3 days or lasting longer than 14 days of age
- total serum bilirubin greater that 15 mg/dL
- direct serum bilirubin greater that 2 mg/dL

2   Hyperbilirubinemia

Alterations in any step of bilirubin metabolism (numbers in Fig 1 correlate with the numbers in the following outline) may cause jaundice in excess of physiologic jaundice. Potential alterations in steps in bilirubin metabolism (see Fig. 23.1):

1   Increased bilirubin production can be due to an increase in the release of heme from red blood cells:

- hemolysis due to Rh incompatibility, ABO incompatibility or other minor blood group incompatibilities

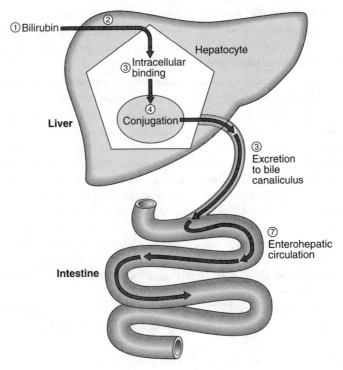

Fig. 23.1   Steps in bilirubin metabolism

- increased fragility of erythrocytes in congenital spherocytosis, hereditary eliptocytosis; polycythemia, red blood cell enzyme defects like glucose 6-phosphate, pyruvate kinase, and hexosekinase deficiencies
- enclosed hematoma

2 Decreased bilirubin uptake into hepatocyte may be caused by hypothyroidism or gestational hormones that may inhibit uptake of bilirubin across the hepatocyte membrane. Thyroxine is important for liver plasma membrane function. A decrease in the amount of bilirubin bound to serum proteins also results in decreased uptake by hepatocytes. This may be due to hypoalbuminemia, generalized hypoproteinemia, or displacement from these proteins by drugs, including sulfonamides, salicylates, heparin, and caffeine

3 Abnormalities of intracellular binding or storage of bilirubin within hepatocytes are rare and include deficiencies or alterations in glutathione S-transferase (GST), the primary intracellular binding protein for bilirubin. **Rotor syndrome** represents deficient intracellular storage of bilirubin and is characterized by direct and indirect hyperbilirubinemia without hemolysis and without alterations in liver enzymes; liver histology is normal. There is an increase in urinary coproporphyrin levels, especially type III, secondary to biliary dysfunction. Treatment is not indicated, as there is no associated morbidity or mortality

4 Inefficient conjugation of bilirubin within the hepatocyte. Within the hepatocyte, bilirubin is conjugated with glucuronic acid by bilirubin UDP-glucuronyl transferase (BGT) to form bilirubin mono- or diglucuronide. A decrease in BGT activity is seen

in **Gilbert's syndrome**, resulting in benign elevations in serum bilirubin levels, especially during stresses such as viral illnesses. **Crigler–Najjar syndrome** is characterized by absence of BGT leading to severe hyperbilirubinemia with associated neurologic effects secondary to kernicterus

- *Note*: neonatal hemochromatosis, alpha-1 antitrypsin deficiency, Wolman's disease, Niemann–Pick disease and cystic fibrosis can cause hyperbilirubinemia in the neonatal period, presumably secondary to hepatocyte damage (see below)

5 Alterations in secretion of bilirubin through the canalicular membrane into the biliary tract can lead to hyperbilirubinemia. Bilirubin diglucuronide is excreted into the canaliculus by an undescribed carrier protein. Alterations in this protein are thought to be the cause of **Dubin–Johnson syndrome**. While this syndrome has no associated morbidity or mortality, it is characterized by elevated levels of conjugated and unconjugated serum bilirubin. Hyperbilirubinemia is accentuated during pregnancy or with use of oral contraceptives. It is likely an autosomal recessive disorder. These patients have an increase in urinary coproporphyrin I levels. Liver biopsy shows a characteristic melanin-like pigment deposited in liver cells but is otherwise histologically normal. Due to the benign nature of this syndrome, no treatment is required

6 Structural abnormalities of the biliary tree can prevent drainage of bile from the canaliculus into the intestine, causing accumulation of bile and reflux of bilirubin into the systemic circulation

- **extrahepatic biliary atresia (BA)** is a progressive disease characterized by inflammation and fibrosis of the extrahepatic biliary tract resulting in partial or complete obliteration of the extrahepatic bile ducts. BA typically presents between 2 and 6 weeks of age as cholestasis (conjugated hyperbilirubinemia). Liver biopsy shows fibrosis and bile duct proliferation. BA may be syndromic (<15% of cases) associated with cardiac anomalies, polysplenism, and malrotation or situs inversus, or nonsyndromic (majority of cases) – etiology unknown. This anomaly is treated initially with a **portoenterostomy** which allows drainage of bile directly from the liver to the intestine. While this is not curative, it often delays progression of disease. **End-stage liver disease secondary to BA is the most common reason for orthotopic liver transplant in children**

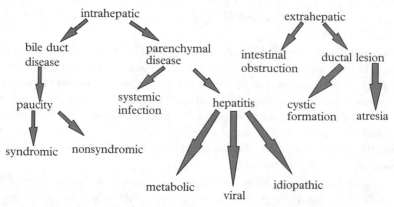

Fig. 23.2   Conjugated hyperbilirubinemia

- **intrahepatic cholestasis** may be associated with the histological finding of bile duct paucity, defined as a reduced ratio of interlobular bile ducts to portal tracts (normal = 0.9–1.8; paucity < 0.5). Paucity of bile ducts may be syndromic (Alagille's syndrome which is associated with peripheral pulmonic stenosis, butterfly vertebrae, and characteristic facies) or nonsyndromic. Treatment is symptomatic with special consideration given to nutrition and pruritus. Liver transplantation may be required in some cases
- **choledochal cyst**, a cystic dilation of the biliary tree, may be exclusively extrahepatic or include dilations of the intrahepatic biliary tree. The etiology of this entity is unknown. It appears to be most common in East Asia, with over 50% of the reported cases coming from Japan. Most patients present as infants with abdominal pain and jaundice with or without a palpable abdominal mass. The diagnosis can be made by ultrasound, computed tomographic (CT) scan, or endoscopic retrograde cholangiopancreatography (ERCP). Treatment is by surgical excision of the dilated segment, rather than bypass or drainage, due to an increase in the incidence of malignancy in the epithelium of the cyst.

7 Alterations in the **enterohepatic circulation** can result in an increase in reabsorption of bilirubin from the intestine. This can be due to obstruction as in intestinal atresia, intestinal obstruction as in Hirschsprung's disease, or alterations in the bacterial flora of the intestine by the use of antibiotics.

8 Complications of hyperbilirubinemia
  a Unconjugated hyperbilirubinemia
    - kernicterus – staining of the basal ganglia with bilirubin resulting in neurologic manifestations including seizure
  b Cholestasis
    - malnutrition secondary to fat malabsorption leading to failure to thrive and fat-soluble vitamin deficiencies
    - intractable pruritus
    - xanthomatosis secondary to alterations in cholesterol metabolism

A   Treatment of unconjugated hyperbilirubinemia

- double volume exchange transfusion – lowers the risk of kernicterus in the newborn by rapidly decreasing the serum bilirubin concentration
- phototherapy – photoisomerization of bilirubin to a more polar compound allowing excretion in the urine
- inducing more rapid bilirubin metabolism can be accomplished by phenobarbital administration which induces microsomal enzymes, thus facilitating bilirubin metabolism

B   Treatment of cholestasis

- surgical correction of anatomic lesions may be effective

- ursodeoxycholic acid, a choleretic bile acid, can be used to augment bile flow during cholestasis (see also Ch. 14)
- liver transplantation may be necessary

3 Hepatomegaly

Hepatomegaly can have multiple etiologies including cell swelling, venous congestion, infiltration with fat, or the accumulation of substances not normally present in the liver

Causes of hepatomegaly

- cellular hyperplasia/hypertrophy:
  - hepatocytes
  - Kupffer's cells
  - inflammatory cells
- fibrosis
- venous congestion
- biliary tract dilation
- accumulation of metabolic substances:
  - fat
  - cholesterol
  - glycogen
  - sphingolipid
  - sphingomyelin
  - abnormal alpha-1 antitrypsin
  - copper
- tumor infiltration

A Inflammatory cell infiltration and Kupffer's cell proliferation

- viral hepatitis (see Chs 3 and 4) may present with tender hepatomegaly secondary to inflammation. The histology of autoimmune hepatitis includes an intense inflammatory infiltrate which may manifest as hepatomegaly on examination. Juvenile rheumatoid arthritis can also present with a periportal inflammatory infiltrate as well as Kupffer's cell hyperplasia resulting in hepatomegaly. The latter two often resolve as the disease process is controlled with antiinflammatory medication

B Fibrosis

- congenital hepatic fibrosis may present with hepatomegaly and splenomegaly secondary to portal hypertension. Other diseases discussed in this section present with hepatomegaly secondary to infiltration of other substances or cells and result in fibrosis. As fibrotic material replaces the hepatocytes, the liver may "shrink"

C   Venous congestion

- any decrease in cardiac function can result in passive congestion of the liver, which may manifest as hepatomegaly (see Ch. 20)

D   Accumulation of metabolic substances

1 Fat accumulation causing hepatomegaly is seen in many disorders, the most common being obesity, malnutrition, and diabetes mellitus (see Ch. 7)

- **diabetes mellitus** (DM) can cause hepatomegaly due to poor insulin control. **Mauriac's syndrome** is characterized by the triad of poorly controlled DM, growth retardation, and hepatomegaly. Liver histology demonstrates fatty infiltration. This syndrome resolves with improvement in glycemic control. Additionally, the Somogyi effect resulting from excess insulin administration can result in fat storage in the liver

- **fatty acid oxidation defects** such as medium-chain acyl-CoA dehydrogenase deficiency (MCAD) and long-chain acyl-CoA dehydrogenase deficiency (LCAD) present with hepatomegaly, hypoglycemia, and increased serum aminotransferase levels. These defects result in an inability to utilize stored fat, which builds up in the liver. Episodes of decompensation are often precipitated by common childhood illnesses such as otitis media or acute gastroenteritis and are characterized by lethargy and severe hypoglycemia. Such episodes respond rapidly to fluid and glucose replacement. The diagnosis is suggested by an abnormal urine organic acid profile. The ratio of ketone bodies to dicarboxylic acid is low, signifying inability to metabolize stored fats. Additionally, total serum carnitine is low, although the fraction of acylcarnitine is unusually high

- **galactosemia** due to a deficiency of galactose 1-phosphate uridyltransferase usually presents within the first few days of life. This deficiency leads to accumulation of galactose 1-phosphate and galactitol and fatty liver. If not treated these infants will succumb to hepatic failure. Treatment is by removal of lactose (and galactose) from the diet, because lactose is broken down to glucose and galactose

- **oxidative phosphorylation defects** as in **Alper's syndrome** result in profound lactic acidosis. This defect manifests as an elevated lactate-to-pyruvate ratio and an increase in 3-hydroxybutyrate. These disorders usually present with neurologic disease, myopathy, and/or seizures and progressive hepatic failure. It is frequently difficult initially to differentiate the hepatotoxic side effects of seizure medications from Alper's syndrome.

- **Reye's syndrome (RS)** (see below) may present with a rapidly enlarging liver secondary to triglyceride accumulation and hypertrophy of the smooth endoplasmic reticulum. It is associated with a typical prodrome of viral illness, most commonly an upper respiratory tract infection or varicella, and has been linked to aspirin use. It presents as protracted vomiting, disorientation and varying degrees of liver failure. Treatment is supportive

2 Cholesterol accumulates in **cholesterol ester storage disease** (CESD) and **Wolman's disease**. CESD is otherwise asymptomatic. Wolman's disease is characterized by a decrease in the lysosomal enzyme acid lipase, resulting in decreased degradation of cholesterol. Poor nutritional status is also seen secondary

to accumulation of lipid in the intestinal epithelium. Neurologic deterioration and death occurs by 6–12 months of age. Treatment consists primarily of parenteral nutrition. Bone marrow transplantation, which may normalize acid lipase activity, has been proposed

3 **Glycogen storage disease (GSD) type I and type IV** present with hepatomegaly secondary to accumulated glycogen in hepatocytes. In GSD I there is absent or abnormal activity of glucose 6-phosphatase; therefore, gluconeogenesis cannot proceed. Patients develop profound hypoglycemia after short fasting periods with lactic acidosis, hyperuricemia, hypophosphatemia, and hyperlipidemia. Treatment includes a high-starch diet often in the form of corn starch or continuous feedings to provide a continuous source of glucose. Patients may be more susceptible to hepatic adenomas. GSD IV is a rare disease presenting in infancy with hepatosplenomegaly and poor weight gain secondary to a debranching enzyme deficiency. Like GSD I this results in defective gluconeogenesis, and accumulation of glycogen. Treatment is with liver transplantation

4 Sphingolipid accumulation is characteristic of **Gaucher's disease** which results from an autosomal recessive deficiency of glucocerebrosidase, the lysosomal enzyme responsible for degrading sphingolipids. There are three forms. Type I typically presents with hepatosplenomegaly and is a chronic nonneuropathic form of disease. Type II also presents with hepatosplenomegaly but has neuropathic features and is often fatal by age 2 years. Type III is associated with hepatosplenomegaly and a later onset of neuropathic features

5 **Niemann–Pick disease** is characterized histologically by lipid-laden "foam cells" and stored sphingomyelin in macrophages. This disorder is caused by decreased sphingomyelinase, resulting in accumulation of sphingomyelin and cholesterol in the reticuloendothelial system in many organs, including the liver

6 **Alpha-1 antitrypsin deficiency** (see Ch. 18) presents with hepatomegaly due to intracellular accumulations of abnormal alpha-1 antitrypsin molecules along the endoplasmic reticulum. The abnormal homozygous PiZZ alpha-1 antitrypsin-deficient phenotype can be determined electrophoretically. Liver transplantation has been used to treat liver disease associated with this disorder

7 Copper storage diseases
   • **Wilson's disease** (WD) (see Ch. 17) is a genetic disease of copper overload; the abnormal gene is located on chromosome 13. The carrier rate is 1 in 90. There appears to be variable expression of the disease even within the same family. While the precise mechanism is unknown, defective copper excretion results in excess accumulation in the liver with subsequent accumulation in the central nervous system and other organs. Presents in the second to fourth decades of life. Earlier presentation usually relates to hepatic manifestations with elevated aminotransferase levels and hepatomegaly. Later presentation tends to be neurologic or psychiatric. WD is diagnosed by a serum ceruloplasmin < 20 mg/dL, liver copper > 25 µg/g, and urinary copper > 100 µg/day. Liver biopsy shows steatosis early in the course progressing to inflammation and fibrosis with cirrhosis. Copper stain of the liver may be helpful in the diagnosis, but is not specific, and absence of stainable copper does not exclude the possibility of WD. The disease is fatal due to hepatic failure without treatment but controllable with copper chelation. Penicillamine and trientine are chelators

which increase urinary excretion of copper. Zinc, which blocks intestinal absorption of copper, has also been used. Some cases present with fulminant hepatic failure; the only effective treatment option in this situation is liver transplantation, which is curative

- Indian childhood cirrhosis is a copper storage disease seen in young children. The etiology is unknown and has been attributed to excessive copper intake as well as to a defect in copper excretion. Presents earlier than WD with hepatic failure leading rapidly to death within weeks to months of presentation. This disease is often fatal by age 4. Patients present with nonspecific complaints of anorexia and irritability but develop hepatomegaly and jaundice followed by secondary manifestations of liver disease. Hepatic copper content is often >1000 μg/g. Copper accumulation appears to inhibit transport of intracellular proteins resulting in hepatocyte swelling. Treatment, like that of WD, is by chelation.

E Tumor infiltration

Tumor infiltration of the liver can contribute to hepatomegaly. Primary tumors, include embryonal rhabdomyosarcoma of the biliary tree, teratomas, hepatoblastoma, and hemangioendothelioma. Tumors which may secondarily infiltrate the liver include neuroblastoma, Wilm's tumor, and lymphoma. These tumors can be identified initially by CT scan as focal abnormalities rather than diffuse infiltration. Diagnosis is by biopsy. Treatment depends on tumor type

4 Acute Liver Disease

Many of the previously discussed diseases present after an indolent course or with subtle findings. Acute liver diseases such as viral hepatitis and Reye's syndrome present with a more sudden onset

A Viral hepatitis

The most common forms of viral hepatitis are hepatitis A and hepatitis B. While both may present as an acute febrile illness with jaundice and hepatomegaly, the courses may differ (see Ch. 3). Additionally, the presentation and course can differ from those in adults

1 Hepatitis A is transmitted by the fecal–oral route, and outbreaks can often be traced to daycare centers (DCC) where hygiene may be suboptimal. Adults who work with DCC children are at an increased risk for contracting this disease. While the disease is often asymptomatic (75–95%) in children, adults are more commonly symptomatic (75–95%), and a small percentage develop severe liver disease. Administration of the recently approved hepatitis A vaccine to children and adults at high risk should decrease the frequency of hepatitis A.

2 Hepatitis B is transmitted parenterally. Children acquire this disease in much the same manner as adults and exhibit a similar clinical course. Rarely there is associated immune complex-mediated extrahepatic disease, such as membranous glomerulonephritis or papular acrodermatitis of childhood (Gianotti–Crosti syndrome). A unique situation in children, however, is perinatal transmission.

Infants born to mothers who are positive for hepatitis B surface antigen (especially those positive for hepatitis B e antigen) are at high risk of becoming chronic carriers and developing hepatocellular carcinoma. Hepatitis B immune globulin administration within 4 to 6 hours of birth followed by the hepatitis B vaccine can prevent this disease. Hepatitis B vaccination is now routine in infants born in the USA

B Reye's syndrome

This is a rare cause of fulminant hepatic failure in children. Typically presents following a prodromal febrile illness such as an upper respiratory tract infection or varicella and is often associated with aspirin treatment. Protracted vomiting occurs 5–7 days after the onset of the initial illness, usually as the first illness is improving. Progression to hepatic failure with associated neurologic deterioration seizures, and coma may occur quite rapidly. Serum aminotransferase levels are typically more than three to four times normal. A significantly elevated ammonia or prothrombin time indicates a greater likelihood of progressive disease. The liver demonstrates hepatocytes with foamy accumulation of triglyceride. Electron microscopy demonstrates alterations in mitochondria. Similar alterations are seen in the mitochondria in brain. Treatment is supportive and focuses on controlling intracranial pressure. Survival depends on early diagnosis; those treated before severe neurologic involvement have a greater chance for complete recovery

5 Cystic Liver Disease (see Ch. 33)

Cystic liver disease results from lack of normal embryonic development of the biliary tree. There is a spectrum of diseases depending on the size of bile duct involved. **Caroli's disease** is the name given to cystic liver disease involving the large intrahepatic bile ducts. Because of bile stasis in the cysts, these patients are predisposed to recurrent cholangitis. Caroli's disease along with most of the other polycystic liver diseases may be associated with extrahepatic decrease, particularly cystic disease of the kidneys

6 Systemic Diseases Affecting the Liver

A Cystic fibrosis (CF)

A disease of altered chloride secretion, most commonly affecting the lungs and pancreas. However, many patients with CF have associated focal and multilobular biliary cirrhosis and associated complications such as portal hypertension. The presence of liver disease does not appear to depend on the genotype of CF, nor is it related to the severity of pulmonary disease. Patients present with hepatomegaly, which may be erroneously attributed to hyperinflation of the lungs. Patients with CF are also known to have a higher than usual incidence of biliary sludge, cholelithiasis, bile duct strictures, microgallbladder, and prolonged neonatal cholestasis. Ursodeoxycholic acid has been shown to improve the abnormal laboratory findings in CF associated liver disease; however, it is unclear whether prophylactic therapy would be beneficial in all CF patients

B Sickle cell disease

Patients with sickle cell disease commonly have, hepatomegaly, apparently secondary to sinusoidal dilatation and Kupffer's cell hyperplasia. The etiology is unclear but may be related to chronic low-level hypoxia. An increased incidence of cholelithiasis is seen in this population secondary to rapid hemoglobin turnover

C   Obesity

In children as well as adults can lead to hepatomegaly. This is associated with steatosis, mild inflammation, and Kupffer's cell hyperplasia. Progression to fibrosis and cirrhosis is rare. These histologic changes usually normalize with weight loss (see Ch. 7)

D   Parenteral nutrition (PN)

In children, especially neonates, this is associated with cholestasis. This may progress to cirrhosis and liver failure. The precise etiology is unknown and likely multifactorial, including toxic substrates in the PN, nutrient/micronutrient deficiency, or toxic bacterial by-products crossing the atrophic intestinal mucosal barrier. The only effective treatment is administration of enteral feedings

E   Muscular dystrophies

These are not particularly associated with liver disease, but often present with an elevated AST leading one to believe that the liver is involved. Further evaluation reveals an elevated creatine kinase level, confirming that the AST originates from muscle

References

1   Balistreri WF. *A new vaccine for an old disease* (Viral Hepatitis Rev 1996) 2: 49–59

2   Balistreri WF, Schubert WK. *Liver disease in infancy and childhood*. In Schiff L, Schiff ER, (eds). *Disease of the Liver*, 7th edn. (Philadelphia: Lippincott, 1993)

3   Colombo C, Crosignani A, Assaisso M, et al. *Ursodeoxycholic acid therapy in cystic fibrosis-associated liver disease: a dose–response study*. (Hepatology 1992) 16: 924–30

4   Suchy FJ (ed). *Liver Disease in Children*. (Mosby-Year Book, Inc., 1994)

5   Kriuit W, Frese D, Chan KW, Kulkarni R. *Wolman's disease: a review of treatment with bone marrow transplantation and considerations for Wolman's disease and bone marrow transplantation: the future*. (Bone Marrow Transplant 1992) 10 (Supp: 1): 97–101

Liver disease in the elderly

KENNETH D. ROTHSTEIN, M.D.
JOSÉ PROENZA, M.D.
SANTIAGO J. MUÑOZ, M.D.

▼

Key Points

1 The clinical presentation, prognosis, and management of several liver disorders can be different in patients with advanced age compared to younger persons

2 Hepatic blood flow, liver size, and hepatic regenerative capacity decrease with age; this may cause decreased metabolism of certain medications and decreased ability to recover promptly from processes such as acute viral hepatitis

3 Certain disease processes, such as fulminant hepatic failure and drug-induced hepatitis, are more severe and have a worse prognosis in elderly patients

4 The development of hepatocellular carcinoma is directly related to duration of cirrhosis; therefore, elderly patients with cirrhosis should be routinely screened for the presence of hepatocellular carcinoma

5 In patients with end-stage liver disease, advanced age is no longer a contraindication to orthotopic liver transplantation, which should be considered for selected elderly patients with irreversible end-stage liver disease. Conversely, livers can be accepted from elderly donors, albeit with some risk of poor graft function

▲

1 Cellular and Biochemical Aspects of the Aging Liver

A Overview

1 The aging process affects the liver, but to a lesser degree than the rest of the body

2 Both hepatic size and blood flow diminish with advancing age, which may result in changes in cellular function and biochemical pathways in the liver

3 These alterations are of considerable importance, given the aging of our population and the fact the elderly use approximately one-third of all prescribed medications, many of which are metabolized by the liver

B Cellular and biochemical changes in the aging liver

1 Aging of liver cells is characterized primarily by decreased production of hepatic proteins; some abnormal proteins accumulate in aging liver cells (Table 24.1)

Glucose-6-phosphate dehydrogenase
Phosphoglycerate kinase
NADP cytochrome c reductase
Cathepsin D
Superoxide dismutase
Aminoacyl-tRNA synthetases

Modified with permission from Dice & Goff (1988)[1]

(Table 24.1: Proteins that accumulate in aging livers)

2 Histopathologic changes seen in aging livers include increases in cell size, the number of abnormal nuclei, and the frequency of chromosomal abnormalities, as described by Van Thiel et al. (1991).[2] There is also, often, an increase in the number and size of lysosomes

3 Lipofuscin, the "wear and tear" pigment, is a common finding on liver biopsies performed on elderly patients. Pongor et al. (1984)[3] described lipofuscin as representing extensive nonenzymatic glycosylation and cross-linking of heterogeneous cellular components, including nucleic acids, proteins, and lipids. Recent evidence suggests that lipofuscin may represent, at least in part, accumulation of retinyl palmitate. While it is thought that lipofuscin is biologically inert, it may interfere with intracellular biochemical reactions and may not be just a marker of aging cells

4 As individuals age, hepatocytes are less sensitive to insulin and glucocorticoids. There is a decrease in protein breakdown as well as both transcriptional and translational processes. This altered breakdown of cellular protein may have important consequences for the cell life cycle and may be a major feature of the aging process

2 Pathophysiology of the Human Aging Liver

A Overview

1 Routine biochemical blood tests of liver function, such as serum albumin, aminotransferases, and bilirubin, do not change significantly as individuals grow old

2 Age-related changes include decreases in liver weight and blood flow, metabolism of drugs, and responsiveness to hormonal and growth factors and delayed regeneration

B Changes in Drug Metabolism

1 The systemic clearance of many drugs (e.g., midazolam, phenytoin, propranolol, and acetaminophen), metabolized by the hepatic cytochrome P-450 system are decreased in the elderly. However, the enzymatic activities of cytochrome $P-450_{IIIA}$ and $P-450_{IIE1}$, do not change with aging. This suggests that elderly individuals may be just as susceptible as younger subjects to the hepatotoxic effects of drugs such as acetaminophen and ethanol

2 Other mechanisms must be present to explain the reduced clearances of the above-mentioned drugs. There is a 40% decrease in hepatic volume and a 50% reduction in liver blood flow in elderly subjects, as described by Wynne et al. (1989).[4] This accounts for the reduction in systemic clearance of drugs that have a high first-pass hepatic uptake, such as propranolol. The decrease in liver volume is most likely responsible for the impaired clearance of medications that do not undergo significant first-pass hepatic uptake

3 The volume of distribution of water-soluble drugs is generally reduced in elderly patients, due to an increase in the ratio of body fat to body water. Although the metabolism of ethanol is essentially unaltered by aging, elevated ethanol blood levels can be observed in elderly subjects after an acute dose due to a reduced volume of distribution

4 The age-related reduction in hepatic blood is due mostly to a decrease in portal vein flow, as demonstrated by Zoli et al. (1989).[5] Using sensitive Doppler techniques, portal blood flow was shown to decrease from 740±150 mL/min in individuals less than 40 years of age, to 595±106 mL/min in healthy individuals over the age of 71. The reason for the decrease in portal vein blood flow is unknown but may relate to atherosclerosis, with a resultant decrease in mesenteric arterial blood flow

C Alterations in cholesterol metabolism

1 The cholesterol content of bile increases with advancing age, as does the lithogenic index. This is due to the combination of increased hepatic secretion of cholesterol and decreased bile acid production. It is also possible that the elderly gallbladder is less responsive to endogenous cholecystokinin (CCK), resulting in a decreased postprandial contraction of the gallbladder. Valdivieso et al. (1978)[6] demonstrated that supersaturated bile was four times more frequent in elderly women than in younger women

2 The frequency of gallstones increases with age. Approximately 40–60% of individuals in their eighth decade will have gallstones. Complications of gallstone disease are more severe in the elderly (see also Ch. 32)

3 Hepatic Diseases in the Elderly

A   Acute viral hepatitis (see also Ch. 3)

1 In elderly patients, acute viral hepatitis may have a course that is more prolonged, severe, and indolent than in younger patients. This is probably due to an aged-related decline in immune function

2 **Hepatitis A**

- relatively uncommon in the elderly due to the high rate of pre-existing immunity. However, it has been shown recently that an increasing proportion of the elderly in Western Countries are not immune to hepatitis A

- the mortality of acute hepatitis A clearly increases with advancing age. Mortality rate is 0.4% in patients between ages 15 and 39 years but 1.1% in those age 40 years and older (Fig. 24.1). In patients over 65, the mortality rate is 4%

- Vaccines against hepatitis A are now available for clinical use (e.g., Havrix™). Elderly individuals who plan to travel to areas where hepatitis A is endemic should be assessed for pre-existing immunity and vaccinated if necessary

3 **Hepatitis B and D**

- Uncommon forms of acute viral hepatitis in the elderly populations because they are generally not in high-risk groups (male homosexuals, intravenous drug users)

- presentation is generally more cholestatic, and patients are frequently oligosymptomatic and have a long recovery interval

- while the clearance of hepatitis B surface antigen (HBsAg) takes somewhat longer in the elderly, their overall prognosis is similar to that of young patients. However, the elderly are more likely to progress to chronic hepatitis

- unfortunately, the elderly do not respond as well to hepatitis B vaccination, probably because of a decrease in the number of antibody-producing B cells. Higher doses or booster immunization may be necessary for successful hepatitis B vaccination of older persons

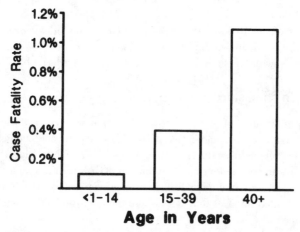

Fig. 24.1   Age-dependent case fatality rates for hepatitis A (Reproduced with permission from the AGA Clinical Teaching Project, Unit 3, *Viral Hepatitis*, 2nd edition, 1994)

4 Hepatitis C
- one study in Italy by Floreani et al. (1992)[7] has suggested that the prevalence of hepatitis C is similar in both the young and old. As with hepatitis A and B, cholestasis may be a prominent feature

5 Other causes of hepatitis
- At the present time, there is no information pertinent to elderly patients infected with the newly identified hepatitis G virus. In individual patients, the possibilities of herpesvirus and cytomegalovirus hepatitis may be considered and appropriately investigated
- in the elderly patient who presents with apparent acute viral hepatitis, the differential diagnosis must include shock liver (resulting from anoxic injury to the liver in the setting of congestive heart failure, cardiac arrythmia, myocardial infarction, or sepsis, see Ch. 20) and widespread hepatic metastases. Conversely, older patients with jaundice and elevated liver enzymes presumed to be due to extrahepatic biliary obstruction may require evaluation for acute viral hepatitis

B Chronic viral hepatitis (see also Ch. 4)

1 The clinical presentation of chronic hepatitis B and C is generally similar to that seen in younger patients. However, many elderly patients with chronic hepatitis B are hepatitis B e antigen (HBeAg) negative. This denotes a lesser degree of infectivity and results in a decreased need for interferon therapy

2 Interferon alpha is the only medication currently approved for the treatment of chronic hepatitis due to hepatitis B or C viruses. The morbidity associated with use of interferon is increased in the elderly, who have difficulties tolerating interferon

3 An important complication of chronic hepatitis B and C is the development of hepatocellular carcinoma (HCC). Because the development of HCC correlates with the duration of chronic hepatitis, elderly patients with cirrhosis due to chronic hepatitis B or C should be screened twice yearly with ultrasound of the liver and serum alpha fetoprotein testing

C Drug-induced hepatotoxicity (see also Ch. 8)

1 The risk of drug-induced hepatotoxicity has been shown to increase with advancing age for many medications, most notably isoniazid (see Table 24.2). Eastwood (1971)[8] found approximately 20% of cases of jaundice in the elderly to be secondary to medications, compared with approximately 2–5% of patients of all ages requiring hospitalization for jaundice

2 Benoxaprofen is a nonsteroidal anti-inflammatory agent in which a clear association between age and hepatotoxicity was demonstrated. Nine patients taking the medication developed fulminant hepatic failure and died; all were over the age of 70. The drug was taken off the market and is no longer available

3 Elderly patients are more likely to be on multiple medications. Williamson & Chopin (1980)[9] found that the frequency of adverse drug reactions was three times higher in patients taking six medications compared with those taking a single agent. This state of "polypharmacy" allows for the greater likelihood of an increase or decrease in cytochrome P-450 activity, leading to drug–drug interactions

| Benoxaprofen |
| Dantrolene |
| Fluoxacilin |
| Halothane |
| Isoniazid |
| Methyldopa |
| Sulindac |

(Table 24.2: Some medications for which hepatotoxicity increases with age)

4 Drug-induced hepatotoxicity should be a major diagnostic consideration in all elderly patients who present with elevated liver enzymes and/or jaundice. All unnecessary medications should be discontinued, and necessary agents should be switched to a different class. Table 24.2 lists some drugs for which hepatotoxicity increases with age

D   Autoimmune liver disease

1 **Primary biliary cirrhosis** (see also Ch. 14)
   - extensive studies by Dickson et al. from the Mayo Clinic (1989)[10] have clearly identified advancing age as a poor prognostic indicator in patients with primary biliary cirrhosis. (This is in direct contrast to a previous study by Lehmann, 1985,[11] who found that individuals presenting with primary biliary cirrhosis after 65 are less likely to have advanced disease)

2 **Autoimmune hepatitis** (see also Ch. 5)
   - Typically occurs in middle-age females, but can be present in older individuals. Management in the elderly can be difficult, due to the adverse effects of long-term corticosteroid use in a group (postmenopausal females) already at high risk for osteoporosis, glaucoma, arterial hypertension, and obesity

3 **Primary sclerosing cholangitis** (see also Ch. 15)
   - usually occurs in the third or fourth decade; it is therefore unusual to make this diagnosis in an elderly patient

E   Alcoholic liver disease (see also Ch. 6)

1 The perception is that most alcoholics who acquire alcoholic liver disease will do so in middle age. However, recent studies from Europe and the USA have demonstrated that a significant proportion of patients with alcoholic liver disease will present in their fifth and sixth decades.

2 Older patients are more likely than younger patients to exhibit the classic signs of hepatic decompensation – ascites, jaundice, and lower extremity edema. Overall mortality due to alcoholic liver disease is higher in patients over age 60 – 34% at 1 year as compared with 5% in younger patients. In patients over age 70, 1-year mortality rate increases dramatically to 75%

F Inborn errors of metabolism

1 **Hereditary hemochromatosis** (see also Ch. 16)
   - while most patients present by middle age, some patients first seek medical attention at an advanced age for hepatocellular carcinoma or another complication of end-stage liver disease
   - females typically become symptomatic approximately a decade after their male counterparts, due to the iron-depleting effects of regular menses and childbirth
   - common symptoms include fatigue and arthritis, both of which are common in the elderly anyway
   - the diagnosis is suggested by a fasting transferrin saturation (serum iron/total iron binding capacity (TIBC) × 100) greater than 60% in males or 50% in females and an elevated serum ferritin. Early diagnosis is crucial for two reasons: (1) complications can be prevented by phlebotomy, and (2) family members can be screened
   - a major cause of death in patients with cirrhosis due to hemochromatosis is HCC; screening with serum alpha fetoprotein testing and ultrasonography should be done every 6 months

2 **Alpha-1 antitrypsin deficiency** (see also Ch. 18)
   - patients with homozygous alpha-1 antitrypsin deficiency (α-1 ATD) usually present before age 65
   - heterozygous α-1 ATD has been thought to be a cause of cirrhosis in approximately 5% of patients with cirrhosis over age 65.[12] However, this condition is frequent in the overall population, and no evidence exists that intracellular accumulation of α-1AT globular inclusions are hepatotoxic
   - although no effective treatment exists, diagnosis is important for family members so that they can avoid risky behavior (such as alcohol, smoking, and intravenous drug use) that may further jeopardize their hepatic and pulmonary function

3 **Wilson's disease** (see also Ch. 17)
   - de novo diagnosis of this entity is extremely rare in elderly patients. Most patients have clinical disease well before the fifth decade

G Cryptogenic cirrhosis (see also Chs 9 and 10)

1 A significant number of elderly patients with cirrhosis have cryptogenic cirrhosis (cause unknown). The percentage of cases of cirrhosis of unknown cause is expected to decrease as serologic assays for hepatitis C, as well as other viruses, become part of routine testing

2 In a postmortem study Ludwig and Baggenstoss (1970)[13] described 77 cases of cryptogenic cirrhosis in patients over age 70 in whom the diagnosis was unsuspected when they were alive. While this raises the possibility of a specific form of cryptogenic cirrhosis in the elderly, further research is needed before the existence of such an entity can be established

H Liver abscess (see also Ch. 28)

1 The majority of patients with pyogenic liver abscesses in the northern hemisphere are over age 60

2 The diagnosis is more difficult to make than in younger patients, since the typical presentation of fever, jaundice, and right-upper-quadrant pain is frequently absent. Elderly patients are more likely to have nonspecific symptoms, such as epigastric pain, weakness, fatigue, and shortness of breath

3 While approximately one-half of infections originate from the biliary tree (most often as a result of ascending cholangitis), other intra-abdominal and gastrointestinal sources should be investigated. They include:

- penetrating gastric or duodenal ulcers
- pancreatitis
- perihepatic abscess
- portal vein thrombosis
- peritonitis (of any cause)
- inflammatory bowel disease
- colon cancer
- diverticulitis and/or diverticular abscess

4 A retrospective study of Sridharan et al. (1990)[14] demonstrated that almost a third of elderly patients with hepatic abscesses at autopsy were misdiagnosed in life as having a hepatic malignancy. Confirmation of tumor by needle biopsy should be obtained, especially if a primary site of malignancy is not present

5 Pyogenic abscesses can be successfully treated by percutaneous aspiration and drainage in conjunction with systemic intravenous antibiotics

I Gallstones (see also Ch. 32)

1 Gallstones are an age-related phenomenon. Unfortunately, the mortality of untreated biliary tract disease also increases with age. Cancer of the gallbladder is also more likely to occur in older patients

2 The management of biliary disease with respect to age has been summarized by James (1991)[15] as outlined in Table 24.3
- with the advent of laparoscopic cholecystectomy early operative intervention has brought the mortality and morbidity for young and old closer together. ERCP with sphincterotomy has been shown to have insignificant differences in morbidity and mortality between old and young, despite a longer hospital admission in the elderly
- incidental appendectomy during cholecystectomy should not be performed in elderly patients due to the risk of wound infection and the relatively low lifetime risk of acute appendicitis

J Hepatic tumors

1 **Hepatocellular carcinoma** (see also Ch. 27)
- elderly patients with cirrhosis are at increased risk of HCC; there is a clear association between HCC development and the duration of cirrhosis

Condition	Treatment
Acute or chronic cholecystitis	Early cholecystectomy (preferably laparoscopic) and perioperative exploration of the bile duct (in acute cholecystitis)
Cholangitis with choledocholithiasis	ERCP with sphincterotomy and stone extraction
Choledocholithiasis with gallstones in the gallbladder	ERCP with sphincterotomy. If symptoms persist, then cholecystectomy or percutaneous cholecystostomy with removal of the gallstones
Asymptomatic gallstones	Controversial: observation generally preferred over prophylactic intervention

ERCP, endoscopic retrograde cholangiopancreatography

(Table 24.3: Management of biliary disease in the elderly[15])

- screening protocols for the detection of HCC should be performed as described previously; early detection of a small tumor may result in prolongation of survival by resection, ethanol injection, embolization, or liver transplantation

2 Metastatic tumors

- most common malignant tumor found in the liver
- the incidence of hepatic metastases is greatest for those tumors arising within the drainage area of the portal vein (colon, pancreatic, and stomach cancer), but other tumors, such as lung and breast cancer, can also metastasize to the liver
- while the prognosis for patients with hepatic metastases is poor (with an average survival of 6 months), identification and localization can be important. Survival is directly correlated with extent of hepatic involvement; patients with solitary metastases have a survival time almost double that of patients with widespread hepatic metastases
- therapy exists which may prolong survival. There are data to suggest that 20% of patients who undergo surgical resection of a solitary hepatic metastasis may be alive 5 years after resection

K   Fulminant hepatic failure (FHF) (see also Ch. 2)

- No matter what the etiology, FHF has a higher mortality rate in the elderly (Table 24.4)

Age group	Survival (%)	
	Hepatitis B	**Non-A, non-B hepatitis**
15–24	40	20
25–44	35	5
45 +	15	0

Modified with permission from the American Gastroenterological Association Teaching File (1988)

(Table 24.4: Age-specific survival rates)

- FHF due to hepatitis A is particularly devastating in the elderly, with a mortality rate much greater than that in individuals between ages 15 and 24
- the best treatment for FHF in the elderly is to prevent its occurrence. Vaccination against hepatitis A and B should be considered in all susceptible elderly individuals. Hepatotoxic drugs, such as isoniazid, should not be used unless absolutely necessary. Frequent monitoring of liver enzymes should be performed in elderly patients who require treatment with medications known to have potential hepatotoxicity

4 Complications of Liver Disease in the Elderly

A Portal hypertension (see also Chs 9–13)

1 Surprisingly, elderly patients admitted with bleeding esophageal varices have short-term mortality rates similar to those of younger patients. However, their 1-year survival is less than that of their younger counterparts

2 Older patients are more likely to be unable to tolerate the effects of vasopressin (with or without nitroglycerin) during an acute variceal bleed. The use of continuous infusion of octreotide is preferable to vasopressin in the medical treatment of bleeding varices in the elderly

3 Chronic sclerotherapy, band ligation, and beta blockers can be used to prevent recurrent bleeding, although some older patients may be unable to tolerate the adverse effects (fatigue, dizziness, depression, etc.) of beta blockers

4 Both portacaval shunts and transjugular intrahepatic portosystemic stent (TIPS) can be used for recurrent variceal bleeding; however, their usefulness is limited by the high incidence of post-shunt hepatic encephalopathy. With TIPS, the incidence of hepatic encephalopathy is directly related to the shunt diameter. It is recommended that small-caliber stents of 7–8 mm be used in patients over age 60, in order to decrease the chances of hepatic encephalopathy. Lowering the hepatic venous pressure gradient to just below 12 mmHg may also minimize the chances of post-TIPS hepatic encephalopathy in elderly cirrhotic patients

5 Elderly patients with refractory ascites and/or recurrent variceal bleeding, who are otherwise healthy, should be considered for liver transplant evaluation

B Hepatocellular carcinoma (HCC) (see also Ch. 27)

1 As stated above, the development of HCC is directly related to the presence of cirrhosis, especially in the Western world. MacMahon and James (1994)[12] noted that 50% of their patients with cirrhosis who developed HCC were over age 60 years, and 40% were over age 70.

2 HCC should be suspected in any patient who presents initially with a complication of cirrhosis

3 If HCC is detected in an early stage, survival and palliation may be enhanced by a variety of interventions (resection, chemoembolization, alcohol injections, chemotherapy)

C   Orthotopic liver transplantation (OLT) (see also Ch. 31)

1   Advanced age is not a contraindication to OLT. Recent studies have shown that in patients older than age 60–65, survival after OLT is comparable to that of younger patients. The decision to proceed with liver transplantation should be based on the overall health of the patient, not chronological age

2   It has also been shown that donor livers can be used safely in individuals over age 50. Previously, there had been concern over the theoretical loss of liver function with advancing age and many donor livers went unused based solely on age. Questions had also been raised as to whether older livers are less resistant to ischemia, preservation, and reperfusion injuries. The increasing demand for donor livers has led to the increasing use of livers from elderly donors.

- several groups have reported that patient and graft outcomes are identical regardless of the age of the donor livers. (This was true even though older livers had significantly increased steatosis and were more likely to be used in patients requiring urgent liver transplantation.)

- The older liver may have a slightly worse performance in the early postoperative period, as evidenced by higher peak serum alanine aminotransferase and bilirubin levels, along with slightly lower bile outputs

3   Yersiz et al. (1995)[16] demonstrated a significant increase in delayed function of livers from donor over age 50 as compared to donors below age 30. Recipients experiencing delayed nonfunction were three times as likely to require retransplantation. However, early recognition of delayed nonfunction with subsequent retransplantation led to similar 1-year patient survival rates in both groups

4   Currently, livers from donors older than age 65 are used only in patients with an urgent need for liver transplantation (e.g., a patient with hepatorenal syndrome or FHF). Ischemic time should be kept to a minimum when an older donor liver is used, to lessen preservation injury and postoperative hepatic graft dysfunction

5   That livers from older donors are able to withstand the often extreme physiologic conditions imposed by liver transplantation (harvesting, implantation, reperfusion, rejection, toxic effects of drugs, infection, etc.) and ultimately provide excellent function is a clear demonstration that the human liver is highly resilient to the aging process[17]

References

1   Dice JF, Goff SA. *Aging and the liver*. In: Arias IM, Jakoby WB, Popper H, Schachter D, Shafritz DA, (eds). *The Liver: Biology and Pathobiology*. (New York: Raven Press, 1988) 1245–58

2   Van Thiel DH, Stauber R, Gavaler J, Francavilla A. *Hepatic regeneration effects of age, sex hormone status, protein and cyclosporine*. (Dig Dis Sci 1991) 36: 1309–12

3   Pongor S, Ulrich P, Bencsath A, Cerami A. *Aging of proteins: isolation and identification of a fluorescent chromophore from the reaction of peptides with glucose*. (Proc Natl Acad Sci USA 1984) 81: 2684–8

4   Wynne HA, Cope LH, Mutch E, Rawlins MD, Woodhouse KW, James OFW. *The effect of age upon liver volume and apparent liver blood flow in healthy man*. (Hepatology 1989) 9: 297–301

5   Zoli M, Iervese T, Abbati S, Bianchi GP, Marchesini G, Pisi E. *Portal flow velocity and flow in aging man*. (Gerontology 1989) 35: 661–5

6   Valdivieso V, Palma R, Wunkhaus R, Antezana C, Severin C, Contreras A. *Effect of aging on biliary lipid composition and bile acid metabolism in normal Chilean women.* (Gastroenterology 1978) 74: 871–4

7   Floreani A, Bertin T, Soffiati G, Naccarato R, Chiaramonte M. *Anti-hepatitis C virus in the elderly: a sero-epidemiological study in a home for the aged.* (Gerontology 1992) 38: 214–16

8   Eastwood HOH. *Causes of jaundice in the elderly: a survey of diagnosis and investigation.* (Gerontol Clin 1971) 13: 69–81

9   Williamson J, Chopin JM. *Adverse reactions to prescribed drugs in the elderly: a multicentre investigation.* (Age Ageing 1980) 9: 73–80

10   Dickson ER, Grambsch P, Fleming TR. *Prognosis in primary biliary cirrhosis. Model for decision making.* (Hepatology 1989) 10: 1–7

11   Lehmann AB, Bassendine MF, James OFW. *Is primary biliary cirrhosis a different disease in the elderly?* (Gerontology 1985) 31: 186–94

12   MacMahon M, James OFW. *Liver disease in the elderly.* (J Clin Gastroenterol 1994) 18: 330–4

13   Ludwig J, Baggenstoss AH. Cirrhosis of the aged and senile cirrhosis: are there two conditions? (J Gerontol 1970) 25: 244–8

14   Sridharan GV, Wilkinson SP, Primrose WR. *Pyogenic liver abscess in the elderly.* (Age Ageing 1990) 19: 199–203

15   James OFW. *Liver disease in the elderly.* In: McIntyre N, Benhamou JP, Bircher J, Rizzetto M, Rodes J (eds). *Oxford Textbook of Clinical Hepatology.* (Oxford: Oxford University Press, 1991) 1305–9

16   Yersiz H, Shaked A, Olthoff K, Imagawa D, Shackleten C, Martin P, Busuttil RW. *Correlation between donor age and the pattern of liver graft recovery after transplantation.* (Transplantation 1995) 60: 790–4

17   Munoz SJ, Friedman LS. *The liver and aging.* In: Rustgi VK, Van Thiel OH, (eds). *The Liver in Systemic Disease.* (New York: Raven Press, 1993) 251–66

HIV and the liver

K. RAJENDER REDDY, M.D., F.A.C.P

Key Points

1 Abnormalities in hepatic biochemical tests are common in patients with acquired immunodeficiency syndrome (AIDS). Jaundice is infrequent

2 Acute HIV infection itself can occasionally cause a mononucleosis-like syndrome associated with hepatic dysfunction. Hepatitis B, C, and D viruses may coinfect with HIV. HIV-related immunosuppression may alter the expression of hepatitis B markers and the severity of liver disease. HIV-infected individuals respond poorly to hepatitis B vaccination. In persons coinfected with HIV and HCV, an increase in HCV viremia may be observed, and such individuals may have a more rapidly progressive course compared with HCV infection alone

3 Drug-induced hepatitis and/or cholestasis should be a consideration in all HIV-infected patients with hepatic dysfunction

4 Opportunistic bacterial and fungal infections of the liver may occur in patients with AIDS. Of these, *Mycobacterium avium* complex (MAC) is most common

5 A spectrum of hepatic sinusoidal abnormalities that include sinusoidal dilation, perisinusoidal fibrosis, and bacillary peliosis hepatis have been observed in AIDS. Bacillary peliosis hepatis is caused by the fastidious, Gram-negative bacillus *Rochalimaea henselae*

6 A unique syndrome of AIDS cholangiopathy, which can mimic bacterial cholangitis, is often caused by opportunistic infections such as *Cryptosporidium* species, *cytomegalovirus*, microsporidia species, MAC, and *cyclospora*, and rarely Kaposi's sarcoma or lymphoma

7 The development of lymphoma, chiefly non-Hodgkin's lymphoma of the B cell and non-B, non-T cell types is well recognized in AIDS patients, particularly male homosexuals, with liver involvement in 10%

---

1   HIV Infection of the Liver and Associated Viral Infections

A   HIV (human immunodeficiency virus)

1 Occasionally, HIV infection may present as an acute mononucleosis-like syndrome. Symptoms and signs include fever, sweating, malaise, myalgias, and hepatosplenomegaly with elevations of serum aminotransferase and alkaline phosphatase levels

2 HIV has been identified immunohistochemically in the liver. Using an anti-P24 antibody, HIV has been noted in Kupffer's cells, granulomas, histiocytes, and sinusoidal endothelial cells

3 By in situ hybridization, HIV DNA has also been found in sinusoidal endothelial cells, hepatocytes, and lymphocytes. Both macrophages and endothelial cells in the liver have been demonstrated to express a CD4 receptor for HIV

B   HAV (hepatitis A virus)

1 The seroprevalence of anti-hepatitis A virus (anti-HAV) is high among homosexuals and intravenous drug users. The severity of acute HAV infection in intravenous drug users, as in homosexual men, may be greater, particularly if they have underlying chronic liver disease related to other viruses such as hepatitis B and C.

2 Prophylaxis of HIV-positive individuals with the hepatitis A vaccine may be worthwhile

C   Hepatitis B and D

1 Most patients with AIDS have serologic markers of hepatitis B virus (HBV) infection, more often of past infection rather than ongoing viral replication

2 HIV-positive individuals who do not have evidence of immunity to HBV infection should be considered for HBV vaccination. Response to the vaccine in these individuals is suboptimal regardless of their lymphocyte counts

3 An immunosuppressed state is likely to facilitate HBV replication with increased levels of HBV DNA in serum. In such individuals serum aminotransferase levels are lower than in non-HIV-infected persons with chronic hepatitis B and the degree of hepatocellular necrosis is lower. HIV infection may facilitate reactivation of HBV

infection, analogous to HBV reactivation observed with cancer chemotherapy and other immunosuppressed states

4 Seroprevalence of hepatitis D virus (HDV, delta) infection is higher in patients with AIDS compared with those without AIDS. Patients with HIV, HBV, and HDV infections are more likely to have progressive liver disease than patients with HBV and HDV infection alone

5 Treatment of HBV infection with interferon alpha is associated with suboptimal responses in HIV-infected persons

D Hepatitis C

1 HIV and hepatitis C virus (HCV) coinfected patients have higher serum levels of HCV RNA compared with patients with HCV infection alone. Coinfected patients may have a more aggressive clinical course, although this has not been consistently observed

2 Multitransfused HIV and HCV coinfected hemophiliacs and older patients have been observed to have progressive liver disease. Further, coinfection may facilitate sexual and perinatal transmission of HCV infection

E Other viral infections

1 Fulminant hepatitis due to herpes simplex virus type II or adenovirus is rare

2 Cytomegalovirus (CMV) infection is common in patients with AIDS and can range from evidence of past CMV infection to a fulminant and disseminated illness. Both a hepatitis-like illness and biliary tract disease may be seen. Often there is a predominant elevation of the serum alkaline phosphatase. Intranuclear inclusion bodies within the hepatocytes, vascular endothelial cells, and biliary epithelium are observed on liver biopsy and may be associated with a granulomatous reaction

3 In situ hybridization techniques have demonstrated DNA of CMV, herpes simplex virus, and Epstein–Barr virus in nuclei and cytoplasm of hepatocytes, monocytes, and lymphocytes and in perisinusoidal lining cells. Biliary epithelium has also been observed to express the DNA of these viruses

2 Opportunistic Infections

A Mycobacterial infections

1 Mycobacterial infections are found frequently in the liver both ante mortem and at autopsy, in patients with AIDS. *Mycobacterium avium* complex (MAC) is the most common causative pathogen, with occasionally cases due to atypical mycobacteria such as *M. xenopi* and *M. kansasii*

2 A disproportionate elevation of the serum alkaline phosphatase level has been observed but is not a consistent feature

3 Hepatic granulomas are often observed with these infections and are usually ill formed, presumably due to the suppressed T lymphocyte activity seen in AIDS

4 Granulomas associated with MAC infection are composed of foamy blue histiocytes with abundant acid-fast bacilli on special stains

5 Liver biopsy cultures may be positive for mycobacteria but the diagnosis is often established on histopathologic evaluation with special stains

6 Occasionally, acid-fast bacilli may be seen in the liver with special stains in the absence of granulomas

B Fungal infections (see Ch. 29)

1 Fungal agents that involve the liver in patients with AIDS include *Histoplasma capsulatum, Candida albicans, Sporothrix schenckii,* and *Coccidioides immitis,* usually as part of a disseminated disease

2 Special stains and cultures of liver biopsy material are helpful in establishing these diagnoses, as occasionally they may present with atypical clinical features

C Protozoan infections (see Ch. 29)

1 Protozoan infections are relatively uncommon. *Pneumocystis carinii* infection may occasionally involve the liver, particularly in patients on inhaled pentamidine as prophylaxis to prevent pulmonary pneumocystosis

2 Rarely, visceral leishmaniasis may have hepatic involvement

3 Sinusoidal Abnormalities

A Nonspecific findings

- abnormalities include sinusoidal dilation, perisinusoidal fibrosis, and bacillary peliosis hepatis. Often nonspecific sinusoidal dilation is an incidental finding and of no major clinical consequence

- ultrastructurally, abnormalities of the sinusoidal barrier have been observed mainly as a proliferation of hyperplastic sinusoidal macrophages. HIV can be demonstrated by in situ hybridization and immunohistochemistry in the liver, and it has been suggested that endothelial cell injury and sinusoidal dilation may be a direct or indirect consequence of HIV infection of the liver

B Peliosis hepatis

1 Blood filled cystic changes in hepatic parenchyma that may or may not have an endothelial lining; not uncommon in AIDS

2 There is convincing evidence that peliosis hepatis associated with HIV infection is caused by a bacillus and is therefore termed **bacillary peliosis hepatis**

3 Histopathologic and ultrastructural studies have demonstrated clumpy, granular, purple material on Warthin-starry stain that have morphologic features consistent with bacilli

4 According to murine antiserum studies, electrophoretic patterns of outer membrane proteins, and restriction in the nucleus digestion patterns of DNA, the bacillus has been designated *Rochalimaea henselae*, a fastidious Gram-negative bacillus

5 Occasionally patients may present with abdominal pain associated with hepatomegaly, but peliosis hepatis is more likely to be an incidental finding on a liver biopsy. A clinical response to erythromycin has been observed

6 The pathogenetic mechanisms involved in the development of peliosis hepatis are unclear. One speculation is that the bacillus elaborates an angiogenic factor similar to a factor elaborated by *Bartonella bacilliformis*

C Other findings

Lipid-laden perisinusoidal cells, along with hypertrophy of Kupffer's cells and endothelial cell inclusions have been observed in AIDS. Hypervitaminosis A has been suggested as the cause, but it may only represent a nonspecific finding related to various drugs or to systemic or hepatic infections

4 AIDS Cholangiopathy

A AIDS-related biliary tract disease

1 AIDS cholangiopathy is a unique syndrome that mimics bacterial cholangitis. Signs and symptoms are fever, right-upper-quadrant abdominal pain, nausea, vomiting, jaundice, and hepatomegaly. The origin is nonbacterial

2 Most often AIDS cholangiopathy is due to *Cryptosporidium*, CMV, microsporidia (*Encephalitozoon bieneusi, E. intestinalis*), MAC, or cyclospora. Occasionally it may be noninfectious in etiology, due for example to Kaposi's sarcoma or noncleaved cell lymphoma infiltrating the biliary tree. In some cases, the etiology is unknown; direct HIV infection of the biliary epithelium has been suggested as a cause, perhaps as a direct extension of HIV infection of the small and large bowel mucosa

3 The predominant hepatic biochemical test abnormality is elevation of the serum alkaline phosphatase level. Mild elevations of the serum aminotransferases are common but jaundice is uncommon. A few patients may have normal hepatic biochemical tests (20% of cases documented by cholangiography in one series). The CD4 lymphocyte count is usually very low ($<100/mm^3$). Ultrasonography may demonstrate dilated intrahepatic and extrahepatic biliary ducts, and computed tomography (CT) is seldom needed. Ultrasonography has a sensitivity of 75–85%. Endoscopic retrograde cholangiopancreatography (ERCP) is the preferred cholangiographic approach for diagnosis.

4 Cholangiographic abnormalities can be characterized into four groups:
  - sclerosing cholangitis and papillary stenosis (most common)
  - sclerosing cholangitis alone
  - papillary stenosis alone
  - long, extrahepatic bile duct strictures

5 Use of ERCP rather than transhepatic cholangiography allows an opportunity for biopsy of the ampulla and for sphincterotomy, which is all that may be needed for treatment of ampullary stenosis alone

6 Endoscopic ampullary biopsies have revealed *Cryptosporidium* in most cases. Multiple pathogens may be occasionally identified. Microsporidia (*E. bieneusi,*

E. intestinalis) are a common cause if blood cultures and multiple stool studies are negative. In some cases, CMV intranuclear inclusions and associated chronic inflammatory changes are identified. CMV dissemination appears to precede the development of cholestasis and cholangiopathy, but ganciclovir and foscarnet do not influence the course of cholestasis. Similarly, MAC organisms have been recovered from periampullary and duodenal biopsy specimens in some cases

7 Placement of biliary stents may provide pain relief, but the serum alkaline phosphatase may continue to rise progressively after stent placement and a decrease in large duct dilation; this is a consequence of progressive disease involving the intrahepatic bile ducts

B Gallbladder disease

1 Occasionally acute acalculous cholecystitis may be a feature of AIDS-related cholangiopathy. *Isospora belli*, CMV, cryptosporidia, and microsporidia are often implicated. Less often, *Candida albicans* and *Salmonella typhimurium* have been recovered. Rarely, Gram-negative bacteria, including *Klebsiella pneumoniae* and *Pseudomonas aeruginosa*, have been cultured from the gallbladder

2 Patients present with right-upper-quadrant abdominal pain and fever. Ultrasound may demonstrate a thickened gallbladder wall, pericholecystic fluid, stones, or ductal abnormalities. Nuclear scanning of the gallbladder is often diagnostic by demonstrating absence of gallbladder uptake

3 Laparoscopic cholecystectomy can be performed with acceptable morbidity. Some patients may require open cholecystectomy

5 Ascites and Peritoneal Disease

1 Ascites with a high protein content may be a presenting feature of AIDS in some patients. Laparoscopy is often helpful in determining the cause of ascites. Most often the cause is peritoneal and liver involvement by non-Hodgkin's lymphoma, Kaposi's sarcoma, or opportunistic infections

2 Plaque-like lesions of the peritoneum have been observed in non-Hodgkin's lymphoma but are not specific for this condition. Differential diagnosis should include disseminated cryptococcosis and *Pneumocystis carinii* infections. Tiny (less than 5 mm in diameter) nodular lesions are suggestive of mycobacterial infections. Histologically, both caseating and noncaseating granulomas have been observed

3 Chylous ascites has been an infrequent observation and, along with multiple intraabdominal adhesions with the appearance of "violin strings", is suggestive of *Mycobacterium tuberculosis*

4 Unusual causes of peritonitis in AIDS include toxoplasmosis and coccidiodomycosis. Other fungal causes include aspergillosis and *Histoplasma capsulatum*. Rare causes of peritonitis are the microsporidian *Encephalitozoon cuniculi* and the bacterium *Nocardia brasiliensis*

5 A chronic nonspecific peritonitis without a clear-cut cause has been observed in some patients. Despite extensive evaluation, an etiology may not be found. It has been suggested that HIV infection itself may cause nonspecific peritonitis

6 In some patients, either alcoholic cirrhosis or postviral hepatitic cirrhosis may be responsible for low-protein ascites. Infrequently, *Salmonella enteritidis* group B has been a cause for spontaneous bacterial peritonitis

6   Liver Disease in Pediatric AIDS

1 To a large part, liver disease seen in pediatric AIDS is similar to that reported in adult AIDS. There are, however, a few differences. For example, giant cell hepatitis is more frequently observed in pediatric AIDS

2 Biliary tree abnormalities are uncommon in pediatric AIDS; this may be due in part to decreased recognition because of the difficulty of performing cholangiographic studies in children

3 Observed histologic abnormalities, either singly or in combination, include giant cell transformation, CMV inclusions, Kaposi's sarcoma, diffuse lymphoplasmacytic infiltrate, granulomatous hepatitis, mild portal inflammation, necrosis around central veins, steatosis, and cholestasis

7   Lymphoma and Kaposi's Sarcoma

A   Lymphoma

1 It is well recognized that AIDS is associated with the development of lymphoma, chiefly non-Hodgkin's lymphoma. The tumors occur most often in male homosexuals and are of the B cell and non-B, non-T cell types. Hodgkin's lymphoma is infrequently seen

2 The frequency of extranodal involvement of multiple organs is significantly higher than seen with lymphomas in the general population. About 10% of patients with lymphomas appear to have liver involvement. The CD4 count is usually less than $200/mm^3$. Jaundice may be a manifestation of lymphoma and is associated with high short-term mortality

3 Hepatic involvement may be detected on ultrasound or CT. The latter is preferred because it also vizualizes the spleen and retroperitoneum

4 Diagnosis can be established laparoscopically or via CT-guided biopsy. Since bone marrow involvement is frequent, a bone marrow aspirate and biopsy should be considered before the more invasive liver or retroperitoneal lymph node biopsy

5 Lymphomas are highly aggressive and respond poorly to treatment

B   Kaposi's sarcoma

1 Also seen predominantly in male homosexuals. Frequently, hepatic involvement is part of disseminated disease and is diagnosed post mortem

2 Abdominal pain and hepatomegaly with disproportionate elevation of the serum alkaline phosphatase may be a clinical feature in the occasional case diagnosed ante mortem

3 Ultrasonography and CT demonstrate defects in the liver and spleen which, however, are not specific for Kaposi's sarcoma

8 Drug-induced Liver Disease (Table 25.1)

Type of drug	Hepatocellular	Cholestatic	Granulomas	Mixed
Analgesics	Acetaminophen Ibuprofen Indomethacin Salicylates	Propoxyphene		Naproxen Piroxicam Sulindac
Anticonvulsants	Diphenylhydantoin Valproate[a]	Diphenylhydantoin	Diphenylhydantoin	Carbamazepine Phenobarbital
Antimicrobials	Amphotericin B Clindamycin Ethionamide Isoniazid Ketoconazole Metronidazole Oxacillin Aminosalicylic acid Pentamidine Pyrazinamide Quinacrine Rifampin[b] Sulfonamides Sulfones (dapsone) Tetracycline[a] Trimethoprim-sulfamethoxazole 2',3'-deoxyinosine Zidovudine	Carbenicillin Erythromycin Ketoconazole Rifampin Thiabendazole Trimethoprim-sulfamethoxazole Zidovudine	Trimethoprim–sulfamethoxazole	Trimethoprim–sulfamethoxazole
Miscellaneous agents	5-Fluorocytosine Disulfiram Vitamin A Prochlorperazine Acyclovir Fluphenazine	Anabolic steroids Chlorpromazine Contraceptive steroids Prochlorperazine		Chlordiazepoxide Diazepam

[a]Microvesicular steatosis may occur
[b]Cholestasis predominates, but hepatocellular damage may also occur.
Adapted from Lewis & Zimmerman (1989),[1] Schwarz & Greene (1992),[2] and Bach et al. (1992)

(Table 25.1 Drugs used in AIDS that may produce hepatotoxicity)

1 It is not uncommon for a patient with AIDS to be on multiple potentially hepatotoxic drugs. These drugs may be used to treat an opportunistic infection or may be directed primarily at HIV

2 **Isoniazid, rifampin, and trimethoprim–sulfamethoxazole** are the most common of the potentially hepatotoxic drugs that may be responsible for hepatic dysfunction in patients with AIDS

3 The abnormalities may range from subtle, nonspecific, and aymptomatic elevations

of liver function tests to severe hepatitis. **The most common cause of jaundice in AIDS is drug-induced hepatitis**. Cholestasis is less frequent, and some cases are characterized by mixed hepatitis and cholestasis. Fulminant hepatic failure is rare. Patients with severe hepatitis often have CD4 counts of less than $100/mm^3$

4 **Zidovudine** may cause a mixed hepatitis/cholestasis pattern, and 2', 3'-deoxyinosine (ddI) may cause a hepatitis-like illness. Rarely ddI has been implicated in fuliminant hepatic failure

5 An underlying poor nutritional status with concomitant use of drugs that induce cytochrome P-450 system may increase susceptibility to various drug hepatotoxicity

6 The decision to continue or discontinue a drug depends on the likelihood of drug-induced liver disease, severity of underlying illness necessitating the use of the implicated drugs, severity of hepatic manifestations, and availability of alternative drugs. Regardless, with severe hepatic disease associated with jaundice, it is prudent to stop one or several implicated drugs and switch to alternative medications

7 The role of newer nucleoside analogs and protease inhibitors in causing serious liver disease is unclear at this time

9 Miscellaneous Considerations

1 Macrovesicular fatty infiltration of the liver is a common histologic finding in patients with AIDS. Fatty change may cause clinically significant hepatomegaly associated with a predominant elevation of the serum alkaline phosphatase. CT scan demonstrates decreased density of the liver

2 Microscopically, macrovesicular fat is randomly distributed throughout the lobule without any zonal predilection. It may be caused by a variety of associated conditions such as cachexia, hyperalimentation, various medications or infections, alcoholism, or HCV infection. Steatohepatitis is uncommon, and liver failure or portal hypertension does not ensue. A case of microvesicular steatosis has been reported in an adult with AIDS but is rare

3 There are sparse reports on ultrastructural changes in the liver in AIDS. A severe case of hepatitis due to a microsporidian protozoan of the genus *Encephalitozoon* (*E. cuniculi*) has been reported in a patient with AIDS

10 Liver Biopsy in Patients with AIDS

Liver biopsy should be considered with caution, as there are rare reports of exsanguinating hemorrhage. Laparoscopy and radiologically guided biopsies may be helpful in patients with ascites and focal lesions in the liver or the retroperitoneum. Because of the disseminated nature of most diseases, it is prudent to consider less invasive procedures such as bone marrow biopsy or bronchoscopy prior to performing a percutaneous liver biopsy

11 Summary (see Table 25.2)

Viral hepatitis		
Hepatitis A	Hepatitis B	Hepatitis C
Hepatitis D	CMV	EBV
HSV	HIV	

Opportunistic infections		
MAC	*Coccidioides immitis*	*Cryptosporidium*
Pneumocystis carinii	*Histoplasma capsulatum*	
Cryptococcus neoformans	*Candida albicans*	
Mycobacterium tuberculosis		

AIDS cholangiopathy	
Acalculous cholecystitis	Sclerosing cholangitis
Papillary stenosis	Lymphoma of the biliary tree
Kaposi's sarcoma	

Neoplasms	
Kaposi's sarcoma	Non-Hodgkin's lymphoma

Drug-induced hepatitis
(See Table 25.1)

Histologic findings		
Steatosis (fatty liver)	Granulomatous hepatitis	Portal inflammation
Sinusoidal dilatation	Peliosis hepatis	

(Table 25.2: Diseases affecting the hepatobiliary systems and histologic changes in AIDS)

References

1 Lewis JH, Zimmerman HJ. *Drug-induced liver disease.* (Med Clin North Am 1989) 73: 775–92

2 Schwarz ED, Greene JB. *Diagnostic considerations in the human immunodificiency virus-infected patient with gastrointestinal or abdominal symptoms.* (Semin Liver Dis 1992) 12: 142–53

3 Bach N, Theise ND, Schaffner F. *Hepatic histopathology in the acquired immunodeficiency syndrome.* (Semin Liver Dis 1992) 12: 205–12

4 Cappell MS. *Hepatobiliary manifestations of the acquired immune deficiency syndrome.* (Am J Gastroenterol 1991) 86: 1–15

5 Cappell MS, Schwartz MS, Biempica L. *Clinical utility of liver biopsy in patients with serum antibodies to the human immunodeficiency virus.* (Am J Med 1990) 88: 123–9

6 Cello JP. *Acquired immunodeficiency syndrome cholangiopathy: spectrum of disease.* (Am J Med 1989) 86: 539–46

7 Cello JP, Chan MF. *Long-term follow-up of endoscopic retrograde cholangiopancreatography sphincterotomy for patients with acquired immune deficiency syndrome papillary stenosis.* (Am J Med 1995) 99: 600–3

8 Chalasani N, Wilcox CM. *Etiology, evaluation, and outcome of jaundice in patients with*

acquired immunodeficiency syndrome (Hepatology 1996) 23: 728–33

9   Housset C, Pol S, Carnot F, et al. *Interaction between human immunodeficiency virus-1, hepatitis delta virus and hepatitis B virus infections in 260 chronic carriers of hepatitis B virus.* (Hepatology 1992) 15: 578–83

10   Jacobson MA, Cello JP, Sande MA. *Cholestasis and disseminated cytomegalovirus disease in patients with the acquired immunodeficiency* syndrome. (Am J Med 1988) 84: 218–24

11   Margulis SJ, Honig CL, Soave R, et al. *Biliary tract obstruction in the acquired immunodeficiency syndrome.* (Ann Intern Med 1986) 105: 207–10

12   Perkocha LA, Geaghan SM, Yen TS, et al. *Clinical and pathological features of bacillary peliosis hepatis in association with human immunodeficiency virus infection.* (N Engl J Med 1990) 323: 1581–6

13   Reddy KR, Jeffers LJ. *Acquired immunodeficiency syndrome and the liver.* In: Schiff L, Schiff ER, (eds). *Diseases of the Liver.* (Philadelphia: Lippencott, 1991) 1362–72

Granulomatous liver disease

JAY H. LEFKOWITCH, M.D.

▼

Key Points

1 Granulomas consist of activated macrophages (epithelioid macrophages) accompanied by lymphocytes, which infiltrate liver tissue as nodular lesions in reaction to foreign or indigestible antigen or as a hypersensitivity reaction

2 The major causes of hepatic granulomas include infectious agents (especially tuberculosis), sarcoidosis, primary biliary cirrhosis, systemic diseases (e.g., Crohn's disease) and neoplasms (e.g., Hodgkin's lymphoma)

3 An elevated alkaline phosphatase level is the chief abnormality in serum liver function tests

4 The cause of hepatic granulomas may remain unknown in up to 50% of cases

5 The work-up for hepatic granulomas includes a complete history of therapeutic drugs, tests for antimitochondrial antibodies and angiotensin converting enzyme and staining liver specimens with acid-fast and silver stains for mycobacteria and fungi, respectively

▲

1 Pathogenesis of Granulomas

A Definition

1 Granulomas are rounded, 1–2 mm collections of activated macrophages and other immune cells which infiltrate a host of tissues, including the liver, in response to a foreign or indigestible antigen (Fig. 26.1)

2 As examples of cell-mediated immunity, the principal components of granulomas include activated macrophages resembling epithelial cells (epithelioid macrophages), T lymphocytes, and, sometimes, multinucleated giant cells which develop from macrophage fusion

3 Granulomas evolve as a result of the elaboration of secretory products (cytokines) by their constituent cells (interferon gamma and interleukin 2 from T helper lymphocytes), expansion of macrophage and T lymphocyte pools, and specialization of macrophages for antigen digestion (Fig. 26.2).

4 Granulomas ultimately either resolve or undergo fibrosis and/or calcification

B Morphologic types of granulomas

Several types of granulomas are described in liver disease and are based on their histologic features and constituents. These have been reviewed by Ferrell (1990)[1] (see Table 26.1)

C Incidence and location of hepatic granulomas

1 Granulomas are found in 2.4–14.6% of liver biopsies, according to a survey by McCluggage and Sloan (1994),[2] although the figure of 10% is often quoted[3]

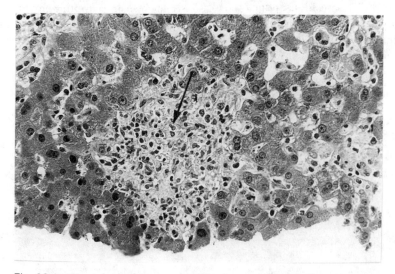

Fig. 26.1   Example of a noncaseating hepatic granuloma, seen here in leishmaniasis. Epithelioid macrophages (arrow) are the main constituents, with small lymphocytes scattered around the periphery (H&E, ×255)

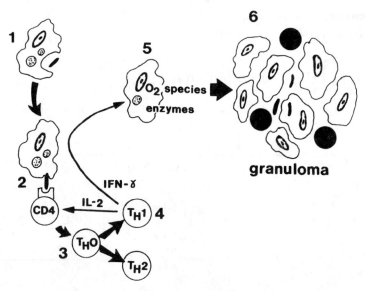

Fig. 26.2   Development of a granuloma (dark rod-shaped structures represent mycobacteria). Step 1: macrophage engulfs mycobacterium. Step 2: macrophage presentation of mycobacterial protein product(s) to a receptor on CD4 lymphocytes. Step 3: CD4 lymphocytes differentiate to precursor T helper lymphocytes ($T_H 0$), later differentiating into $T_H 1$ lymphocytes. Step 4: $T_H 1$ lymphocytes secrete interleukin 2 (IL-2), a clonal expander of CD4 cells, as well as interferon gamma (IFN-γ), which upregulates enzymes and oxygen (O_2) species in macrophages in step 5. Step 6: further recruitment of macrophages and lymphocytes with ongoing digestion of mycobacteria

Type of granuloma	Histologic features	Example(s)
Caseating	Peripheral macrophages ± giant cells; central necrosis	Tuberculosis
Noncaseating	Cluster of macrophages ± giant cells	Sarcoidosis Drugs
Lipogranuloma	Lipid vacuole(s) surrounded by macrophages and lymphocytes	Fatty liver Mineral oil
Fibrin-ring (doughnut granuloma)	Central lipid vacuole or empty space; macrophages and lymphocytes; ring of fibrin	Q fever Allopurinol Hodgkin's lymphoma

(Table 26.1: Types of granuloma)

2   Granulomas are found in any of the following sites, or in combination:[4]

- lobular (sarcoidosis, drugs)
- portal/periportal (sarcoidosis)
- periductal (primary biliary cirrhosis)

- perivenous (mineral oil lipogranulomas)
- peri-/intra-arterial (phenytoin)

2   Causes of Hepatic Granulomas

Etiology is multifactorial, but the major causes and examples are shown in Table 26.2

Etiology	Example(s)

Infectious	Viral:
	    cytomegalovirus
	    infectious mononucleosis
	Bacterial:
	    brucellosis
	    tuberculosis
	Rickettsial:
	    Q fever
	Spirochetal:
	    Treponema pallidum
	Parasitic:
	    schistosomiasis

Primary biliary cirrhosis	More common in early stages
Foreign body	Suture, talc
Systemic disease-related	Sarcoidosis, Crohn's disease
Drug	Allopurinol, diphenylhydantoin, penicillin
Neoplasia	Hodgkin's lymphoma

(Table 26.2: Etiologies of hepatic granulomas)

3   Clinical Features

A   Signs and symptoms

Often include:

- abdominal pain
- weight loss
- fatigue
- chills
- hepatomegaly
- splenomegaly
- lymphadenopathy
- fever of unknown origin (FUO)

B   Liver function tests

1   Liver function test pattern is that of infiltrative disease
   - elevated alkaline phosphatase is typical: 3–10 times normal
   - aminotransferases usually normal or only mildly raised
2   Liver function tests may be normal[5]

C   Other laboratory tests

1   Angiotensin converting enzyme (ACE) is elevated in sarcoidosis, primary biliary cirrhosis, silicosis, and asbestosis[6]
2   Serum globulins elevated in sarcoidosis, berylliosis, and chronic granulomatous disease of childhood[3]
3   Peripheral blood eosinophilia may be present with drug or parasite-related granulomas

4   Specific Causes of Granulomatous Liver Disease

A   Sarcoidosis

1   Sarcoid granulomas preferentially cluster in portal/periportal regions and are associated with hyaline fibrosis (Fig. 26.3)
2   Granulomas are noncaseating, may contain inclusions (asteroid and Schaumann bodies), and can be located within lobular parenchyma as well as in or near portal tracts

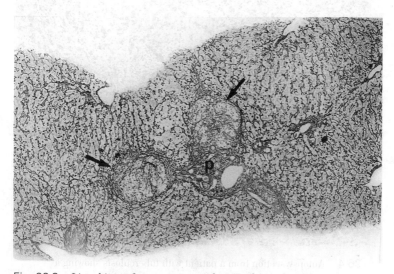

Fig. 26.3   Liver biposy from a patient with sarcoidosis, shown here with reticulin stain to demonstrate tendency of granulomas (arrows) to cluster in and around portal tracts (p). (Reticulin stain, ×68)

3 Other pathologic features may be seen, as described by Devaney et al. (1993)[7]
- chronic intrahepatic cholestasis due to bile duct destruction (originally described by Rudzki et al. 1975)[8]
- bile duct damage resembling primary biliary cirrhosis
- periductal fibrosis resembling primary sclerosing cholangitis
- suppurative cholangitis
- hepatitis, including portal and lobular lymphocyte and plasma cell infiltrates with liver cell necrosis
- cirrhosis occurs, but is rare

B Tuberculosis

1 Caseation is seen in 29% of biopsy specimens and 78% of autopsy specimens in *Mycobacterium tuberculosis* infection[9] (Fig. 26.4)

2 Acid-fast stain is often not positive (see above)[9]

3 Tuberculous granulomas may be found throughout the liver parenchyma

4 Rupture into bile ducts may result in tuberculous cholangitis

C AIDS

1 The frequency of infectious granulomas in the liver in patients with AIDS is sufficiently high as to warrant routine acid-fast and silver staining of all liver specimens from patients with AIDS

2 Granulomas due to *M. avium* complex (MAC) in AIDS characteristically show pale staining epithelioid macrophages containing linear structures (mycobacteria) on

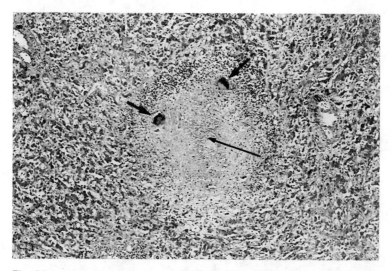

Fig. 26.4 Autopsy section from a patient with tuberculosis showing a caseating granuloma at center. There is central necrosis (thin arrow), a peripheral rim of small lymphocytes, and two multinucleated giant cells (thick arrows). (H&E, ×68)

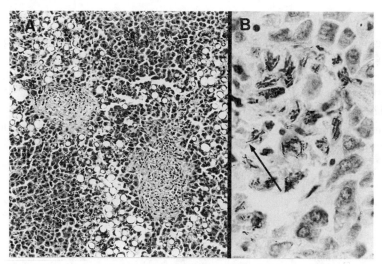

Fig. 26.5   Autopsy liver specimen from a patient with AIDS and *M. avium* complex granulomas. **A**: Several granulomas are seen in the lobule (H&E, ×213. **B**: Ziehl–Neelsen (acid-fast) stain shows abundant darkly stained mycobacteria within the macrophages. Individual mycobacteria can also be discerned (arrow). (Ziehl–Neelsen stain, ×680, oil immersion)

routine hematoxylin and eosin stain, with abundant, packed organisms in each macrophage on acid-fast stain (Fig. 26.5)

3 Cytomegalovirus (CMV) hepatic infection occasionally results in small noncaseating granulomas

4 Other infections identified in hepatic granulomas in AIDS include histoplasmosis, cryptococcosis, and toxoplasmosis

5 Drugs used in AIDS therapy (e.g., sulfonamides, isoniazid) may cause hepatic granulomas[10]

D   Primary biliary cirrhosis (PBC)

1 Granulomas are seen in approximately 25% of patients with PBC[11]

2 Granulomas are usually seen in early stages of PBC, in portal tracts near damaged bile ducts

3 Occasionally granulomas may be found within the lobular parenchyma[12]

E   Lipogranulomas

1 These are due to fatty liver or dietary mineral oil ingestion (laxative or in food products)

2 Consist of fat vacuoles, scattered lymphocytes and macrophages and strands of connective tissue

3 Mineral oil lipogranulomas are seen in portal tracts or near central veins, or both

4 This type of granuloma has no major clinical consequences

F   Fibrin-ring ("doughnut") granulomas

1   These granulomas consist of a central vacuole or empty space, a surrounding pink ring of fibrin, epithelioid macrophages and lymphocytes (Fig. 26.6)

2   Fibrin strands in these granulomas can be stained with the PTAH (phosphotungstic acid–hematoxylin) or Lendrum methods

3   Fibrin-ring granulomas were first described in Q fever

4   These granulomas have been considered as nonspecific by Murphy et al. (1991)[13] because of their diverse causes:

- Q fever
- Hodgkin's lymphoma
- allopurinol
- CMV
- leishmaniasis
- toxoplasmosis
- hepatitis A
- systemic lupus erythematosus
- giant cell arteritis

G   Drug-related granulomas

1   Approximately one-third of hepatic granulomas may be due to drugs, according to McMaster and Hennigar (1981)[14]

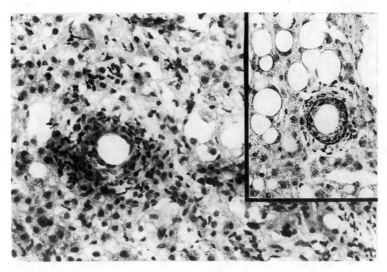

Fig. 26.6   A fibrin-ring ("doughnut") granuloma is seen at left in a patient with AIDS and CMV infection. There is a characteristic central vacuole surrounded by macrophages and lymphocytes with intermixed fibrin. (H&E, ×319) Inset: a dark ring of fibrin has been stained in another fibrin-ring granuloma using the PTAH (phosphotungstic acid–hematoxylin) method. (PTAH stain, ×319)

2 Drug-related granulomas may be found throughout the hepatic parenchyma, may show eosinophils, and may be accompanied by other evidence of drug hepatitis (cholestasis, fat, hepatocyte ballooning, and acidophilic degeneration)

3 The list of causative drugs is extensive[1]

4 Drug-related granulomas usually heal without sequelae[14]

H Miscellaneous granulomatous conditions

1 In children, Collins et al. suggest in a recent study[15] that histoplasmosis is an important etiologic consideration, particularly in endemic geographic regions

2 Idiopathic granulomatous hepatitis, described by Simon & Wolff (1973),[16] is seen in patients with fever of unknown origin and no established cause for the granulomas found on liver biopsy

3 Patients with chronic hepatitis C may have small, noncaseating granulomas in their liver biopsies, but they may be coincidental findings[17]

5 Therapy

1 Should be directed toward the causative agent, when known, including antibiotics for microbial infection, removal of the implicated drug in drug-related cases, and steroids in sarcoidosis

2 In idiopathic granulomatous hepatitis, disease may resolve spontaneously, with steroid treatment, or, in a recent trial of seven patients conducted by Knox et al. (1995),[18] with methotrexate

References

1 Ferrell LD. *Hepatic granulomas: a morphologic approach to diagnosis.* (Surg Pathol 1990) 3: 87–106

2 McCluggage WG, Sloan JM. *Hepatic granulomas in Northern Ireland: a thirteen year review.* (Histopathology 1994) 25: 219–28

3 Ishak KG. *Granulomas of the liver.* In: Ioachim HL, (ed.). *Pathology of Granulomas.* (New York: Raven, 1983) 307–70

4 Denk H, Scheuer PJ, Baptista A, et al. *Guidelines for the diagnosis and interpretation of hepatic granulomas.* (Histopathology 1994) 25: 209–18

5 Cunningham D, Mills PR, Quigley EMM et al. *Hepatic granulomas: experience over a 10-year period in the West of Scotland.* (Q J Med 1982) 51: 162–70

6 Nunez-Gornes JE, Tewksbury DA. *Serum angiotensin-converting-enzyme in Crohn's disease.* (Am J Gastroenterol 1981) 75: 384–5

7 Devaney K, Goodman ZD, Epstein MS, Zimmerman HJ, Ishak KG. *Hepatic sarcoidosis. Clinicopathologic features in 100 patients.* (Am J Surg Pathol 1993) 17: 1272–80

8 Rudzki C, Ishak KG, Zimmerman HJ. *Chronic intrahepatic cholestasis of sarcoidosis.* (Am J Med 1975) 59: 373–87

9 Guckian JC, Perry JE. *Granulomatous hepatitis: an analysis of 63 cases and review of the literature.* (Ann Intern Med 1966) 65: 1081–100

10 Schneiderman DJ, Arenson DM, Cello JP, Margaretten W, Weber TE. *Hepatic disease in patients with the acquired immune deficiency syndrome (AIDS).* (Hepatology 1987) 7: 925–30

11 Portmann BC, MacSween RNM. *Diseases of the intrahepatic bile ducts.* In: MacSween RNM, Anthony PP, Scheur PJ, Burt AD, Portmann BC. *Pathology of the Liver, 3rd Edition.* (Edinburgh: Churchill Livingstone, 1994) 477–512

12 Klatskin G. *Hepatic granulomata: problems in interpretation.* (Mount Sinai J Med 1977) 44: 798–812

13 Murphy E, Griffiths MR, Hunter JA, Burt AD. *Fibrin-ring granulomas: a non-specific reaction to liver injury?* (Histopathology 1991) 19: 91–3

14 McMaster KR, Kennigar GR. *Drug-induced granulomatous hepatitis.* (Lab Invest 1981) 44: 61–73

15 Collins MH, Jiang B, Croffie JM, Chong SKF, Lee C-H. *Hepatic granulomas in children. A clinicopathologic analysis of 23 cases including polymerase chain reaction for Histoplasma.* (Am J Surg Pathol 1996) 20: 332–8

16 Simon HB, Wolff SM. *Granulomatous hepatitis and fever of unknown origin: a study of 13 patients.* (Medicine 1973) 52: 1–21

17 Emile JF, Sebagh M, Féray C, David F, Reynès M. *The presence of epithelioid granulomas in hepatitis C virus-related cirrhosis.* (Hum Pathol 1993) 24: 1095–7

18 Knox TA, Kaplan MM, Gelfand JA, Wolff SM. *Methotrexate treatment of idiopathic granulomatous hepatitis.* (Ann Intern Med 1995) 122: 595–5

Hepatic tumors

ADRIAN M. DI BISCEGLIE, M.D., F.A.C.P.

Key Points

1 Hemangioma of the liver is found in up to 1% of the normal population and is rarely of clinical consequence

2 Other benign tumors of the liver are rare, including hepatic adenoma. Hepatic adenoma usually requires surgical resection because of the risks of rupture and the development of malignancy

3 In the presence of cirrhosis, hepatocellular carcinoma (HCC) accounts for approximately 75% of all liver tumors. The most important risk factors for development of HCC are cirrhosis and chronic hepatitis B virus (HBV), and hepatitis C virus (HCV) infection

4 Although surgical resection or liver transplantation offers the best chance of cure in HCC, few patients are suitable for surgery

5 Cholangiocarcinoma (CCC) is not usually associated with cirrhosis. It has a poor prognosis. CCC of the central type is often associated with primary sclerosing cholangitis

1 Benign Tumors of the Liver

A Hepatocellular adenoma

- this is a benign proliferation of hepatocytes.[1] It is a rare tumor which occurs largely in females. Its incidence has increased in the last few decades, probably related to introduction and increased use of oral contraceptives
- etiologic factors include hormones (estrogen, particularly in the form of oral contraceptives) and glycogen storage diseases
- patients typically present with pain or discomfort in the right upper quadrant, although occasional tumors are found incidentally. Adenomas may rupture, resulting in hemoperitoneum
- adenomas are usually single but may be multiple; rarely more than five lesions. Size is variable but typically greater than 5 cm in diameter at diagnosis; sometimes massive
- liver histology shows benign hepatocytes organized in cords, but with no portal triads
- the presence of a mass in the liver may be confirmed by computed tomography (CT) or ultrasound. Technetium (^{99m}Tc) radioisotope scan may show a defect within the liver. Diagnosis must be confirmed by liver biopsy
- treatment includes discontinuing the use of estrogens. Surgical resection is usually advisable, to obtain tissue to confirm the diagnosis and because of the risk of rupture. Liver transplantation should be considered for adenoma found in association with type I glycogen storage disease because of the high risk of malignant transformation

B Tumor-like lesions of hepatocytes

1. **Focal nodular hyperplasia (FNH)** represents an abnormal proliferation of hepatocytes around an abnormal hepatic artery. The artery is usually embedded in a characteristic central stellate scar[2]
   - usually clinically silent. Typically found incidentally, often at the time of abdominal surgery for some other reason
   - in comparison to adenoma, FNH tends to be smaller, is less likely to be multiple, and carries little risk of rupture
   - hepatic arteriogram may suggest the diagnosis if a tumor can be found surrounding a large hepatic artery. The diagnosis may be difficult to make on needle biopsy. Excisional biopsy may be required and is usually curative

2. **Nodular regenerative hyperplasia (NRH)** is characterized by the diffuse formation of nodules comprised of hepatocytes throughout the liver.[3] This is similar to cirrhosis except that these nodules do not have a surrounding rim of fibrosis
   - often associated with identifiable systemic diseases such as autoimmune disorders, rheumatoid arthritis (including Felty's syndrome), and myeloproliferative disorders
   - pathogenesis is unknown but often appears to be related to obliterative venopathy involving portal vein branches
   - the incidence of NRH increases with age and is most commonly found among patients older than age 60

- NRH is often complicated by the development of presinusoidal portal hypertension. Patients may present with splenomegaly and hypersplenism or bleeding esophageal varices
- no specific therapy is available, but patients may require portal decompression to prevent rebleeding from varices. Generally, patients with NRH tolerate variceal bleeding better than those with cirrhosis, presumably because they have relatively well-preserved hepatic synthetic function

3 **Adenomatous hyperplasia (macroregenerative nodule)**

- term used for regenerative nodules of hepatocytes greater than 1 cm in diameter found in association with cirrhosis or, rarely, in submassive hepatic necrosis
- in the context of cirrhosis, adenomatous hyperplasia is suspected as being the site of development of hepatocellular carcinoma[4]
- no specific therapy is needed. In patients with cirrhosis, the presence of adenomatous hyperplasia should signal the need for intensive screening for development of HCC

4 **Partial nodular transformation**

- a rare condition characterized by the presence of nodules of hepatocytes located in the perihilar region and associated with portal hypertension

C   Hemangioma

- hemangiomas of the liver are relatively common, identified in at least 1% of autopsies
- comprised of an endothelial lining on a thin fibrous stroma making up cavernous, blood-filled spaces
- usually small. If larger than 10 cm in diameter, they are referred to as "giant" hemangiomas
- usually asymptomatic, but if large enough may cause some discomfort. Occasionally, thrombosis within a giant hemangioma may result in consumption of platelets and thrombocytopenia. They have been documented to increase in size over time, but have no potential to become malignant[5]
- usually do not require any specific therapy. May be resected if they are associated with significant symptoms. Percutaneous needle biopsy should be avoided because of the risk of bleeding

D   Benign hepatic tumors of cholangiocellular origin

1 **Bile duct adenoma**

- typically solitary subcapsular tumors, composed of a proliferation of small, round, normal-appearing bile ducts with cuboidal epithelium

2 **Biliary microhamartoma (von Meyenberg complex)**

- part of the spectrum of adult polycystic disease but may also be found together with polycystic disease (adult or childhood type), congenital hepatic fibrosis, or Caroli's disease (see Chs 23 and 28)

3 **Biliary cystadenoma**

- multiloculated cyst, analogous to mucinous cystadenomas of the pancreas. Has significant potential for development of malignancy

4 Biliary papillomatosis

- a rare condition consisting of multicentric biliary tract adenomatous polypoid tumors which sometimes develop into adenocarcinoma (similar to polyposis coli)

E Benign hepatic tumors of mesenchymal origin

These are listed in Table 27.1.

Tumor	Comment
Mesenchymal hamartoma	Childhood tumor with a mixture of elements (bile ducts, vessels, and mesenchyma)
Infantile hemangioendothelioma	Tumor of infancy; may be complicated by thrombocytopenia, high-output heart failure; may require resection or ablation
Lipoma	Collection of lipocytes; distinct from focal fatty change within hepatocytes
Lymphangiomatosis	Masses of prominent, dilated lymphatic channels
Angiomyolipoma	Has distinct radiographic appearance
Leiomyoma	Extremely rare
Fibroma	Solid fibrous tumor of the liver
Inflammatory pseudotumor	Chronic inflammation and fibrosis; may cause pain, fever
Myxoma	Myxomatous connective tissue

(Table 27.1: Benign hepatic tumors of mesenchymal origin[1])

2 Malignant Tumors of the Liver

A Metastatic disease

- The liver is a common site of metastasis. **Metastases are by far the most common form of hepatic malignancy**. The most frequent sites of origin for hepatic metastases are lung, breast, and gastrointestinal and genitourinary tracts

B Hepatocellular carcinoma (HCC)

HCC is a malignant tumor of hepatocytes.

1 Epidemiology

- one of the most common malignancies worldwide. The incidence varies considerably around the world. High incidence areas include China, Taiwan, Korea, and other parts of Southeast Asia as well as most of sub-Saharan Africa, where the incidence may be as high as 120 per 100,000 population per year. Areas of intermediate incidence include Japan and the countries of southern Europe (particularly Italy and Spain) and the Middle East. Regions of low incidence include northern countries of Europe, the USA and South America, where the rate may be as low as 5 per 100,000 population[6]

- much more common in males than females
- median age at diagnosis is in the fourth decade of life in high incidence areas; it presents at a somewhat older age in other regions

2 Etiologic factors

- one of the few human cancers for which an etiologic factor can be identified in most cases. Known and possible risk factors are shown in Table 27.2

Known risk factors

Cirrhosis (of any cause)
Chronic hepatitis B
Chronic hepatitis C
Metabolic disorders:
    Alpha-1 antitrypsin deficiency
    Hemochromatosis
    Hereditary tyrosinemia
Carcinogens:
    Aflatoxin
    Thorotrast[a]

Possible risk factors

Alcohol (in absence of cirrhosis)
Smoking
Anabolic or estrogenic steroids

[a]Thorotrast is a contrast agent that was used for arteriography for a period after the Second World War. It contains thorium dioxide, a low level emitter of alpha particles, which is retained in Kupffer's cells

(Table 27.2: Known and possible etiologic factors in HCC)

- **chronic HBV infection is the most common etiologic factor in high incidence areas, while chronic HCV infection plays the most important role in areas of intermediate incidence**
  - the precise mechanism by which chronic viral hepatitis results in HCC is not known but may be through the presence of liver regeneration and injury characteristic in cirrhosis
  - in addition, HBV is a DNA virus whose genome may become integrated within the genome of hepatocytes, thereby possibly interfering with actions of oncogenes or tumor suppressor genes. The X protein of HBV is known to be a transactivator; i.e., it is capable of turning on DNA, again thereby possibly activating growth factors or oncogenes
  - HCV is an RNA virus which does not become integrated. Almost all cases of HCV-related HCC are associated with cirrhosis.[7] Alcohol may be an important co-factor with HCV in development of HCC
- certain metabolic diseases may be associated with development of HCC, but virtually always in the presence of cirrhosis (e.g. hemochromatosis, alpha-1

antitrypsin deficiency). Hereditary tyrosinemia is a rare inborn error of metabolism associated with severe liver injury and regeneration with development of HCC in childhood

- environmental toxins play a role in pathogenesis of HCC in some parts of the world. Aflatoxin is formed as a product of fungal comtamination of stored foodstuffs. It is directly hepatocarcinogenic in rodents and, in humans, interacts with HBV to cause HCC

3 Clinical features

- abdominal pain or discomfort and weight loss are the most frequent presenting symptoms. HCC may occasionally rupture, presenting as an acute abdomen. Increasingly, many patients diagnosed with HCC are asymptomatic, the tumor being detected incidentally or during screening of at-risk subjects
- HCC may also be associated with a variety of nonmetastatic manifestations including hypoglycemia, erythrocytosis, hypercholesterolemia, and feminization

4 Diagnosis

- use of imaging studies is critical. Ultrasound and CT are the mainstays of diagnosis. Small HCCs are seen on ultrasound as hypodense lesions. Tumors as small as 0.5–1 cm may be detected by ultrasound. While CT scanning may not have the sensitivity of ultrasound, it is useful in confirming the presence of tumors greater than 2–3 cm in diameter and assessing the extent of tumor within the abdomen
- arteriography may be useful, as HCC is a highly vascular tumor, but its use is usually limited to preparation for surgery
- lipiodol CT involves injection of the oily contrast medium at the time of arteriography, followed by CT scanning 10–14 days later. HCC tissue typically retains the Lipiodol, making even small tumors readily detectable. Lipiodol CT scanning is recommended when HCC is suspected (e.g., raised serum alpha fetoprotein (AFP) level) but cannot be confirmed
- radioisotope scans are of little value in diagnosing HCC, and seems to have little advantage over CT scanning
- serological markers are useful. Approximately 80–90% of patients with HCC have elevated serum levels of AFP, although the majority with small tumors (<5 cm in diameter) have normal or minimally elevated levels
  - AFP values may be raised in patients with chronic viral hepatitis and cirrhosis without HCC, causing diagnostic confusion
  - abnormal forms of prothrombin (des-gamma carboxyprothrombin, DCP) may be manufactured by HCC, and elevated levels may be found in the serum of patients with HCC. Unfortunately, tests for this abnormal protein are not widely available
- liver biopsy is often required to confirm a diagnosis of HCC. There is a slightly increased risk of bleeding after liver biopsy in HCC and other forms of malignancy. Biopsy of the nontumorous portion of the liver is advisable to evaluate the severity of underlying liver disease
- fibrolamellar HCC is a variant of HCC usually not associated with cirrhosis or any of the other known etiologic factors. It has a better prognosis than other forms of HCC

5 Management

- the outlook is generally poor. In Africa and Asia, HCC is associated with mean survival times measured in weeks to months. Only surgery provides any chance of cure, but most patients are not amenable to surgery at the time of diagnosis because of the extent of the tumor or severity of underlying liver disease
- Table 27.3 offers a scheme for management of patients with HCC

Extent of tumor	Cirrhosis	Treatment options
Confined to liver	No	Large-scale resection
Confined to liver	Yes, but compensated	Segmentectomy. Consider ethanol injection or transplantation
Confined to liver	Decompensated	Liver transplantation
Spread beyond liver	Yes or no	Chemotherapy, chemoembolization

(Table 27.3: Scheme for managing patients with HCC based on extent of tumor and underlying liver disease)

- **surgery**: large resections of the liver are possible if cirrhosis is not present. However, only small resections, segmentectomy, or enucleation may be possible in a cirrhotic liver. Rate of recurrence or development of new tumors is very high
- **liver transplantation** appears to result in a survival rate similar to that of resection in cirrhotics but with a lower recurrence rate. Unfortunately, liver transplantation is only available in a small number of countries, and limitations on the supply of donor organs prevent widespread applicability of this form of treatment
- **injection of absolute ethanol** is associated with tumor necrosis and is easy to perform, with few side effects. Its use should be confined to tumors less than 4 cm in diameter and may be most useful in patients with decompensated cirrhosis who will not tolerate surgery or in cases of recurrent HCC after surgery
- **chemoembolization**, in which chemotherapeutic agents are injected into the hepatic artery, which is subsequently occluded, is effective in shrinking tumors but confers little beneficial effect on survival. It can perhaps best be used as a prelude to surgical resection or liver transplantation
- **systemic chemotherapy** has not been as effective as regional chemotherapy (administered via the hepatic artery). Cis-platinum, in combination with other agents, appears to be the most effective agent

6 Prevention

- HCC is potentially a preventable form of cancer. The widespread use of HBV vaccination is expected to decrease the rate of HCC in many of the high-incidence areas of the world. HCV infection may also decline due to increased awareness and screening of donated blood. At present, an effective vaccine is not available against HCV, although it has been suggested that interferon therapy may decrease the risk of HCV-related HCC

C Cholangiocarcinoma (CCC) (see also Ch. 33)

1 Epidemiology
- much less common than HCC and distributed more evenly around the world. CCC tends to occur at an older age than HCC and has a more even sex distribution[8]

2 Etiologic factors (see Table 27.4)

Primary sclerosing cholangitis and IBD[a]
Clonorchis sinensis infestation
Intrahepatic lithiasis, cholelithiasis
Congenital anomalies (e.g., Caroli's disease)
Exposure to Thorotrast
Benign cysts, von Meyenberg complex

[a]IBD, inflammatory bowel disease   (Table 27.4: Risk factors for cholangiocarcinoma)

3 Clinical features
- divided into two basic types – peripheral and central. They tend to have differing pathogenesis and clinical manifestations
- the peripheral type is rarely associated with cirrhosis or sclerosing cholangitis. Often presents with abdominal pain and weight loss
- the central type arises in major bile ducts and is often associated with chronic inflammation in bile ducts, as in primary sclerosing cholangitis.[9] Klatskin tumor arises in the bifurcation of the common bile duct. Central type CCC often presents with obstructive jaundice

4 Diagnosis
- can be made by needle biopsy of peripheral type tumor. Central tumors may be more difficult to diagnose, as they arise in the presence of primary sclerosing cholangitis so that the bile ducts are already anatomically abnormal. Cytological examination of material obtained by endoscopic brushing may make the diagnosis. Elevated serum levels of CA 19–9 may also be useful in establishing the diagnosis of malignancy
- cholangiocarcinoma may be difficult to distinguish from other forms of adenocarcinoma, and the diagnosis may only be confirmed at laparotomy or autopsy. Mixed HCC/CCC may be found in association with cirrhosis

5 Management
- peripheral CCC are sometimes amenable to resection. Central CCC may also be resected particularly when very small, as with Klatskin tumors
- with both types, however, the recurrence rate after resection is high and survival is poor
- liver transplantation is currently not a viable therapeutic alternative because of the high recurrence rate

D   Pediatric tumors of the liver (see also Ch. 23)

- some tumors of the liver occur specifically in children.[10] Furthermore, they often occur at a specific age, as shown in Figure 27.1
- hepatoblastoma is a malignant tumor of hepatocytes that occurs in children under age 2 years. It is not associated with cirrhosis. Virtually all patients have elevated serum AFP levels. Hepatoblastoma is considered potentially curable with a combination of surgery and chemotherapy
- although HCC is typically a disease of adults, it has been recorded in children as young as 4 years of age in association with HBV infection

E   Other tumors of the liver

1 Epithelioid hemangioendothelioma

- a tumor of vascular endothelial origin with low-grade malignant behavior. It may arise in organs other than the liver, particularly the lung
- it has a distinctive histologic appearance with dense fibrotic masses containing pleiomorphic epithelioid cells. Vascular invasion is a prominent feature. Malignant cells in this tumor stain positively for factor VIII
- it must be distinguished histologically from angiosarcoma and cholangiocarcinoma
- approximately one third of patients have metastases. Nonetheless, examples of prolonged survival with this tumor have been documented

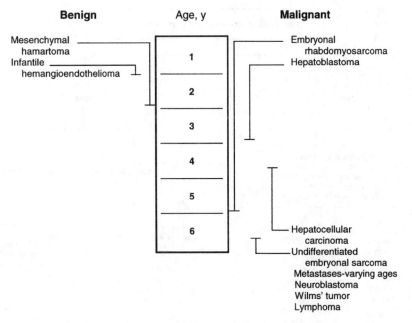

Fig. 27.1   Tumors which occur in chidren at specific ages (From Di Bisceglie AM, Buetow PC. Tumors of the liver. In: Feldman M, (ed.). *Gastroenterology and Hepatology: The Comprehensive Visual Reference*, Vol. 1: *The Liver* (Philadelphia: Current Medicine, 1996))

- this tumor is important to recognize because of its malignant behavior and because it is potentially curable with extensive resection or even liver transplantation

2 Primary hepatic lymphoma

- although secondary involvement of the liver by lymphoma is common, primary lymphoma may also arise in the liver
- these tumors are often of B cell origin and occur at increased frequency in patients with HIV infection and AIDS
- responds poorly to chemotherapy and is associated with a poor prognosis

3 Angiosarcoma

- a high-grade malignancy of blood vessels arising within the liver
- predisposing factors are exposure to vinyl chloride monomers or the intravenous contrast agent Thorotrast
- it grows rapidly, responds poorly to radiation or chemotherapy, and has a poor prognosis

3 Diagnostic Approach to Liver Masses or Tumors

The approach is very different depending on whether the patient has cirrhosis or not. A scheme for evaluating the noncirrhotic patient is shown in Figure 27.2 and the patient with cirrhosis in Figure 27.3

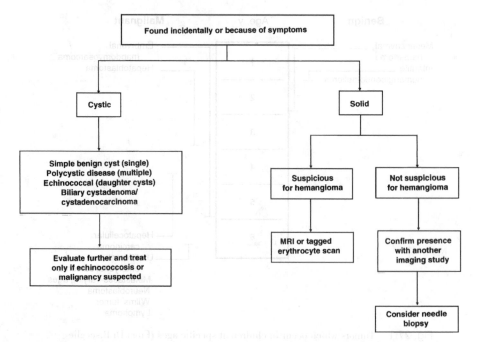

Fig. 27.2   Evaluation in the noncirrhotic patient (From Di Bisceglie AM, Buetow PC. Tumors of the liver. In: Feldman M, (ed.). *Gastroenterology and Hepatology: The Comprehensive Visual Reference*, Vol. 1: The Liver (Philadelphia: Current Medicine, 1996))

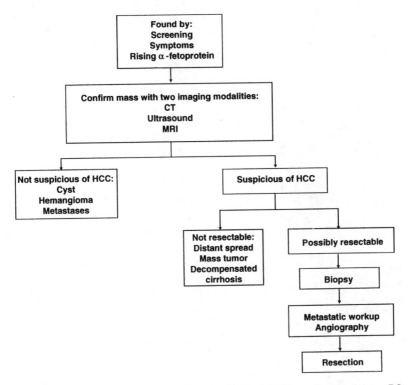

Fig. 27.3   Evaluation in the patient with cirrhosis (From Di Bisceglie AM, Buetow PC. Tumors of the liver. In: Feldman M, (ed.). *Gastroenterology and Hepatology: The Comprehensive Visual Reference*, Vol. 1: *The Liver* (Philadelphia: Current Medicine, 1996))

References

1   Okuda K, Ishak KG, (eds). *Neoplasms of the Liver*. (Berlin: Springer-Verlag, 1987)

2   Kerlin P, Davis GL, McGill DB, Weiland LH, Adson MA, Sheedy PF. *Hepatic adenoma and focal nodular hyperplasia: clinical, pathologic, and radiologic features.* (Gastroenterology 1983) 84: 994–1002

3   Stromeyer FW, Ishak KG. *Nodular transformation (nodular "regenerative" hyperplasia) of the liver.* (Hum Pathol 1981) 12: 60–71

4   Furuya K, Nakamura M, Yamamoto Y, Togei K, Otsuka H. *Macroregenerative nodule of the liver.* (Cancer 1988) 61: 99–105

5   Trastek VF, Van Heerden JA, Sheedy PF, Adson MA. *Cavernous hemangioma of the liver: resect or observe?* (Am J Surg 1983) 145: 153

6   Di Bisceglie AM, Rustgi VK, Hoofnagle JH, Dusheiko GM, Lotze MT. *Hepatocellular carcinoma.* (Ann Intern Med 1988) 108: 390–401

7   Colombo M, Rumi MG, Donato MF, et al. *Hepatitis C antibody in patients with chronic liver disease and hepatocellular carcinoma.* (Dig Dis Sci 1991) 36: 1130–3

8   Altaee MY, Johnson PJ, Farrant JM, Williams R. *Etiologic and clinical characteristics of peripheral and hilar cholangiocarcinoma.* (Cancer 1991) 68: 2051–5

9   Rosen CB, Nagorney DM, Wiesner RH, Coffey RJ, LaRusso NF. *Cholangiocarcinoma complicating primary sclerosing cholangitis.* (Ann Surg 1991) 213: 21–5

10 Boechat MI, Kangarloo H, Gilsanz V. *Hepatic masses in children.* (Semin Roentgenol 1988) 23: 185–193

CHAPTER 28

Hepatic abscesses and cysts

HELEN M. AYLES, M.B.B.S., M.R.C.P.
KEVIN M. De COCK, M.D., F.R.C.P., D.T.M.&H.

▼

Key Points

1 Hepatic abscesses are pyogenic or amebic in nature. Lack of consideration of the diagnosis and failure to perform simple imaging may delay the diagnosis and thus increase the associated morbidity and mortality of these conditions

2 A history of dysentery or diarrhea is present in only 20% of patients with an amebic liver abscess. Diagnosis is by hepatic imaging and serology, and treatment is with antibiotics.

3 Pyogenic liver abscess is a life-threatening condition, resulting from infected blood or bile. Diagnosis is by hepatic imaging, blood cultures, and aspiration of the abscess, and treatment is with antibiotics and drainage.

4 Worldwide, the most common infective cause of hepatic cysts is *Echinococcus granulosus* – hydatid disease; other causes include simple cysts, tumors, congenital biliary diseases and polycystic disease.

▲

1 Amebic Liver Abscess

A Overview

1 480 million people worldwide are infected with *Entameba histolytica*

2 Amebic infection may be asymptomatic or may present as dysentery, hepatic amebic abscess, or other (rarer) manifestations

3 The diagnosis and management of hepatic amebic abscess have been revolutionized by advances in imaging and interventional radiology

4 Treatment now relies almost entirely on drug therapy

B Parasitology

1 Amebic liver abscess is caused by the protozoan *Entameba histolytica*. The reservoir of infection is man (Fig. 28.1)

2 The infective form is the cyst (12 μm in diameter), which is ingested. Excystation occurs in the small intestine. The trophozoite (10–60 μm) infects the colon and may cause inflammation and dysentery. Amebae spread to the liver via the portal circulation

3 The cyst is able to survive outside the body for weeks or months, whereas the trophozoite degenerates in minutes

4 Amebae may be pathogenic or nonpathogenic. The nonpathogenic form has now been reclassified as *E. dispar*. Pathogenic species can be differentiated from non-pathogenic by:

  • zymodene analysis; 22 distinct isoenzyme patterns on electrophoresis (zymodenes) have been isolated

  • RNA and DNA probes

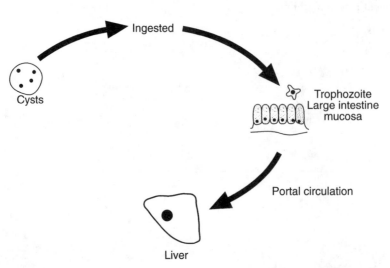

Fig. 28.1 Life cycle of *Entameba histolytica*

C Epidemiology

1 Infection with *E. histolytica* affects 10% of the world's population, causing 40,000 deaths per year

2 The prevalence of infection varies from <1% in industrialized countries to 50–80% in some tropical regions. One study in the Gambia found a 100% infection rate

3 Spread is by fecal–oral route and is increased by:
   - poor sanitation
   - contamination of food by flies
   - unhygienic food handling
   - unclean water
   - the use of human feces as fertilizer

4 High-risk groups include:
   - lower socioeconomic status in endemic areas
   - immigrants from endemic areas
   - institutionalized populations, e.g., inpatients of mental hospitals
   - male homosexuals
   - travelers

D Pathogenesis

1 In the liver, *E. histolytica* lyses the host's tissue with proteolytic enzymes contained in cytoplasmic vacuoles

2 The hepatic lesion is a well-demarcated "abscess" consisting of necrotic liver, usually affecting the right lobe. The initial host response to the ameba is neutrophil migration, but the ameba can also lyse neutrophils, thus releasing their enzymes and assisting in the process of tissue destruction

3 The abscess contains acellular debris; amebic trophozoites are found only at the periphery of the lesion, where they can invade further

4 Host factors contributing to the severity of disease:
   - age (children>adults)
   - pregnancy
   - malnutrition and alcoholism
   - corticosteroid use
   - malignancy

   - HIV/AIDS does not appear to increase the incidence or severity of disease

E Clinical features

   - amebic liver abscess presents with amebic colitis in only 10% of cases

- 20% of cases have a past history of diarrhea or dysentery
- the parasite can be isolated from the stool in about 50% of cases

1 **History: socioeconomic and demographic**
- emigrant from or resident in endemic area
- traveler to endemic area
- men > women (3–10×)
- young adults > children or elderly

2 **Symptoms**
- fever, rigors, night sweats
- nausea, anorexia, malaise
- right-upper-quadrant abdominal discomfort
- weight loss
- chest symptoms: dry cough, pleuritic pain
- diaphragmatic irritation: shoulder tip pain, hiccups

3 **Physical examination**
- patient appears unwell
- fever
- tender hepatomegaly
- chest signs: dull right base (usually from raised hemidiaphragm); crackles at right base; pleural rub

- jaundice, peritonitis or pericardial rub are rare and are **poor prognostic signs**

F Diagnosis

1 **Laboratory findings** (see Table 28.1)

Laboratory finding	% of patients
Leukocytosis	80
Anemia	>50
↑ Serum alkaline phosphatase	80
↑ Serum aminotransferases	Poor prognostic sign
↑ Erythrocyte sedimentation rate (ESR)	Common
Proteinuria	Common

(Table 28.1: Laboratory findings in amebic liver abscess)

- ↑ bilirubin is **uncommon**

2 Diagnostic imaging

  a Chest x-ray (CXR):

- elevation of right hemidiaphragm
- blunting of right costophrenic angle
- atelectasis

  b ultrasonography:

- round or oval single lesion (sometimes multiple)
- lack of significant wall echoes, so that there is an abrupt transition from abscess to normal liver
- hypoechoeic appearance compared with normal liver; diffuse echoes throughout abscess
- peripheral location, close to liver capsule
- distal enhancement

  c Computed tomography (CT)

- well-defined lesions, round or oval, mostly single (sometimes multiple)
- low density compared with surrounding liver tissue
- nonhomogeneous internal structure

  d Magnetic resonance imaging (MRI):

- the abscess has low signal intensity on T1-weighted image and high signal intensity on T2 images

  e Radioisotope scanning:

- indicates filling defect; has been largely superseded by other imaging modalities

3 Serological tests

The mainstay of diagnosis of invasive amebiasis. Standard techniques include the indirect hemagglutination assay (IHA) with a sensitivity of 90–100%. A combination of the immunofluorescent antibody test (IFAT) and the cellulose acetate precipitin test (CAP) gives 100% correlation between positive results and invasive amebic disease. These tests are positive in *all* forms of invasive amebic disease (including dysentery). Positive IFAT tests may persist for more than 6 months after treatment, and IHA titers may be raised for more than 2 years. The CAP may become negative within 1 week of the start of effective treatment; therefore, combined tests are necessary for accurate diagnosis. A latex agglutination test for extraluminal amebiasis has also been developed and may prove useful in rapid screening for invasive disease[1]

- positive serological tests are found in 95–100% of patients with amebic liver abscess

4 Aspiration of abscess (only when diagnosis is uncertain or for imminent rupture)

- yellow to dark brown "anchovy sauce"
- odorless
- "pus" consists mainly of acellular debris; most amebae are found in abscess wall

G Complications

1 Rupture of abscess into:

   a chest, causing:

- hepatobronchial fistula (± expectoration of "anchovy" pus)
- lung abscess
- amebic empyema

   b pericardium, causing:

- heart failure
- pericarditis
- cardiac tamponade (often fatal; may be followed by constrictive pericarditis)

   c peritoneum, causing:

- peritonitis
- ascites

2 Secondary infection is usually iatrogenic following aspiration

3 Other (rare):

- fulminant hepatic failure
- hemobilia
- inferior vena cava obstruction
- Budd–Chiari syndrome
- hematogenous spread causing cerebral abscess

4 Factors predisposing to complications:[2]

- Age > 40
- concomitant corticosteroid use
- multiple abscesses
- large abscess > 10 cm in diameter
- ESR and C-reactive protein reported to be very high in those patients who presented with or went on to develop systemic complications

2 Pyogenic Liver Abscess

A Overview

1 Pyogenic liver abscess is a life-threatening condition

2 Incidence varies but accounts for approximately 1 in 7000 hospital admissions in the USA

3 Delays in or failure to recognize this condition result in high morbidity and mortality

4 Often associated with other medical conditions

B Microbiology

Cultures of blood and/or abscess contents are positive in most cases

- *Escherichia coli* is the most commonly reported single bacterium
- microaerophilic organisms, particularly *Streptococcus milleri*, are increasingly common causes but need careful culture for isolation
- anaerobic organisms account for one third to one half of abscesses
- lesions may be polymicrobial
- unusual organisms include: *Salmonella, Haemophilus,* and *Yersinia* spp. Tuberculosis, actinomycosis, and melioidosis also occur especially in patients with defective immunity, e.g., AIDS, post-transplant

C   Epidemiology

- pyogenic liver abscess is rare; 1 case per 7000 hospital admissions
- originally reported as common in young patients following intra-abdominal sepsis; now more common in middle-aged and older people

- liver abscess often occurs in patients with predisposing medical conditions:
  - malignancy
  - previous abdominal surgery or endoscopic procedure
  - diabetes
  - Crohn's disease
  - diverticulitis
  - following trauma

- equal sex distribution
- no geographic or racial differences

D   Pathogenesis

1 Pyogenic infection is carried to the liver via the blood or bile. Frequently no infective source is found; however, when one can be identified, common sources include:
   - cholangitis, secondary to biliary stricture, stones, or endoscopic intervention
   - intra-abdominal sepsis, e.g., diverticulitis, peritonitis
   - generalized septicemia
   - trauma, including liver biopsy or surgery
   - secondary infection of a pre-existing liver cyst or rarely of an amebic abscess
2 The right lobe of the liver is the most frequently involved
3 Abscesses may be single or multiple; those caused by hematogenous spread are frequently multiple
4 The abscess contains polymorphonuclear neutrophils and necrotic liver cells surrounded by a fibrous capsule

E   Clinical features

1   History
- Table 28.2 shows the results from a recent retrospective study of 142 patients[3]

Symptom	% of patients
Fever	79
Chills	60
Abdominal pain	55
Nausea	37
Vomiting	30
Weight loss	28
Pleuritic chest pain	21
Cough or dyspnea	21
Diarrhea	20
Abdominal distention	5

(Table 28.2: Symptoms found in a recent retrospective study of 142 patients with pyogenic liver abscess[3])

2 Physical examination
- patient appears unwell
- fever
- anemia in long-standing cases
- finger clubbing (rare)
- jaundice (in 33%)
- tender hepatomegaly

In their study, Seeto and Rockey found the "classic triad" of fever, jaundice, and tender hepatomegaly in less than 10% of patients

F   Diagnosis
1 Laboratory findings (see Table 28.3)

2 Diagnostic imaging
a CXR abnormal in 50%:
- elevation of right hemidiaphragm
- blunting of right costophrenic angle
- atelectasis

If gas-forming organism is cause of abscess, fluid levels may be seen below the diaphragm

b ultrasonography
- round, oval, or elliptoid lesion
- margin irregular
- hypoechoic with variable internal echoes

Laboratory finding	% of patients
Anemia	50
Leukocytosis	75
↑ ESR	100
↑ Serum bilirubin	Common
↑ Serum alkaline phosphatase	Common
↑ Serum aminotransferases	Common
↓ Serum albumin	Poor prognostic sign
↑ Prothrombin time	Common

(Table 28.3: Laboratory findings in pyogenic liver abscess)

  c CT scanning
- highly sensitive; detects up to 94% of lesions. Lesions show reduced attenuation and may enhance with contrast

  d MRI
- more sensitive at detecting small lesions than CT.[4] The lesions have low signal intensity on T1-weighted images and very high signal intensity on T2-images. Lesions enhance with gadolinium

  e Radioisotope
- gallium is avidly taken up by abscesses

3 Microbiology
- blood cultures should be taken prior to antibiotic use
- positive blood cultures occur in 50–100%
- aspiration of abscess increases yield of positive microbiological diagnosis
- in polymicrobial abscesses, all the causative organisms may not be present in the blood

G   Complications
- septicemia
- metastatic abscess
- septic shock
- adult respiratory distress syndrome
- renal failure
- rupture

3   Hepatic Cysts

A   Overview
- causes of cystic lesions in the liver are diverse

1 Congenital

- polycystic disease
  - Infantile polycystic disease is a rare autosomal recessive condition which results in cyst formation in liver and kidneys. Hepatomegaly is often present at birth but renal damage is usually the cause of reduced lifespan. Adult polycystic disease is an autosomal dominant condition predominantly affecting the kidneys but with hepatic cysts in 33% of patients
- choledochal cysts (see also Ch. 33)
  - Many disease entities present with cystic dilatation of the biliary tree. Caroli's disease is one of these conditions in which non-obstructive dilatation of intrahepatic bile ducts occurs.

2 Acquired

- benign tumors e.g., hamartomas
- simple cysts
- infective: most common is hydatid disease (caused by *Echinococcus granulosus*)

4 Hydatid Disease of the Liver

A Overview

- hydatid cystic disease has a worldwide distribution and is endemic in many sheep- and cattle-rearing regions of the world
- hydatid disease is a chronic and potentially dangerous condition which is often overlooked as a cause of abdominal pain and hepatic disease

B Parasitology

Hydatid cystic disease is caused by *Echinococcus granulosus*

- *E. granulosus* is a 3–6 mm tapeworm
- carnivorous host, usually a dog, becomes infected by eating the viscera of infected sheep containing hydatid cysts
- scolices from the cysts adhere to the small intestine of the dog and develop into the tapeworm
- each worm produces up to 500 ova in the host bowel
- infected dogs excrete *Echinococcus* eggs in feces. Eggs are viable in the environment for several weeks
- eggs are ingested by humans, either from contamination of soil and foodstuffs or from the dogs's coat, and hatch in the intestine to form oncospheres which invade tissue to enter the portal circulation
- each oncosphere matures into a vesicle and subsequently a cyst, the metacestode
- cysts can form in any organ, most commonly the liver (50–70%). Cysts consist of a germinal layer that buds asexually to form daughter cysts, which contain protoscolices, the infective form to be ingested by the definitive host (Fig. 28.2)

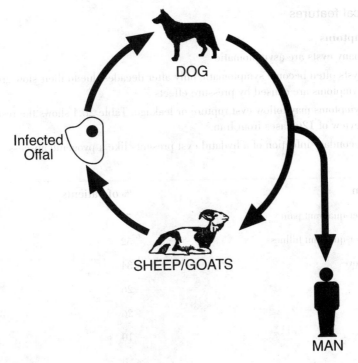

Fig. 28.2   Life cycle of *Echinococcus granulosus*

C Epidemiology

Infections with *E. granulosus* occur worldwide. The scale of human disease is not fully documented but rural communities face a significant health problem from infection.

Areas with a documented high prevalence of disease include sheep farming areas:

- Mediterranean countries
- northern Kenya (Turkana district)
- areas of South America
- Wales
- New Zealand

D Pathogenesis

1 Spread of oncospheres is via the bloodstream, usually the portal circulation, and results in hepatic disease in 50–70% of cases. Other sites of disease:

- lung (20–30%)
- bone (<10%)
- brain
- heart

2 Cysts enlarge slowly and cause tissue damage directly or by compromising blood supply. The parasite causes a host response to form a collagenous capsule around the germinal layer. This capsule may calcify. There is often no host inflammatory response

E   Clinical features

1 Symptoms

- many cysts are asymptomatic
- cysts often become symptomatic only after decades due to their slow growth. Symptoms are caused by pressure effects
- symptoms may follow cyst rupture or leakage. Table 28.4 shows the results from a review of 126 cases from Iran.[5]
- secondary infection of a hydatid cyst presents like a pyogenic abscess

Symptom	% of patients
Right-upper-quadrant pain	74
Right-upper-quadrant fullness	52
Both of above	34
Fever	26
Jaundice	26
Anorexia	10
Weight loss	8
Vomiting	7
Pruritus	5

Duration of symptoms was >12 months in 39% of cases

(Table 28.4: Symptoms found in a review of 126 cases from Iran[5])

2 Physical examination

- tender mass
- chest signs, especially at right base
- fever
- jaundice (rare)

F   Diagnosis

1 Laboratory findings

- ↑ serum alkaline phosphatase
- ↑ peripheral eosinophils (>7%) in 30% of patients, usually indicating leakage or rupture of cyst
- ↑ serum bilirubin is uncommon

2 Diagnostic imaging

a CXR

- elevation of right hemidiaphragm
- cysts may be seen in the lung
- calcification of hepatic cyst may be seen below the diaphragm

b ultrasonography
- cysts may be anechoic
- typically round
- septate or daughter cysts often seen
- separation of germinal membrane: "water-lily sign"
- collapsed cysts may be seen
- calcification of wall
- hydatid "sand"

c CT
- germinal layer seen clearly
- daughter cysts readily visualized
- identifies extrahepatic disease
- lesion is of low attenuation: 3–30 Hounsfield units

d MRI
- characteristic low-intensity rim 4–5 mm thick, best seen on T2-weighted images
- lesion center is nonhomogeneous
- lesion is hypointense on T1 images, hyperintense on T2

3 Serological tests

IHA and enzyme-linked immunosorbent assay (ELISA) are 75–94% sensitive. Specificity is lower, necessitating confirmatory test, e.g., molecular biological methods or immunoblotting

4 Molecular biological tests

Polymerase chain reaction (PCR)-derived probes allow diagnosis and species differentiation

G Complications

1 Leakage or rupture of cyst (sometimes iatrogenic from aspiration of undiagnosed hydatid) may cause
- allergic reaction, including anaphylaxis (may be fatal)
- dissemination of disease
- cholangitis if cyst ruptures into biliary tree
- hemoptysis and secondary infection if bronchial rupture

2 Secondary infection of cyst behaves like pyogenic abscess

5 Diagnostic Approach and Therapy of Hepatic Abscesses and Cysts

- The patient's history may give important clues to the diagnosis (See Table 28.5)
- **A geographic history is of vital importance**
- Figure 28.3 summarizes our suggested diagnostic approach

Parameter	Amebic liver abscess	Pyogenic liver abscess	Hydatid cyst
Age	Any, mostly younger	Any; mostly older	Any; mostly older
Sex	Male > female	Equal	Equal
Epidemiologic features	Residence or travel in endemic area; poverty, poor hygiene	None; occasional association with helminth infection	Residence in endemic area; farm animal exposure
Associated medical conditions	Rare	Common (e.g., surgery; biliary tract disease; diverticulitis)	Rare
Significant jaundice	Rare	Common	Rare
Multiple abscesses (cysts)	Infrequent	Common	Septate and daughter cysts
Liver tests	Mildly abnormal	More markedly abnormal	Mildly abnormal
Amebic serology	Positive	Negative	Negative
Hydatid serology	Negative	Negative	Positive
Blood cultures	Negative; positive result indicates superinfection	Frequently positive	Negative; positive results indicates superinfection
Abscess contents	Thick fluid; variable color, yellow-brown, odorless	Pus; creamy yellow, foul smelling	Aspiration not recommended; thin fluid
Effectiveness of medical therapy	Almost always	Often	Usually in combination with surgery
Surgery required	Almost never	Sometimes	Usually

(Table 28.5: Comparison of amebic and pyogenic liver abscess and hydatid cyst)

A Serological tests and blood cultures

- serological tests are positive in cases of amebic liver abscess in 90–100% of cases
- serological tests are positive in 75–95% of cases of hepatic hydatid disease
- blood cultures should be performed on all febrile patients; amebic and hydatid cavities may become superinfected
- blood cultures alone are positive in at least 50% of patients with pyogenic liver abscesses

B Imaging

- **imaging confirms the diagnosis of a cyst or abscess**
- **ultrasonography is the investigation of choice** due to good sensitivity, low radiation dose, low cost, and ready availability

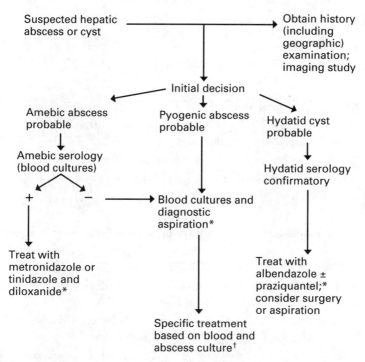

Fig. 28.3 Suggested diagnostic approach to suspected hepatic abscess or cyst.
*Indications for diagnostic aspiration: diagnosis of pyogenic abscess, critically ill
patient requiring urgent diagnosis, failure of intial therapy. †Presumptive treatment is
usually begun on the basis of clinical suspicion pending test results

- CT may provide further information, especially in pyogenic liver abscess (contrast
  enhanced) and in hydatid disease
- MRI may be more sensitive than ultrasonography and CT in detecting small
  lesions
- radioisotope scanning has largely been superseded by other imaging modalities

C Aspiration

- required for diagnosis and treatment in cases of suspected pyogenic abscess
- gives microbiological diagnosis in >80% of patients with pyogenic abscess.
  Combined aspiration and blood culture gives positive identification of causative
  organism in >85% of cases
- may be performed in cases of suspected amebic abscess if the abscess is large
  and rupture is imminent or if the diagnosis is in doubt. Usually aspiration is *not*
  required for diagnosis
- in general aspiration should *not* be carried out in cases of suspected hydatid
  disease. It may be indicated if the cyst appears to be infected. In the event of
  aspiration of a hydatid cyst, efforts should be taken to prevent leakage of cyst
  contents, which has potentially serious sequelae. Aspiration should be carried out
  by experienced operators under imaging guidance through as thick a rim of
  normal liver as possible

D   Management and prognosis

1 Amebic liver abscess

a Treatment is usually with drugs alone

> • Commonly used regimens:
>   – metronidazole 750 mg t.i.d. for 5–10 days (pediatric 35–50 mg/kg/day in three divided doses for 5 days)
>   – tinidazole 2 g/day for 3 days (pediatric 50–60 mg/kg daily for 5 days)
>   – chloroquine 1 g loading dose for 1–2 days, then 500 mg/day for 20 days (pediatric 10 mg/kg base)

- **luminal amebicides must always be used following these regimens**:
  - diloxanide furoate 500 mg t.i.d. for 10 days (pediatric 20 mg/kg/day in three divided doses)
  - diiodohydroxyquin 650 mg tid for 20 days (pediatric 30–40 mg/kg/day in three divided doses; maximum 2 g/day)
  - paromomycin sulfate 25–35 mg/kg/day in three divided doses for 5–10 days (pediatric 25–35 mg/kg/day in three divided doses)
  - patients with suspected amebic abscess should be started on therapy while awaiting serological confirmation. Response will usually be rapid, with defervescence occurring in 48–72 hours
- critically ill patients or those who do not respond to initial drug therapy may require radiologically guided fine-needle aspiration to exclude a pyogenic abscess
- complications such as rupture of the abscess may be managed medically but often require percutaneous drainage. Surgical drainage is seldom required

b Prognosis

- amebic liver abscess is an eminently treatable condition
- in uncomplicated disease mortality is < 1%
- delay in diagnosis may result in abscess rupture, causing higher mortality:
  - rupture into chest or peritoneum – 20% mortality rate
  - rupture into pericardium – 32–100% mortality rate

2 Pyogenic liver abscsess

a Treatment

- in the past, standard treatment involved open surgical drainage of the abscess in combination with broad-spectrum antibiotics. Recent studies have shown equally good results with either percutaneous drainage or aspiration in combination with antibiotics.[3] Some patients can be managed medically without surgery or aspiration
- it is usually possible to combine diagnostic and therapeutic aspiration in these patients
- complications of drainage include hemorrhage, perforation of a viscus, infection from the drain, and catheter displacement

- antibiotic therapy should include coverage against Gram-negative organisms as well as microaerophilic and anaerobic organisms
- antibiotic therapy will usually be intravenous initially. The duration of intravenous antibiotic therapy and decision to and change to oral medication are governed by the individual clinical response. We recommend a total duration of antibiotics of 2–3 weeks
- surgical intervention may be required if the patient fails to respond rapidly to therapy; a flexible approach must be adopted

b Prognosis
- untreated pyogenic liver abscess has a mortality rate approaching 100%
- recent series report mortality rates of the order of 10–30% depending on the underlying cause of the abscess and associated medical conditions

3 Hydatid cyst

- surgery remains the mainstay of treatment
- drug therapy should be employed first to minimize the risk of dissemination

a Drug therapy includes:
- albendazole 10–14 mg/kg/day for 3 months initially (may continue for 1 year)[6]
- mebendazole 30–70 mg/kg/day for 3 months (may require up to 200 mg/kg/day)
  - these benzimidazole agents act on the germinal layer
- praziquantel (40 mg/kg/day for 14 days) has recently been used as a protoscolicide and, as such, has an important role preoperatively
- until recently, standard surgical intervention involved radical cystopericystectomy with or without cyst evacuation and local instillation of scolicidal agents. Increasingly radiologically guided cyst aspiration and instillation of scolicides is being used with good results[7,8]
- the scolicidal agents used include:
  - 0.5% silver nitrate
  - 15–20% hypertonic saline
  - 80% ethanol
  - 0.5% cetrimide
- complications of surgery are high: 57% in a series of 59 patients (H. Ayles, unpublished data) – dissemination of infection, secondary infection, fistula formation, and complications from seepage of scolicidal agents into the biliary tree (causing a sclerosing cholangitis-like syndrome)
- hydatid cysts presenting with secondary infection carry a high mortality and should be treated as pyogenic abscesses; however, aspiration of hydatid cysts is more hazardous

b Prognosis
- hydatid cysts may remain asymptomatic throughout a person's life
- cyst rupture or infection is associated with considerable mortality

References

1 Cummins AJ, Moody AH, Lalloo K, Chiodini PL. *Rapid latex agglutination test for extraluminal amoebiasis.* (J Clin Pathol 1994) 47: 647–8

2   Ahmed M, McAdam KP, Sturm AW, Hussain R. *Systemic manifestations of invasive amebiasis.* (Clin Infec Dis 1992) 15: 974–82

3   Seeto RK, Rockey DC. *Pyogenic liver abscess, changes in etiology, management and outcome.* (Medicine 1996) 75: 99–113

4   Mendez RJ et al. Hepatic abscesses: MR Imaging findings. (Radiology 1994) 190(2): 431–6

5   Bastani B, Dehdashti F. *Hepatic hydatid disease in Iran, with review of the literature.* (Mt Sinai J Med 1995) 62: 62–9

6   Horton RJ. *Chemotherapy of Echinococcus infection in man with albendazole.* (Trans Royal Soc Trop Med Hygiene 1989) 83: 97–102

7   Morris DL. *Echinococcus of the liver.* (Gut 1994) 35: 1517–18

8   Akhan O, Ozmen MN, Dincer A, Savek I, Gocmen A. *Liver hydatid disease: long-term results of percutaneous treatment.* (Radiology 1996) 198: 259–64

9   Barnes PF, DeCock KM, Reynolds TN, Ralls PW. *A Comparison of amebic and pyogenic abscess of the liver.* (Medicine 1987) 66: 472–83

10   DeCock KM, Reynolds TB. *Amebic and pyogenic liver abscess.* In: Schiff L, Schiff E, (eds). *Diseases of the Liver.* (Philadelphia: Lippincott, 1993)

11   Gottstein B, Reichen J. *Echinococcosis/hydatidosis.* In: Cook GC, (ed.). *Manson's Tropical Diseases.* (London: Saunders, 1996)

CHAPTER 29

Other infections involving the liver

RAYMOND T. CHUNG, M.D.

▼

Key Points

1 Primary bacterial infection of the liver is rare. However, a number of systemic infections can cause hepatic derangements, ranging from mild liver function test abnormalities to frank jaundice and, rarely, hepatic failure

2 A variety of spirochetal, protozoal, helminthic, and fungal organisms can involve the liver

3 Schistosomiasis, capillariasis, toxocariasis, and strongyloidosis evoke strong host inflammatory responses and fibrosis that contribute to their hepatic manifestations

4 Leishmaniasis and malaria lead to disease primarily through disruption of reticuloendothelial system function.

5 The liver flukes and ascariasis cause cholangitis, biliary hyperplasia, and, in some cases, cholangiocarcinoma

6 Echinococcosis causes significant cystic disease and should be considered in the differential diagnosis of hepatic cysts

7 Advances in drug therapy have rendered nearly all nonviral infections of the liver readily treatable; therefore, prompt diagnosis in the appropriate clinical context is essential

▲

1 Bacterial Infections Involving the Liver

A *Legionella pneumophila*

- pneumonia is the predominant clinical manifestation; abnormalities of liver function tests occur frequently, usually without jaundice
- involvement of the liver in systemic infection does not influence clinical outcome
- liver histology is characterized by microvesicular steatosis and focal necrosis; occasional organisms can be seen

B *Staphylococcus aureus* (toxic shock syndrome)

- a multisystem disease caused by the staphylococcal toxic shock syndrome toxin (TSST-1). Originally described in association with tampon use, the syndrome is now more frequently a complication of *Staphylococcus aureus* infections in surgical wounds
- typical findings include a scarletiniform rash, mucosal hyperemia, hypotension, vomiting, and diarrhea. Hepatic involvement is nearly always present, can be extensive, and is marked by deep jaundice and high serum aminotransferase levels
- histologic findings in the liver include microabscesses and granulomas
- the diagnosis is confirmed by culture of toxigenic *S. aureus* from the wound, blood, or other body sites

C *Clostridium perfringens*

- associated with myonecrosis, or gas gangrene; usually a mixed anaerobic infection that results in rapid development of local wound pain, abdominal pain, and diarrhea
- jaundice may develop in up to 20% of patients with gas gangrene and is predominantly a consequence of massive intravascular hemolysis caused by the bacterial exotoxin
- liver involvement may include abscess formation and gas in the portal vein. The presence of hepatic involvement does not appear to affect mortality

D *Listeria monocytogenes*

- hepatic invasion in adult human infection is uncommon
- in nearly all cases with overt hepatic involvement, underlying chronic liver disease is present
- hepatic histologic findings include multiple abscesses and granulomas

E *Gonococcal infection*

- half of patients with disseminated gonococcal infection have abnormal liver function tests – elevated serum alkaline phosphatase levels in nearly all of these and elevated aspartate aminotransferase (AST) levels in 30–40%. Jaundice is uncommon
- the most common complication of gonococcal infection is the Fitz-Hugh–Curtis

syndrome, a perihepatitis believed to result from direct spread of infection from the pelvis

- clinically, patients describe the sudden onset of sharp right-upper-quadrant pain, which may be confused with acute cholecystitis or pleurisy. Most patients have a history of pelvic inflammatory disease
- the syndrome is distinguished from gonococcal bacteremia by a characteristic friction rub over the liver and negative blood cultures. The diagnosis is made by vaginal cultures for gonococcus
- the overall prognosis of disseminated gonorrhea appears to be unaffected by the presence of perihepatitis

F   *Pseudomonas pseudomallei* (melioidosis)

- *Pseudomonas pseudomallei* is a soil- and water-borne Gram-negative bacterium that causes the syndrome of melioidosis, found predominantly in Southeast Asia. The clinical spectrum ranges from asymptomatic infection to fulminant septicemia
- severe disease involves the lung, gastrointestinal tract, and liver, where histologic changes include inflammatory infiltrates, multiple microabscesses, and focal necrosis. Organisms can be visualized with Giemsa staining of liver biopsy specimens. Granulomas may be seen with chronic disease

G   *Shigella* and *salmonella*

- cholestatic hepatitis can be attributable to enteric infection with *Shigella*
- histologic findings in the liver include portal and periportal polymorphonuclear infiltration and necrosis with cholestasis
- typhoid fever caused by *Salmonella typhi* frequently involves the liver. Some patients may present with an acute hepatitis-like picture, characterized by fever and tender hepatomegaly
- mild elevations of serum bilirubin (in up to 16% of cases) and aminotransferase (in 50%) levels are common in typhoid fever and should not prompt a search for a separate diagnosis
- cholecystitis and liver abscess may also complicate hepatic involvement with *S. typhi*
- hepatic damage appears to be mediated by bacterial endotoxin, which may produce focal necrosis, a periportal mononuclear infiltrate, and Kupffer's cell hyperplasia. These changes resemble those seen in Gram-negative sepsis.
- characteristic typhoid nodules can be scattered throughout the liver and are the result of profound hypertrophy and proliferation of Kupffer's cells
- the hepatic abnormalities do not appear to affect outcome and typically remit after 2–3 weeks of treatment

H   *Yersinia enterocolitica*

- presents as ileocolitis in children and terminal ileitis and mesenteric adenitis in adults

- patients with hepatic involvement have underlying comorbidity such as diabetes, cirrhosis, or hemochromatosis. Excess tissue iron, in particular, may be a predisposing factor to infection with *Yersinia* species
- the subacute septicemic form of the disease resembles typhoid fever or malaria. Multiple abscesses are diffusely distributed in the liver and spleen. The mortality rate approaches 50%

I *Coxiella burnetii* (Q fever)

- characterized by relapsing fevers, headache, myalgias, malaise, pneumonitis, and culture-negative endocarditis; the liver is commonly affected. The predominant abnormality is an elevated serum alkaline phosphatase level
- the histologic hallmark in the liver is the fibrin-ring granuloma. The diagnosis is confirmed by serologic testing for complement-fixing antibodies

J Rocky Mountain spotted fever (RMSF)

- while mortality caused by this systemic tick-borne rickettsial illness has decreased considerably as a result of early recognition, there exists a small subset of patients who present with multiorgan manifestations and in whom the mortality rate has remained high. Hepatic involvement is frequent in multiorgan RMSF and reflects severe microbe-induced vasculitis
- the predominant hepatic manifestation in this group of patients is jaundice, which is likely due to a combination of inflammatory bile ductular obstruction and hemolysis

K *Actinomyces israelii* (actinomycosis)

- while cervicofacial infection is the most frequent manifestation of actinomycosis, gastrointestinal involvement is frequent (13 – 60% of cases)
- hepatic involvement (liver abscess) is present in 15% of cases of abdominal actinomycosis and is thought to result from metastatic spread from other abdominal sites. The course is more indolent than with other causes of pyogenic hepatic abscess. Abscesses may be multiple and in both lobes of the liver
- diagnosis is based on aspiration of an abscess cavity and visualization of characteristic "sulfur granules" or a positive anaerobic culture
- most abscesses resolve with prolonged courses of intravenous penicillin or oral tetracycline

L *Bartonella bacilliformis* (bartonellosis)

- endemic to Colombia, Ecuador, and Peru, bartonellosis is an acute febrile illness accompanied by jaundice, hemolysis, hepatosplenomegaly, and lymphadenopathy
- centrilobular necrosis of the liver and splenic infarction may occur. As many as 40% of patients die of sepsis or hemolysis
- prompt treatment with chloramphenicol or tetracycline prevents fatal complications

M   Brucellosis

- may be acquired from infected pigs (*Brucella suis*), cattle (*B. abortus*), goats (*B. melitensis*), or sheep (*B. ovis*) and presents as an acute febrile illness
- hepatic abnormalities are seen in most cases, and jaundice may be present in severe cases. Typically, liver biopsy shows multiple noncaseating hepatic granulomas; less often, there is focal mononuclear infiltration of the portal tracts or lobules
- diagnosis is confirmed by serologic testing using counter-immunoelectrophoresis (CIE) in combination with an animal exposure history

2   Spirochetal Infections of the Liver

A   Leptospirosis

- one of the most common zoonoses in the world, with a wide range of domestic and wild animal reservoirs. Human disease can occur as one of two syndromes – anicteric leptospirosis or Weil's syndrome
- anicteric leptospirosis accounts for more than 90% of cases and is characterized by a biphasic illness
  - the first phase begins abruptly, with viral illness-like symptoms associated with fever, leptospiremia, and characteristic conjunctival suffusion (an important diagnostic clue)
  - the second phase follows a brief period of improvement and is characterized by myalgias, nausea, vomiting, and abdominal tenderness, and in some cases aseptic meningitis. During this phase, a minority of patients have elevated serum aminotransferase and bilirubin levels with hepatomegaly
- Weil's syndrome is a severe icteric form of leptospirosis and constitutes 5–10% of all cases
  - the first phase is often marked by jaundice, which may last for weeks
  - during the second phase, fever may be high, and hepatic and renal manifestations predominate. Jaundice is marked, with serum bilirubin levels approaching 30 mg/dL. Aminotransferase levels usually do not exceed five times the upper limit of normal. Acute tubular necrosis often develops and can lead to renal failure, which may be fatal
- the diagnosis of leptospirosis is made on clinical grounds in conjunction with a positive blood or urine culture in the first and second phases, respectively. Serologic testing may confirm the diagnosis when cultures are unrevealing.
- doxycyline is effective therapy if given within the first several days of illness. Most patients recover without residual organ impairment.

B   Syphilis

1   Secondary syphilis

- liver involvement is characteristic (up to 50% of cases). Syphilitic hepatitis usually presents with nonspecific symptoms. Jaundice, hepatomegaly, and right-upper-quadrant tenderness are less common. Nearly all patients exhibit generalized lymphadenopathy

- biochemical testing generally reveals low-grade elevations of serum aminotransferase and bilirubin levels, with a disproportionate elevation of the serum alkaline phosphatase; isolated elevation of the alkaline phosphatase is common

- histologic examination of the liver in syphilitic hepatitis reveals focal necrosis, especially in the periportal and centrilobular regions. Spirochetes may be demonstrated by silver staining in up to half of patients

2 Tertiary (late) syphilis

- hepatic lesions are common but typically silent. Occasionally, tender hepatomegaly and nodularity may raise the suspicion of metastatic cancer

- the characterisic lesion in tertiary syphilis is the gumma, which can be single or multiple. Syphilitic gummas are necrotic centrally and often surrounded by granulation tissue consisting of a lymphoplasmacytic infiltrate and endarteritis. These inflammatory processes can lead to exuberant deposition of scar tissue

- if hepatic involvement goes unrecognized, hepatocellular dysfunction and complications of portal hypertension can ensue

C Lyme disease

- a multisystem disease caused by the tick-borne spirochete *Borrelia burgdorferi*. Predominant manifestations are dermatologic, cardiac, neurologic, and musculoskeletal. Hepatic involvement has been described in 20% of affected patients and usually manifests as increased serum aminotransferase and lactate dehydrogenase levels

- in early stages of the illness, the spirochetes are thought to disseminate hematogenously from the skin to other organs, including the liver. The clinical picture is suggestive of acute hepatitis and often accompanies erythema chronicum migrans, the sentinel rash

- histologic examination of the liver in Lyme hepatitis reveals hepatocyte ballooning, marked mitotic activity, microvesicular fat, Kupffer's cell hyperplasia, a mixed sinusoidal infiltrate, and intraparenchymal and sinusoidal spirochetes

- the diagnosis is confirmed by serology in a patient with a typical clinical history. Hepatic involvement does not appear to affect overall outcome, which is excellent in primary disease after insitution of appropriate antibiotic treatment with penicillin or a tetracycline

3 Parasitic Diseases that Involve the Liver

A Protozoal infections (see Table 29.1)

1 Amebic liver abscess (see Ch. 28)

2 Malaria

Malaria remains one of the most important public health problems worldwide, infecting about 200 million persons in over 100 countries

Disease (cause)	Endemic areas	Predisposition	Pathophysiology	Manifestations	Diagnosis
Amebiasis (*E. histolytica*) (Ch. 28)	Worldwide, esp. Africa, Asia, Mexico, S. America	Poor sanitation Sexual transmission	Hematogenous spread and tissue invasion, abscess formation	Fever, RUQ pain, peritonitis, elevated right hemidiaphragm	Cysts in stool serology (CIE, IHA) hepatic imaging
Malaria (*Plasmodium falciparum, P. malariae, P. vivax, P. ovale*)	Africa, Asia, S. America	Blood transfusion Intravenous drug use	Sporozoite clearance by hepatocytes; exoerythrocytic replication in liver	Tender hepatomegaly; splenomegaly (HMS), rarely hepatic failure (*P. falciparum*)	Identification of parasite on blood smear
Leishmaniasis (*Leishmania donovani*)	Old World, Central America, S. America	Immunosuppression (AIDS, organ transplant)	Infection of RE cells	Fever, weight loss, hepatosplenomegaly, secondary bacterial infections, gray hyperpigmentation (kala-azar)	Amastigotes seen in spleen, liver or bone marrow biopsy
Toxoplasmosis (*Toxoplasma gondii*)	Worldwide	Intrauterine infection Immunosuppression (AIDS, organ transplant)	Replication in liver leading to inflammation, necrosis	Fever, lymphadenopathy, occ. hepatosplenomegaly, atypical lymphocytosis	Serology (IF, EIA) isolation of organism in tissue

(Table 29.1: Protozoal infections)

CIE, counter-immunoelectrophoresis; IHA, indirect hemagglutination assay; IF, immunofluorescence; EIA, enzyme immunoassay; RE, reticuloendothelial; RUQ, right-upper-quadrant; HMS, hyperreactive malarial splenomegaly

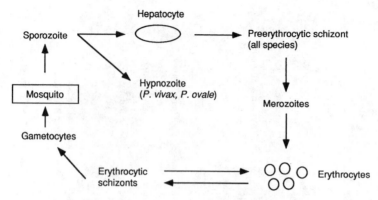

Fig. 29.1   Schematic life cycle of *Plasmodium* species

a   Malarial life cycle (see Fig. 29.1)
  - the liver is affected during two stages of the malarial life cycle, the pre-erythrocytic phase and the erythrocytic phase, which coincides with clinical illness
  - malarial sporozoites injected by an infected mosquito circulate to the liver, enter hepatocytes, and mature to schizonts. When the schizont ruptures, merozoites are released into the bloodstream and enter erythrocytes. The four major species of *Plasmodium* responsible for malaria differ with respect to the number of merozoites released and the maturation times
  - infection by *P. falciparum* and *P. malariae* is not associated with a residual liver stage after release of merozoites, whereas infection by *P. vivax* and *P. ovale* is associated with a persistent exoerythrocytic stage, the hypnozoite, which persists in the liver and can divide and mature into schizont forms
  - the extent of hepatic injury varies with the malarial species (most severe with *P. falciparum*) and the severity of infection. Unconjugated hyperbilirubinemia is most commonly seen as a result of hemolysis, but occasional hepatocyte dysfunction can be seen, leading to conjugated hyperbilirubinemia as well. Moderate elevations of serum aminotransferase and 5′-nucleotidase levels are less common
  - reversible reductions of portal venous blood flow during the acute phase of falciparum malaria may be a consequence of micro-occlusion of portal venous branches by parasitized erythrocytes

b   Histopathology
  - in an acute attack of falciparum malaria, large quantities of malarial pigment (the result of hemoglobin degradation by the parasite) accumulate in Kupffer's cells, which hypertrophy and phagocytose erythrocytes
  - histologic examination of liver biopsies demonstrates Kupffer's cell hyperplasia with pigment deposition and a mononuclear infiltrate. All abnormalities reverse with successful treatment

c   Clinical presentation
  - only the erythrocytic stage of malaria is associated with clinical illness. Symptoms develop 30–60 days after exposure to an infected mosquito and include hectic fever, malaise, anorexia, nausea, vomiting, diarrhea, and

myalgias. Jaundice caused by hemolysis is common in adults, especially in heavy infection with *Plasmodium falciparum*

- hepatic failure is generally seen only in association with concomitant viral hepatitis or with severe *P. falciparum* infection. Tender hepatomegaly with splenomegaly is common. Cytopenias are common in acute infection
- the differential diagnosis includes hepatotropic and nonhepatotropic viral hepatitis, gastroenteritis, amebic liver abscess, yellow fever, typhoid, tuberculosis, and brucellosis

d Diagnosis
- definitive diagnosis of acute malaria rests on clinical history, physical examination, and identification of parasites on peripheral "thick" blood smears. Because the number of parasites in the blood may be small, repeated smear examinations should be performed when the index of suspicion is high
- serologic assays are less useful for acute infection than for chronic infection

e Treatment

- treatment of acute malaria depends on the species of parasite and the pattern of chloroquine resistance for falciparum infection. In general, chloroquine is effective for *P. malariae*, *P. vivax*, *P. ovale* and *P. falciparum* in areas endemic for chloroquine-sensitive species. Resistant falciparum infections can be treated with meflaquine alone or quinine and tetracycline, doxycycline, or pyrimethamine–sulfadoxine (Fansidar)
- for *P. vivax* and *P. ovale* infections, treatment with primaquine (in persons without glucose 6-phosphate dehydrogenase (G6PD) deficiency) is indicated to eliminate the exoerythrocytic hypnozoites in the liver

f Hyperreactive malarial splenomegaly (tropical splenomegaly syndrome)
- repeated exposure to malaria may lead to an aberrant immunologic response with overproduction of B lymphocytes, malarial antibody, increased levels of circulating immune complexes, dense hepatic sinusoidal lymphocytosis, massive splenomegaly, markedly elevated antimalarial antibody levels, and high serum IgM levels
- severe anemia due to hypersplenism, especially in women of childbearing age, can result; variceal bleeding is uncommon
- treatment consists of lifelong antimalarial therapy and supportive care of anemia

3 Leishmaniasis

Visceral leishmaniasis is caused by parasites of the *Leishmania donovani* complex and is endemic in the Mediterranean, the Middle East, Asia, Africa, and Latin America

a Life cycle
- intracellular stage of the parasite (amastigote) is ingested by the sandfly and becomes a flagellated promastigote. Following injection into the human host,

promastigotes are phagocytosed by macrophages in the reticuloendothelial system, where they multiply

b Histopathology

- organisms found in mononuclear phagocytes of the liver and spleen, bone marrow and lymph nodes. Kupffer's cells containing amastigotes proliferate. Occasionally parasite-bearing cells aggregate within noncaseating granulomas
- hepatocyte necrosis is mild compared with that seen with cutaneous leishmaniasis. Healing is accompanied by fibrous deposition, and occasionally the liver looks cirrhotic; however, complications of cirrhosis are rare

c Clinical presentation

- visceral infection begins with a papular or ulcerative skin lesion at the site of the sandfly bite (as with the cutaneous form of the disease). Following an incubation period of 2–6 months, intermittent fevers, weight loss, diarrhea (of bacillary, amebic, or leishmanial origin), and progressive painful hepatosplenomegaly develop, often accompanied by pancytopenia and a polyclonal hypergammaglobulinemia
- secondary bacterial infections resulting from infiltration and suppression of reticuloendothelial cell function include pneumonia, pneumococcal infection, and tuberculosis, and are important causes of mortality
- physical findings include hepatomegaly, often massive splenomegaly, jaundice or ascites in severe disease, generalized lymphadenopathy, and muscle wasting. Cutaneous gray hyperpigmentation, which prompted the name kala-azar ("black fever"), is characteristically seen in India. Oral and nasopharyngeal nodules due to granuloma formation can be seen

d Diagnosis

- based on history, physical examination, and demonstration of tissue amastigotes
- the highest yield comes from aspiration of the spleen; parasites may be seen in 90% of cases. Liver biopsy is nearly as sensitive and carries less risk. Bone marrow aspiration has an 80% yield (higher in individuals with the acquired immunodeficiency syndrome (AIDS), who harbor extremely high levels of amastigote). Lymph node aspiration has a 60% sensitivity
- serologic testing can be used to support a presumptive diagnosis of visceral leishmaniasis. The leishmanin skin test (Montenegro test) is unhelpful in acute visceral disease

e Treatment

- no specific measures are necessary to treat hepatic involvement. Treatment of secondary bacterial infections is essential, and specific antileishmanial chemotherapy should be initiated promptly
- **pentavalent antimonial compounds are the drugs of choice for all forms of leishmaniasis**. Sodium stibogluconate (Pentostam) is available through the Centers for Disease Control (CDC) for treatment of infections in USA. Interferon gamma or allopurinol have been used in combination with antimonials in cases refractory to antimonials alone. Alternative agents include amphotericin B, paromomycin, and pentamidine

- treatment with antimonials should be administered for at least 4 weeks. However, patients with AIDS and leishmaniasis often fail to respond or relapse following treatment with conventional regimens

4 Toxoplasmosis

Infection caused by *Toxoplasma gondii* is found worldwide. In the USA, serologic surveys suggest that 20–40% of the population has been exposed to *T. gondii*. Toxoplasmosis is a congenitally transmitted disease as well as an opportunistic cause of cerebral mass lesions complicating AIDS

a Life cycle

Oocysts of *T. gondii* in soil, water, or contaminated meat are ingested and mature in the intestinal tract of humans to become sporozoites, which penetrate the intestinal mucosa, become tachyzoites, and circulate systemically, invading a wide array of cell types. Hepatic involvement has been observed in severe, disseminated infection

b Clinical presentation

- acquired toxoplasmosis can present as a mononucleosis-like illness with fever, chills, headache, and lymphadenopathy. Uncommonly, hepatomegaly, splenomegaly, and minimal elevations of serum aminotransferase levels are present
- infections of immunocompromised hosts can result in pneumonia, myocarditis, encephalitis, and, uncommonly, hepatitis
- toxoplasmosis can produce atypical lymphocytosis, an otherwise unusual feature of parasitic disease

c Diagnosis

- best made by detecting specific IgM or IgG antibody using indirect immunofluorescence or an enzyme immunoassay, both highly specific

d Treatment

- antibiotic therapy (pyrimethamine for 4 weeks and sulfadiazine for 4–6 weeks, with leucovorin to minimize hematologic toxicity) should be administered to immunocompetent individuals with severely symptomatic infection and immunocompromised or pregnant patients with acute uncomplicated infection

B Helminthic infections nematodes (see Table 29.2)

1 Ascariasis

Ascaris lumbricoides is estimated to infect about 1 billion persons worldwide, especially in areas of lower socioeconomic standing

a Life cycle

- humans are infected by ingesting embryonated eggs, usually in raw vegetables. The eggs hatch in the small intestine, and the larvae penetrate the mucosa, enter the portal circulation, and reach the liver, pulmonary artery, and lungs. The larvae grow in the alveolar spaces, are regurgitated and swallowed, and

Disease (cause)	Endemic areas	Predisposition	Pathophysiology	Manifestations	Diagnosis
Ascariasis (*Ascaris lumbricoides*)	Tropical climates	Ingestion of raw vegetables	Larval migration to liver Adult invasion of bile ducts	Abdominal pain, fever, jaundice biliary obstruction, perioval granulomas	Ova or adult in stool or contrast study
Toxocariasis (*Toxocara cani, T. cati*)	Worldwide	Exposure to dogs or cats, esp. children <5 years	Larval migration in liver (visceral l. migrans)	Granuloma formation with eosinophilia	Larvae in tissue serology (EIA)
Hepatic capillariasis (*Capillaria hepatica*)	Worldwide	Exposure to rodents	Larval migration to liver Inflammatory reaction to eggs	Acute, subacute hepatitis, tender hepatomegaly, occ. splenomegaly, eosinophilia	Adult worms or eggs in liver biopsy
Strongyloidiasis (*Strongyloides stercoralis*)	Asia, Africa, S. America, S. Europe, USA	Immunosuppression (AIDS, chemotherapy, organ transplant)	Larval penetration from intestine to liver	Hepatomegaly, occ. jaundice, larvae in portal tract or lobule	Larvae in stool or duodenal aspirate
Trichinosis (*Trichinella spiralis*)	Temperate climates	Ingestion of undercooked meat	Hematogenous dissemination to liver	Occ. jaundice, biliary obstruction, larvae in hepatic sinusoids	History, eosinophilia, fever, muscle biopsy

(Table 29.2: Helminthic infections – nematodes)

become mature adults in the intestine 2–3 months after ingestion, whereupon the cycle repeats itself

b Clinical presentation

- most infected persons are asymptomatic or minimally symptomatic during larval migration. Symptoms are generally proportionate to the worm burden
- cough, fever, dyspnea, wheezing, and substernal chest discomfort have been reported in the first 2 weeks of infection, as has hepatomegaly, as the larvae pass through the liver
- chronic infection is more frequently characterized by episodic epigastric or periumbilical pain. If the worm burden is particularly heavy, small bowel obstruction, intussusception, volvulus, or perforation, and appendicitis may occur
- fragments of disintegrating worms within the biliary tree can serve as a nidus for biliary calculus formation. Pre-existing disease of the biliary tree or pancreatic duct can predispose to worm migration into the bile ducts, resulting in obstructive jaundice, cholangitis, or intrahepatic abscesses

c Diagnosis

- in the absence of a history of worm passage or regurgitation, the diagnosis is made definitively by identification of characteristic eggs in stool specimens. Larvae have also been identified in sputum and gastric washings as well as liver and lung biopsies
- patients with biliary or pancreatic symptoms can be evaluated by ultrasonography or endoscopic retrograde cholangiopancreatography (ERCP), which may identify the organism. ERCP offers the added potential of extracting the worm

d Treatment

- infected persons may be treated with: (1) a single dose of mebendazole 500 mg; (2) mebendazole 100 mg twice daily for 3 days; (3) pyrantel pamoate 10 mg/kg up to a maximum of 1 g; or (4) piperazine citrate 75 mg/kg for 2 days to a maximum of 4 g for adults or 2 g for children who weigh less than 20 kg

- intestinal or biliary obstruction may require surgical or endoscopic intervention. In the absence of intestinal perforation or ischemia, conservative management may be attempted first for up to 24 hours

2 Toxocariasis

Toxocara canis and *T. cati* infect dogs and cats, respectively; infection occurs worldwide, especially in children

a Life cycle

- infection is acquired when soil or food containing eggs is ingested. The eggs hatch in the small intestine and release larvae that penetrate the intestinal wall, enter the portal circulation, and reach the liver and systemic circulation. The immature worms bore through the vessel walls and migrate through the tissues, leading to secondary inflammatory responses

- When larvae become trapped in tissue, they provoke granuloma formation with a predominance of eosinophils. The liver, brain, and eye are the most frequently affected organs

b Clinical presentation

- most infections are asymptomatic. Two major clinical syndromes are recognized: visceral larva migrans and occult infections associated with nonspecific symptoms that include abdominal pain, anorexia, fever, and wheezing
- visceral larva migrans is seen most commonly in children with a history of pica. Findings include fever, hepatomegaly, urticaria, leukocytosis with a persistent eosinophilia, hypergammaglobulinemia, and elevated blood group isohemagglutinins. Pulmonary, cardiac, neurologic and ocular manifestations are often seen

c Diagnosis

- the diagnosis of visceral toxocariasis should be considered in persons with a history of pica, exposure to dogs or cats, and persistent eosinophilia
- stool studies are not useful for toxocariasis because these organisms do not produce eggs in humans and do not remain in the gastrointestinal tract
- definitive diagnosis is made by identification of the larvae in affected tissues, although blind biopsies are low in yield and not routinely recommended. Liver biopsy may be necessary to differentiate visceral larva migrans from hepatic capillariasis
- a strongly positive enzyme-linked immunosorbent assay (ELISA) result using larval antigens provides supportive evidence of infection

d Treatment

- primarily supportive. Diethylcarbamazine 3 mg/kg three times daily for 21 days or thiabendazole 50 mg/kg/d for 5 days can be given to kill larvae and prevent migration. An alternative, better-tolerated regimen is albendazole 5–10 mg/kg/d for 5 days. Significant pulmonary, cardiac, ophthalmologic, or neurologic manifestations may warrant the use of systemic corticosteroids

3 Hepatic capillariasis

Infection with *C. hepatica* is acquired by ingestion of soil, food, or water contaminated with embryonated eggs

a Life cycle

- larvae released in the cecum penetrate the intestinal mucosa, enter the portal venous circulation, and become lodged in the liver. Later, adult worms disintegrate, releasing eggs into the hepatic parenchyma and producing an intense inflammatory reaction, leading to marked peri-egg fibrosis

b Clinical presentation

- hepatic capillariasis typically presents as acute or subacute hepatitis. Physical examination may show tender hepatomegaly and, occasionally, splenomegaly. Laboratory investigation may reveal prominent eosinophilia, mild elevations of serum aminotransferase, alkaline phosphatase, and bilirubin levels, anemia, and an elevated erythrocyte sedimentation rate

c Diagnosis

- the diagnosis is established by detection of adult worms or eggs in liver biopsy or autopsy specimens. Associated histologic findings in the liver include necrosis, fibrosis, and granuloma formation. Finding *C. hepatica* eggs in stool likely reflects passage of undercooked liver from an infected animal and is not helpful

d Treatment

- treatment of hepatic capillariasis has, in general, been unsuccessful. Anecdotal success has been reported with dithiazanine iodide, sodium stibogluconate, and thiabendazole

4 Strongyloidiasis

Strongyloides stercoralis is prevalent in the tropics and subtropics, southern and eastern Europe, and USA. Infection is usually asymptomatic

a Life cycle

- humans are infected by the filariform larvae, which penetrate intact skin, are carried to the lungs, migrate through the alveoli, and are swallowed to reach the intestine, where maturation ensues
- autoinfection can occur if the rhabditiform larvae transform into infective filariform larvae in the intestine; reinfection occurs by penetration of the bowel wall or perianal skin
- symptomatic infection results from a heavy infectious burden or infection in an immunocompromised patient. In the latter case, a hyperinfection syndrome may result from dissemination of filariform larvae into tissues not ordinarily in the life cycle of the nematode

b Clinical presentation

- as with other helminthic infections, acute infection can lead to a pruritic eruption followed by fever, cough, wheezing, abdominal pain, diarrhea, and eosinophilia
- in immunocompromised patients, the hyperinfection syndrome may be characterized by invasion of any organ, including the liver, lung, and brain
- when the liver is affected, cholestatic liver function abnormalities can be seen. Liver biopsy may show periportal inflammation, eosinophilic granulomatous hepatitis, or both. Larvae may be observed in intrahepatic bile canaliculi, lymphatic vessels, and small branches of the portal vein

c Diagnosis

- based on the identification of larvae in the stool or intestinal biopsy specimens. The presence of an obstructive hepatobiliary picture in a person with established strongyloidiasis suggests the possibility of dissemination

d Treatment

- for acute infection, the drug of choice is albendazole 400 mg/d for 3 days for adults and children over 2 years of age. Retreatment with a second course may be necessary
- following dissemination, treatment options are limited, and mortality rates are

as high as 85%. Hyperinfection syndrome requires longer courses of treatment than primary acute infection

5 Trichinosis

a Life cycle

- humans may be infected with *Trichinella spiralis* by consuming raw or undercooked pork bearing larvae, which are released in the upper gastrointestinal tract, enter the small intestine, penetrate the mucosa, and disseminate through the systemic circulation. Larvae can be found in the myocardium, cerebrospinal fluid, brain, and less commonly, liver and gallbladder. The larvae then re-enter the circulation and finally reach striated muscle, where they become encapsulated

b Clinical presentation

- clinical manifestations occur when the worm burden is high and include diarrhea, fever, myalgias, periorbital edema, and leukocytosis with marked eosinophilia. Rarely, hepatic histology may demonstrate invasion of hepatic sinusoids by larvae. Jaundice may result from biliary obstruction

c Diagnosis

- based on a characteristic history in association with fever and eosinophilia. Serologic studies for antibody to *Trichinella* may not be helpful in the acute phase of infection. Muscle biopsy may help confirm the diagnosis

d Treatment

- consists of corticosteroids to relieve allergic symptoms followed by antihelminthic treatment with mebendazole 200 mg/d for 5 days or albendazole 400 mg/d for 3 days

C Helminthic infections: trematodes (see Table 29.3)

1 Blood flukes: schistosomiasis

Schistosomiasis (bilharziasis) is caused by trematodes of the genus *Schistosoma*. About 200 million persons are infected worldwide. Table 29.4 shows the geographical distribution and clinical diseases caused by individual *Schistosoma* species

a Life cycle

- the infectious cycle is initiated by penetration of the skin by free cercariae in fresh water. Within 24 hours, the cercariae reach the peripheral venules and lymphatics and the pulmonary vessels. They pass through the lungs and reach the liver, where they lodge, develop into adults, and mate

- mated adult worms then migrate to their ultimate destinations in the inferior mesenteric venules (*S. mansoni*), superior mesenteric venules (*S. japonicum*), or the veins around the bladder (*S. hematobium*). These locations correlate with the clinical complications associated with each species. The eggs are deposited in the terminal venules and eventually migrate into the lumen of the involved organ, after which they are excreted in the stool or urine

- eggs remaining in the organ provoke a robust granulomatous response. Excreted eggs hatch immediately in fresh water, liberating early intermediate miracidia, which infect their snail hosts. The miracidia transform into cercariae within the snails and are then released into the water, from which they may again infect humans

Disease (cause)	Endemic areas	Predisposition	Pathophysiology	Manifestations	Diagnosis
Schistosomiasis (*Schistosoma mansoni*, *S. japonicum*)	Asia, Africa, S. America Caribbean	Travelers exposed to fresh water	Fibrogenic host immune response to eggs in portal vein	Acute: eosinophilic infiltrate Chronic: hepatosplenomegaly, presinusoidal portal hypertension Perioval granuloma formation	Ova in stool, rectal or liver biopsy
Fascioliasis (*Fasciola hepatica*)	Worldwide	Cattle or sheep raising Ingestion of freshwater plants (watercress)	Larvae migrate through liver Penetration of bile ducts	Acute: fever, abdominal pain, jaundice, hemobilia Chronic: hepatomegaly, stone formation	Ova in stool, flukes in bile ducts at ERCP or surgery
Clonorchiasis/ opisthorchiasis (*Clonorchis sinensis*, *O. viverrine*, *O. felineus*)	SE Asia, China, Japan, Korea, E. Europe	Ingestion of raw freshwater fish; SE Asian immigrants	Migration through ampulla, egg deposition in bile ducts	Biliary hyperplasia, obstruction, sclerosing cholangitis, stone formation, cholangiocarcinoma	Ova in stool, flukes in bile ducts at ERCP or surgery

(Table 29.3: Helminthic infections – trematodes)

Species	Geography	Clinical disease
S. mansoni	Western hemisphere	Liver disease
S. japonicum	Far East	Liver disease
S. hematobium	Africa, Middle East	Bladder cancer
S. mekongi	Far East	Liver disease
S. intercalatum	Central Africa	Colonic disease

(Table 29.4: Schistosoma species, their distribution and related disease)

b Clinical presentation

- acute toxemic schistosomiasis (Katayama's syndrome) is believed to be a consequence of the host immunologic response to mature worms and eggs. Occurs about 4–6 weeks after exposure. Manifestations include headache, fever, chills, cough, diarrhea, myalgias, arthralgias, tender hepatomegaly, and eosinophilia

- untreated acute schistosomiasis invariably progresses to chronic disease. Mesenteric infection leads to hepatic complications, including periportal fibrosis, presinusoidal occlusion, and, ultimately portal hypertension, as a result of the inflammatory reaction to eggs deposited in the liver. With severe schistosomal infection, portal hypertension becomes progressive, leading to ascites, gastroesophageal varices, and splenomegaly

- chronic schistosomal infection may be complicated by increased susceptibility to *Salmonella* infections. Hepatitis B viral coinfection is also common in persons living in endemic areas and may accelerate the progression of liver disease and the development of hepatocellular carcinoma

- laboratory findings of chronic schistosomiasis include anemia from recurrent gastrointestinal bleeding or hypersplenism, eosinophilia, an elevated erythrocyte sedimentation rate, and increased serum IgE levels. Tests of liver function are generally normal until the disease is advanced

c Diagnosis

- the diagnosis of acute schistosomiasis should be considered in a patient with an exposure history, abdominal pain, diarrhea, and fever. Multiple stool examinations for ova may be required to confirm the diagnosis, because results are frequently negative in the early phases of disease

- serologic testing using CIE or an ELISA has proved useful in facilitating earlier diagnosis. Sigmoidoscopy or colonoscopy may reveal rectosigmoid or transverse colonic involvement and may be useful in chronic disease when few eggs pass in the feces

- ultrasonography and liver biopsy are useful for demonstrating periportal (or "pipestem") fibrosis but not for diagnosing acute infection

d Treatment

- praziquantel 40–60 mg/kg given in 1 day in two or three divided doses is the treatment of choice for infection caused by any schistosomal species. Oxamniquine 15–60 mg/kg for 1–2 days is an effective alternative regimen in patients who cannot tolerate praziquantel

- treatment of acute toxemic schistosomiasis requires an increase in the dose of praziquantel to 75 mg/kg in 1 day in three divided doses and, in some cases, prednisone for the prior 2–3 days in order to suppress immune-mediated helminthicidal or drug reactions

- injection sclerotherapy or band ligation of varices is effective in controlling severe variceal bleeding. Management of advanced chronic schistosomal liver disease may require distal splenorenal shunt with or without splenopancreatic disconnection or esophagogastric devascularization with splenectomy. Fortunately, since the advent of praziquantel, complicated schistosomal liver disease has become uncommon

2 Liver flukes: fascioliasis

Fascioliasis, caused by the sheep liver fluke *Fasciola hepatica*, is endemic in many areas of Europe and Latin America, North Africa, Asia, the Western Pacific, and some parts of the USA

a Life cycle

- the life cycle is spent between herbivores and intermediate aquatic snail hosts. Eggs passed in the feces of infected mammals into fresh water give rise to miracidia that penetrate snails and emerge as cercariae, which encyst on aquatic plants such as watercress. Hosts become infected when they consume plants bearing the encysted organims, which bore into the intestinal wall, enter the abdominal cavity, penetrate the hepatic capsule, and settle in the bile ducts, where they attain maturity

b Clinical presentation

- divided into three phases corresponding to three syndromes: acute or invasive, chronic latent, and chronic obstructive
  - **acute**: migration of young flukes through the liver. Marked by fever, right-upper-quadrant pain, and eosinophilia. Urticaria with dermatographia is common, as are nonspecific gastrointestinal symptoms. Physical examination often reveals fever and a tender, enlarged liver. Splenomegaly reported in up to 25% of cases, but jaundice is rare. Eosinophilia can be profound, (occasionally >80%). Abnormalities of liver function tests are minimal
  - **latent**: corresponds to the settling of the flukes into the bile ducts and lasts months to years. Affected patients may experience vague gastrointestinal symptoms. Eosinophilia persists, and fever can occur
  - **chronic obstructive**: consequence of intrahepatic and extrahepatic bile ductal inflammation and hyperplasia evoked by the presence of adult flukes. May be marked by recurrent biliary colic, cholangitis, cholelithiasis, and biliary obstruction. Blood loss may result from epithelial injury, and rare cases of overt hemobilia have been described. Liver function testing commonly demonstrates an obstructive pattern. Long-term infection may lead to biliary cirrhosis and secondary sclerosing cholangitis. However, there is no convincing association with biliary tract or hepatic malignancy

c Diagnosis

- fascioliasis should be considered in patients with prolonged fever, abdominal pain, diarrhea, tender hepatomegaly, and eosinophilia. During the acute phase, because eggs are not passed, diagnosis depends on the detection of antibody by CIE or ELISA. In the latent and chronic phases, the diagnosis is made definitively by detection of eggs in stool, duodenal aspirates, or bile. On occasion, ultrasonography or ERCP will demonstrate the flukes in the gallbladder and common bile duct
- hepatic histologic findings include necrosis and granuloma formation with eosinophilic infiltrates and Charcot–Leyden crystals. Eosinophilic abscesses,

epithelial hyperplasia of the bile ducts, and periportal fibrosis may also be
seen

d   Treatment

- Unlike other liver fluke infections, praziquantel is not effective for fascioliasis

- The drug of choice is bithionol, a halogenated phenol derivative, in a
  dose of 50 mg/kg/d for 10 doses. Intramuscular dehydroemetine
  1 mg/kg/d for 14 doses is also effective but more toxic (cardiac,
  gastrointestinal, and hepatic reactions).

- both drugs are available only through the CDC. Encouraging preliminary
  reports may support the eventual use of a single dose of the benzimidazole
  derivative triclabendazole

3   Liver flukes: clonorchiasis and opisthorchiasis

Clonorchis sinensis, Opisthorchis viverrine, and *O. felineus* are trematodes of the
family Opisthorchioidea. *C. sinensis* and *O. viverrine* are widespread in East and
Southeast Asia, and infection is linked to lower socioeconomic status. *O. felineus*
infects humans and domestic animals in eastern Europe. All three have similar life
cycles and result in similar clinical manifestations

a   Life cycle

- all require two intermediate hosts, an aquatic snail and freshwater fish. Eggs
  are passed in the feces into fresh water, consumed by snails, and hatch as free-
  swimming cercariae, which seek and penetrate fish or crayfish and encyst in
  skin or muscle as metacercariae. The mammalian host is infected when it
  consumes raw or undercooked fish. The metacercariae excyst in the small
  bowel and migrate into the ampulla of Vater and into the bile ducts, where they
  mature into adult flukes. Infection can be maintained for two decades or longer

b   Clinical presentation

- clinically silent or nonspecific, with fever, abdominal pain, and diarrhea
- chronic manifestations correlate with the fluke burden and are dominated by
  hepatobiliary features, fever, right-upper-quadrant pain, tender hepatomegaly,
  and eosinophilia. With a heavy worm burden in the bile ducts, chronic or
  intermittent biliary obstruction can ensue, with frequent development of
  cholelithiasis, cholecystitis, jaundice, and, ultimately, recurrent pyogenic
  cholangitis
- serum alkaline phosphatase and bilirubin levels are elevated, and mild to
  moderate elevations of serum aminotransferase levels are also seen.
  Longstanding untreated infection leads to exuberant inflammation resulting in
  periportal fibrosis, marked biliary epithelial hyperplasia and dysplasia, and a
  substantially increased risk of cholangiocarcinoma
- cholangiocarcinoma resulting from clonorchiasis or opisthorchiasis tends to be
  multicentric and arises in the secondary biliary radicles of the hilum of the
  liver. The diagnosis should be suspected in infected persons with weight loss,
  jaundice, epigastric pain, or an abdominal mass

c Diagnosis
- based on detection of characteristic fluke eggs in the stool. Stool examination is usually positive except late in the disease, when biliary obstruction supervenes. In these cases, the diagnosis is made by identifying flukes in the bile ducts or gallbladder at surgery or in bile obtained by postoperative drainage or percutaneous aspiration.
- endoscopic or intraoperative cholangiography reveals slender, uniform filling defects within intrahepatic ducts that are alternately dilated and strictured and that may mimic sclerosing cholangitis
- serologic methods of diagnosis are generally unhelpful

Treatment
- all patients with clonorchiasis or opisthorchiasis should be treated with praziquantel, which is uniformly effective in a dose of 75 mg/kg in three divided doses over 1 day. Side effects are uncommon and include headache, dizziness, and nausea. After treatment, dead flukes may be seen in the stool or biliary drainage.
- when the burden of infecting organisms is high, the dead flukes and surrounding debris or stones may cause biliary obstruction, necessitating endoscopic or surgical drainage

D Helminthic infections: cestodes (tapeworms) (see Table 29.5)

1 Echinococcosis (see also Ch. 28)

Disease (cause)	Endemic areas	Predisposition	Pathophysiology	Manifestations	Diagnosis
Echinococcosis (*Echinococcus granulosa*, *E. multilocularis*)	Worldwide	Sheep and cattle raising (*E. granulosa*)	Larval migration to liver encystment (hydatid)	Tender hepatomegaly, fever, eosinophilia, cyst rupture, biliary obstruction	Serology (IHA, EIA) hepatic imaging

(Table 29.5: Helminthic infections – cestodes)

Infections with *Echinococcus granulosus* can be found worldwide in areas where dogs are used to raise livestock. *E. multilocularis* is distributed in northern North America and Eurasia, whereas *E. vogeli* is found in scattered areas of Central and Latin America.

a Life cycle
- infection occurs when humans, an intermediate host, eat vegetables contaminated by dog feces bearing embryonated eggs. The eggs hatch in the small intestine and liberate oncospheres that penetrate the mucosa and migrate to distant sites
- the liver is the most common destination (70%), followed by the lungs (20%), kidney, spleen, brain, and bone. In these organs, the hydatid cyst develops by vesiculation, resulting in the production of thousands of protoscolices
- the cyst wall contains three layers: (1) the outer adventitial layer (host-derived),

which can calcify; (2) the intermediate acellular; and (3) the inner germinal layers (worm-derived). A protoscolex is produced asexually within small secondary cysts that develop from the inner layer. Rupture of the hydatid cyst releases the viable protoscolices, which set up daughter cysts in secondary sites. Dogs acquire the infection by consumption of organs of sheep, cattle, or other livestock bearing the hydatid cyst

b Clinical presentation

- as the cysts of *E. granulosus* grow within the liver, they cause low-grade fever, tender hepatomegaly (usually the right lobe), and eosinophilia
- if the cysts grow large enough, they may rupture into the lungs, leading to dyspnea and hemoptysis. More extensive rupture into the peritoneum or lungs may lead to a life-threatening anaphylactic reaction to the cyst contents. Rupture into the biliary tract can cause cholangitis and obstruction
- superinfection of the hepatic cysts can lead to pyogenic liver abscesses in up to 20% of patients with hepatic disease. Echinococcal disease is the most common cause of pyogenic hepatic abscess in Greece and Spain
- *E. multilocularis* is highly invasive and leads to solid masses in the liver that are easily confused with cirrhosis or carcinoma. Alveolar hydatid disease is the term applied to hepatic nodules that appear on microscopy as alveolus-like microvesicles. Unfortunately, infection is generally not diagnosed until the lesions are inoperable due to extensive invasion or distant metastatic disease, and mortality rates are high, approaching 90%
- Infection with *E. vogeli* has clinical features intermediate between those of the other two species and is characterized by multiple fluid-filled cysts containing daughter cysts and protoscolices

c Diagnosis

- a history of exposure in a patient with hepatomegaly and an abdominal mass is suggestive, but the most important diagnostic tools are radiography and serology
- ring-like calcifications of up to a quarter of hepatic cysts are visible on plain abdominal films in patients infected with *E. granulosus*. The sensitivity and specificity of both ultrasonography and CT in confirming the diagnosis is high. Both modalities can demonstrate intracystic septations and daughter cyst formation in about half the cysts. Contrast-enhanced CT may display avascular cysts with ring enhancement
- percutaneous aspiration of the cyst has traditionally been discouraged due to concern about anaphylactic reactions. However, encouraging reports suggest that under carefully controlled conditions using thin needles and concomitant antihelminthic therapy, aspiration for diagnosis and therapy may be performed safely. The detection of protoscolices, or acid-fast hooklets, in the cyst fluid confirms the diagnosis
- both an ELISA and an indirect hemagglutination assay may also be used for diagnosis, with a sensitivity of 90%. Assays for detecting circulating antigen are likely to be of additional benefit in the future. The Casoni skin test is nonspecific and not currently recommended.
- *E. multilocularis* infection can be diagnosed with high sensitivity using a combination of an ELISA and CT, which often shows scattered areas of

calcified necrotic tissue. In *E. vogeli* infection, CT demonstrates polycystic lesions in the liver or peritoneal space

d Treatment

- approaches to treatment are both surgical and medical. Accessible cysts in younger persons should be treated surgically. The goal should be removal of the cestode without disruption of cyst contents. Successful approaches have included cystectomy, endocystectomy, omentoplasty, and marsupialization

- in complicated cases, hepatic lobectomy or hemihepatectomy may be necessary. If the cyst cannot be safely removed surgically, then aspiration and instillation of a scolicidal agent (silver nitrate) may be considered. However, because nearly half of hydatid cysts communicate with the bile ducts, extreme caution should be exercised before instilling a potentially sclerosing agent. A pretreatment cholangiogram should be performed. The perioperative use of antihelminthics such as albendazole 400 mg twice daily in one to three 4-week courses with a 2-week hiatus between courses is recommended

- surgical resection is curative in up to one third of cases of *E. multilocularis* infection; however, in most cases the disease is advanced at diagnosis. In such cases, palliative drainage procedures or long-term treatment with albendazole may increase survival. Surgery appears to be the most effective approach for *E. vogeli* infection

4 Fungal Liver Disease

A Candidiasis

1 *Candida* species may cause invasive systemic infection in persons who are severely immunocompromised. The liver can become infected by *C. albicans* in the setting of disseminated, multiorgan disease

2 Most disseminated infections occur in leukemic patients undergoing high-dose chemotherapy and become manifest during the period of recovery from severe neutropenia. In several series comprising predominantly leukemic patients, hepatic candidiasis was present in 51–91% of patients. Disease is often overwhelming with high mortality rates

3 Less frequent presentations in the compromised host are isolated or focal hepatic candidiasis or hepatosplenic candidiasis. Focal candidiasis is thought to result from colonization of the gastrointestinal tract by *Candida*, which disseminates locally following the onset of neutropenia and mucosal injury due to high-dose chemotherapy. Resulting fungemia of the portal vein seeds the liver and leads to hepatic micro- and macroabscesses

4 In either focal or disseminated candidiasis involving the liver, clinical features include fever, abdominal pain and distention, nausea, vomiting, diarrhea, and tender hepatomegaly. The serum alkaline phosphatase level is nearly invariably elevated, with variable elevations in serum aminotransferase and bilirubin levels

5 CT of the abdomen is the most sensitive test to detect hepatic and/or splenic abscesses, which are often multicentric. In the majority of cases diagnosed ante mortem, liver biopsy reveals macroscopic nodules, necrosis with microabscess formation, and characteristic yeast and/or hyphal forms of *Candida*. Cultures of

biopsy material are negative in the majority of cases. Laparoscopy may also be employed to confirm the diagnosis

6 If hepatic candidiasis is diagnosed in its focal form, response rates to therapy with intravenous amphotericin B are better (nearly 60% response) than for disseminated disease. However, the success of treatment is currently far from optimal

B   Histoplasmosis

1 Infection with *Histoplasma capsulatum* is acquired through the respiratory tract. In the majority of cases, disease is confined to the lungs. However, severely immunocompromised persons (e.g., with AIDS) in endemic regions are predisposed to disseminated histoplasmosis

2 In both the acute and chronic forms of progressive disseminated histoplasmosis, the liver can be invaded. In addition to fever and oropharyngeal ulcers, hepatomegaly and splenomegaly may be present in chronic disease. In children with acute hepatic disease, marked hepatosplenomegaly is universal and associated with high fever and lymphadenopathy. Serum aminotransferase and alkaline phosphatase levels are often elevated. Hepatosplenomegaly is present in 30% of adults with acute disease (often the AIDS-defining illness)

3 Yeast forms can be identified in sections of liver biopsies on standard hematoxylin and eosin staining. The silver methenamine method is superior for detecting yeast forms in areas of caseating necrosis or granuloma formation. The organism is difficult to culture and almost never grows from biopsy specimens.

4 Serologic testing for complement-fixing antibodies is helpful in confirming the diagnosis. In immunocompromised persons who may not be capable of mounting a significant antibody response, detection of *H. capsulatum* antigens in urine and serum can be useful

5 Disseminated histoplasmosis should be treated with intravenous amphotericin B, as ketoconazole or fluconazole treatment failure is common

References

1   Chung RT, Friedman LS. *Bacterial, parasitic, fungal, and granulomatous liver disease and liver abscess*. In: Scharschmidt B, Feldman M, eds. *Gastrointestinal Disease.* (Philadelphia: Saunders, 1997)

2   Cunha BA. *Systemic infections affecting the liver*. (Postgrad Med 1988); 84: 148–68

3   Brandborg LL, Goldman IS. *Bacterial and miscellaneous infections of the liver*. In: Zakim DS, Boyer TD, (eds). *Hepatology.* (Philadelphia: Saunders, 1990) 1086–98

4   Farid Z, Kilpatrick ME, Chiodini PL. *Parasitic diseases of the liver*. In: Schiff L, Schiff ER, (eds). *Diseases of the Liver.* (Philadelphia: Lippincott, 1993) 1338–55

5   Bryan RT, Michelson MK. *Parasitic infections of the liver and biliary tree*. In: Surawicz C, Owen RL, (eds). *Gastrointestinal and Hepatic Infections.* (Philadelphia: Saunders, 1995) 405–54

6   Abdel Wahab MF. *Schistosomiasis in Egypt*. (Boca Raton, FL: CRC Press, 1982)

7   World Health Organization. *Prevention and control of intestinal parasitic infections: report of a WHO expert committee.* (Geneva: World Health Organization, 1987)

8   *Drugs for parasitic infections*. (Med Lett Drugs Ther 1993) 35: 111–22

9   Canto MIF, Diehl AM. *Bacterial infections of the liver and biliary system*. In: Surawicz C, Owen RL, (eds). *Gastrointestinal and Hepatic Infections.* (Philadelphia: Saunders, 1995) 355–89

CHAPTER 30

Surgery in the patient with liver disease and postoperative jaundice

LAWRENCE S. FRIEDMAN, M.D.

▼

Key Points

1 Minor liver test abnormalities are common after surgery; overt liver dysfunction is uncommon but more likely if there is pre-existing liver disease

2 Hepatic blood flow is reduced by anesthesia, blood loss, and other hemodynamic derangements

3 Operative mortality is increased in patients with acute hepatitis, alcoholic hepatitis, severe chronic hepatitis, and Child's class B and C cirrhosis; additional risk factors include emergency surgery, biliary surgery, liver resection, and ascites

4 Obstructive jaundice is associated with increased surgical risk and an increased risk of renal failure, stress ulcers, disseminated intravascular coagulation and impaired wound healing; the benefit of preoperative biliary decompression is unproven

5 Postoperative jaundice may result from an increased pigment load as a result of transfusions or hemolysis, hepatocellular dysfunction as a result of reduced hepatic blood flow, drug toxicity, or infection, or, rarely, biliary obstruction

---

▲

1 Effects of Anesthesia and Surgery on the Liver

A Overview

- most surgical procedures, whether performed under general or local (i.e., spinal or epidural) anesthesia, are followed by changes in liver biochemical tests
- postoperative elevations of serum aminotransferase, alkaline phosphatase, or bilirubin levels are generally minor, transient, and of questionable clinical significance
- clinically significant hepatic dysfunction is more likely to occur in patients with pre-existing liver disease than in those with normal preoperative liver function

B Effects of anesthetic agents on the liver

- reduction in hepatic blood flow and decreased hepatic oxygen uptake; however, a clinical effect on healthy volunteers has not been demonstrated (see Table 30.1 for the effects of individual agent)

Agent	Effects
Cyclopropane (no longer used)	Sympathetic stimulation ↑ Splanchnic vascular resistance
Methoxyflurane (rarely used)	↓ Mean arterial pressure Portal venoconstriction
Halothane, enflurane, isoflurane	Systemic vasodilatation ↓ Cardiac output (↑ Hepatic artery flow by isoflurane)
Spinal, epidural	↓ Mean arterial pressure
Nitrous oxide	Least depressive effect unless concomitant hypercarbia

(Table 30.1: Effects of anesthetic agents on the liver)

C Other intraoperative factors

Other intraoperative factors that may contribute to decreased hepatic oxygenation by decreasing hepatic blood flow or increasing splanchnic vascular resistance are:

- hypotension, shock
- hemorrhage
- hypoxemia
- hypercapnia
- congestive heart failure
- vasoactive drugs
- intermittent positive pressure ventilation
- traction on abdominal viscera – reflex dilatation of splanchnic capacitance vessels

D   Hepatic metabolism of anesthetic agents

1 Inhalational anesthetic agents are lipid-soluble compounds that require hepatic transformation to more water-soluble compounds for biliary excretion. Degree of hepatic metabolism varies among different agents (see Table 30.2)

Agent	Degree of hepatic metabolism (%)
Methoxyflurane	50
Halothane	20
Enflurane	3
Isoflurane	1

(Table 30.2: Degree of hepatic metabolism of anesthetic agents)

2 Consequences of hepatic metabolism:
- prolonged anesthetic action in patients with liver disease (also caused by hypoalbuminemia and impaired biliary excretion)
- formation of toxic intermediates or oxygen-derived free radicals especially in the presence of hypoxia or reduced hepatic blood flow
    - methoxyflurane → hepatotoxicity and nephrotoxicity
    - halothane → hepatitis (rare)
    - enflurane → hepatitis (even rarer)

3 **Isoflurane** and **nitrous oxide** may be preferable in patients with liver disease because these agents undergo the least hepatic metabolism; only a few cases of isoflurane hepatitis have been reported

E   Other agents in liver disease

1 Narcotics (e.g., meperidine), sedatives (e.g., diazepam), induction agents (e.g., phenobarbital)
- prolonged duration of action in decompensated liver disease
    - narcotics have high first-pass extraction by liver: blood levels increase as hepatic blood flow decreases; orally administered forms have increased bioavailability due to portosystemic shunting; exception – sufentanil (similar durations of action in normals and cirrhotics)
    - benzodiazepines have low first-pass extraction by liver: those eliminated by glucuronidation (oxazepam, lorazepam) are usually not affected by liver disease; those not glucuronidated (diazepam, chlordiazepoxide) have enhanced sedative effects in liver disease
- may precipitate hepatic encephalopathy in patients with severe liver disease
- smaller than standard doses indicated for those drugs whose metabolism is affected by liver disease

2 Curare-like muscle relaxants
- resistance in liver disease in part because of decreased hepatic pseudocholinesterase production

- large doses required in patients with liver disease may cause difficulty in reversing their effect postoperatively
- agents not metabolized by liver preferred, e.g., atracurium

F   Effect of surgery

- may be more important determinant of postoperative hepatic dysfunction than anesthesia
- risk correlates with nature and extent of surgery; greatest with biliary tract and upper abdominal surgery

2   Operative Risk in Patients with Liver Disease

A   Problems in estimating operative risk

- lack of large, prospective studies
- limited data on acute and chronic hepatitis and nonalcoholic cirrhotic patients

B   Acute viral hepatitis

1   Small retrospective studies have conflicting results, but in general an increased operative risk is reported, as in study of Harville and Summerskill (1963)[1] (see Table 30.3)

	42 patients with viral hepatitis
Surgical mortality	4 (9.5%)
Morbidity	5 (11.9%)

(Table 30.3: Operative risk in patients with acute viral hepatitis)

2   Elective surgery can usually be avoided in patients with viral hepatitis. In the past, exploratory laparotomy was often performed to differentiate viral hepatitis from cholestatic disorders. Nowadays, such a distinction can almost always be made by a combination of serologic testing, ultrasonography, cholangiography, and/or percutaneous needle biopsy of the liver

3   Unsuspected preoperative aminotransferase elevation (incidence ~ 1 in 700)
- may be caused by early viral hepatitis which, if it becomes clinically apparent postoperatively, may be mistakenly attributed to anesthetic agent
- best to postpone elective surgery until liver dysfunction is investigated and the course of the disease is observed

C   Chronic hepatitis

1   Surgical risk appears to correlate with disease severity; elective surgery contraindicated in active, symptomatic disease. (Emergency surgery in patients on chronic corticosteroid therapy requires "stress" coverage)

2 Asymptomatic HBsAg carrier
- no increased surgical risk
- unclear whether anesthesia results in activation of virus
- risk that patient may infect medical and surgical personnel (especially if patient is HBeAg+). Control measures
  - proper operating room protocol: gloves, masks, caps, gowns, overshoes, disposable or decontaminated equipment, avoidance of unnecessary venipuncture or injections, minimal necessary personnel
  - hepatitis B vaccine to all personnel at risk
  - immediate hepatitis B immune globulin + vaccine series to unvaccinated personnel who sustain an accidental needlestick exposure to hepatitis B

D   Alcoholic liver disease

1 Alcoholic fatty liver
- elective surgery not contraindicated in presence of normal liver function
- however, it may be desirable to postpone surgery until nutritional deficiencies are corrected and/or acute effects of alcohol have resolved

2 Acute alcoholic hepatitis
- spectrum of severity, but surgical risk generally increased, particularly if liver biopsy specimen contains alcoholic hyaline (Mallory bodies)
- abstinence from alcohol and supportive therapy for 6–12 weeks generally required before elective surgery; repeat liver biopsy may be useful

3 Alcoholism: additional perioperative risks independent of liver disease – altered drug metabolism
- acetaminophen toxicity may occur after regular use of standard doses in alcoholics
- enhancement of halothane hepatotoxicity by alcohol in animal model

E   Cirrhosis

1 Difficulties in detection/diagnosis
- multiple etiologies
- wide spectrum of severity
- lack of correlation between presence of cirrhosis and biochemical tests of liver function
- importance of careful history and physical examination (e.g., cutaneous spiders, telangiectases, palmar erythema)

2 Important consequences in postoperative period
- fluid and electrolyte disturbances, renal failure
- hypoxemia (R → L shunts)
- altered drug metabolism
- increased susceptibility to infection (abdominal abscess, sepsis)
- nutritional wasting
- cardiac complications, shock
- portal hypertension

3 Surgical risk

    a Variety of **risk factors** identified in several, relatively small, retrospective studies of nonportosystemic shunt surgery: emergency surgery, upper abdominal (esp. biliary) surgery, low albumin, prolonged prothrombin and/or partial thromboplastin times, elevated bilirubin, anemia, ascites, encephalopathy, malnutrition, postoperative bleeding, decreased aminopyrine or galactose clearance (quantitative hepatic function tests), indocyanine green clearance, central plasma clearance rate of amino acids (hepatic protein synthesis), portal pressure, Child's class

    b Difficulties in interpreting individual studies

- small numbers of patients
- retrospective – selection bias
- arbitrary choices of parameters examined

    c Garrison, et al. (1984)[2] studied 100 cirrhotics, > 95% alcoholic, mortality 30%, morbidity 30%: 52 parameters were assessed

- risk factors for mortality and morbidity identified: ascites, malnutrition, emergency surgery, infection, bilirubin $\geq$ 3 mg/dL, albumin $\leq$ 3 g/dL white blood cell count (WBC) > 10,000/mm³, prothrombin time (PT) 1.5 s prolonged, partial thromboplastin time (PTT) prolonged, Child's class
- multivariate analysis of risk factors
  - excluding Child's class → **albumin, infection, prolonged PT/PTT**
  - including Child's class → **Child's class**: mortality A 10%, B 31%, C 76%
- Child's class also shown to be best predictor of surgical mortality by Bloch et al. (1985)[3]

    d Child's classification (see Table 30.4)[4]

	A	B	C
Bilirubin (mg/dL)	<2.0	2.0–3.0	>3.0
Albumin (g/dL)	>3.5	3.0–3.5	<3.0
Ascites	None	Easily controlled	Poorly controlled
Encephalopathy	None	Mild	Advanced
Nutritional status	Excellent	Good	Poor

(Table 30.4: Child's classification)

- problems with use of Child's classification:
  - definition of terms (e.g., no ascites = clinically or sonographically absent?)
  - subjective parameters (e.g., encephalopathy – "mild" vs. "advanced")
  - assignment of overall class based on components in different classes (some have used a point system to add greater precision)

    e Conclusions

- **Child's classification** most widely used predictor of surgical risk; usefulness demonstrated in retrospective, but not prospective, studies. Correlates with postoperative mortality and morbidity (liver failure, encephalopathy, bleeding, sepsis, ascites, renal failure, pulmonary failure)

- additional risk factors:
  - **emergency surgery**
  - **biliary tract surgery**: marked vascularity of gallbladder bed in patients with portal hypertension; subtotal cholecystectomy recommended in decompensated cirrhosis and cholecystostomy recommended in emergency
  - **hepatic resection**: generally contraindicated in already compromised (cirrhotic) liver, particularly if decompensated (cirrhotic liver cannot regenerate); additional risk factors for hepatic resection: thoracotomy, pulmonary disease, diabetes mellitus, malignancy, complex intrahepatic inflammatory disease. How to quantitate hepatic reserve remains a challenging problem: methods used include indocyanine green clearance, uptake of radiolabeled gold colloid by Kupffer's cells, quantitative liver function tests (galactose elimination capacity, aminopyrine breath test, drug or amino acid clearance rates) and measurement of hepatic volume (e.g., CT scanning), but these are either not widely available or clearly predictive of outcome
  - **ascites**: abdominal wall herniation and wound dehiscence
- operative guidelines are shown in Table 30.5[5]
- major/complex abdominal surgery should be avoided in potential candidates for liver transplantation

Child's class	Operability
A	No limitations; normal response to surgery
B	Some limitations to liver function; good tolerance to surgery with preoperative preparation: sizeable liver resections contraindicated
C	Severe limitations to liver function; poor response to all surgery regardless of preparation; liver resection contraindicated

(Table 30.5: Operative guidelines for surgery in the patient with cirrhosis)

3   Obstructive Jaundice

A   Surgical risk

1 Mortality 8–20%
2 Risk factors: retrospective review of 373 patients undergoing surgery for relief of biliary obstruction,[6] multivariate discriminant analysis
   - initial hematocrit < 30%
   - initial serum bilirubin > 200 mmol/L (11 mg/dL)
   - malignant cause of obstruction
     - all three present → mortality rate 60%

    – all three absent → mortality rate < 5%

3 Risk factors for surgery of common bile duct (CBD) stones:[7]
- serum bilirubin
- other medical illnesses (however, not a risk for endoscopic sphincterotomy)
- preoperative endoscopic sphincterotomy

4 Situations in which endoscopic sphincterotomy for CBD stones may be preferable to surgery:
- patients at high operative risk
- retained stones after cholecystectomy
- severe acute cholangitis

B   Special perioperative problems in patients with obstructive jaundice –

?result of increased circulating levels of endotoxin due to impaired bile salt delivery to bowel and decreased hepatic reticuloendothelial function; endotoxin toxicity may be mediated in part by tumor necrosis factor

- renal failure
    - ↓ glomerular filtration rate (GFR) in 60–75% (vs. <1% of anicteric surgical patients)
    - frank renal failure in 9% with mortality > 50%
- disseminated intravascular coagulation
- gastric stress ulcers and bleeding
- delayed wound healing, wound dehiscence, and incisional hernias
- ? impaired myocardial contractility

C   Management

- reduction or prevention of endotoxemia: experimental – oral bile salts, oral antibiotics, lactulose, etc.
- preoperative intravenous antibiotic administration to prevent wound infection
- intravenous mannitol to prevent renal dysfunction traditionally advocated, though may cause dehydration if patient is not well hydrated; adequate perioperative hydration may be critical factor

D   Preoperative biliary decompression

- usefulness in reducing postoperative mortality suggested in several retrospective studies
- value not confirmed in recent prospective randomized, controlled studies (predominantly external biliary drainage)
    - no decrease in mortality in three studies; one study suggests benefit when combined with intravenous hyperalimentation
    - complications of transhepatic biliary drainage; cholangitis, sepsis, dehydration, catheter displacement
    - may increase hospital cost and length of stay
    - preoperative **endoscopic internal** biliary drainage, by avoiding percutaneous puncture, preserving enterohepatic circulation of bile salts, and reducing the

frequency of systemic endotoxemia, may improve postoperative wound healing, renal function, and liver function, but has not been shown to improve survival

- useful alternative to surgery for palliation of patients with inoperable malignancy and/or poor surgical risk; however, does not generally prolong survival. Endoprosthesis insertion may also be reasonable alternative to operative bypass in selected patients who are otherwise fit for surgery; endoscopic stenting associated with fewer early complications and surgery with fewer late complications

4 Preoperative Evaluation and Preparation

A General measures

1 History and physical examination
- best screen for unrecognized liver disease (routine liver function tests may be misleading)
- assess status of patients with known liver disease (e.g., Child's class)
- include careful medication and alcohol history and review of previous adverse experiences with anesthesia

2 Liver function tests: aspartate aminotransferase (AST), alanine aminotransferase (ALT), alkaline phosphatase, bilirubin, albumin
- of unclear cost-effectiveness in healthy, asymptomatic patients; may detect occasional case of early or subclinical hepatitis
- indicated in patients with remote history of hepatitis or risk factors for hepatitis (e.g., intravenous drug use); check HBsAg and anti-HCV
- further investigation of any patient with clinical or biochemical evidence of liver disease:
  - hepatocellular dysfunction – serologic testing, possibly liver biopsy;
  - cholestasis – abdominal ultrasound, possibly endoscopic or transhepatic cholangiography and liver biopsy

B Management of coagulopathy

1 Impaired hemostasis in liver disease
- vitamin K deficiency: decreased levels of factors II, VII, IX, and X
- decreased hepatic protein synthesis: decrease in levels of all factors except VIII
- occasional disseminated intravascular coagulation
- pattern of hemostatic abnormalities:
  - prolonged PT
  - low plasma fibrinogen level
  - normal or increased PTT
  - prolonged thrombin time
- thrombocytopenia: result of hypersplenism, folate deficiency, and/or alcohol-induced bone marrow suppression

2 Preoperative preparation
- vitamin K_1 10 mg i.m. (one to three doses): corrects hypoprothrombinemia related to malnutrition or intestinal bile salt deficiency, not hepatocellular disease
- fresh frozen plasma in patients with hepatocellular dysfunction: aim for PT no more than 3 sec longer than control (large volumes, short half-life limit efficacy)
- platelet transfusions: 8–10 U when count is below 50 000/mm³
- experimental: plasmapheresis, desmopressin (factor VIII stimulant, shortens bleeding time)

C Management of fluids and electrolytes (see Ch. 11)

1 Derangements in liver disease
- factors contributing to development of ascites in cirrhosis:
  - portal hypertension
  - decreased plasma oncotic pressure (hypoalbuminemia)
  - increased hepatic lymph
  - secondary hyperaldosteronism
  - stimulation of renin–angiotensin $\rightarrow$ renal vasoconstriction $\rightarrow$ decreased "effective" intravascular volume and avid sodium retention
- associated electrolyte abnormalities:
  - hyponatremia (impaired free water clearance)
  - hypokalemic alkalosis
- hepatorenal syndrome (see Ch. 12)
  - normally, elevated levels of vasodilatory prostaglandins (serum prostacycline and urinary prostaglandin E_2 (PGE_2)) in patients with hepatic insufficiency and stable renal function compensate for vasoconstrictive stimulus of angiotensin
  - in hepatorenal syndrome levels of urinary PGE_2 are decreased (loss of vasodilatory compensation)
  - azotemia, oliguria, hyponatremia, and hypotension unresponsive to volume expansion
  - may be precipitated by sudden volume loss (e.g., bleeding, rapid diuresis, paracentesis)

2 Preoperative management
- diagnostic paracentesis in patients with new or worsening ascites: exclude infection or malignancy, differentiate spontaneous from secondary (surgical) bacterial peritonitis
- control ascites before abdominal surgery to reduce risk of postoperative wound dehiscence or herniation:
  - rigid salt restriction (1–2 g NaCl) (for i.v. use D5W)
  - potassium-sparing, aldosterone-antagonist diuretic: spironolactone 100 $\rightarrow$ 400 mg/day + furosemide 40 $\rightarrow$ 160 mg/day if necessary
  - alternatively, "large-volume" paracentesis of up to 5 L or more with intravenous infusions of albumin in patients with stable renal function; may avoid risks of diuretics

- monitor patient's weight, intake and output, urinary sodium concentration (should increase above 25 mEq/L if diuretics are effective), and, if necessary, central venous pressure
- fluid restriction if hyponatremia is present
- monitor serum creatinine, blood urea nitrogen, (BUN), and, if necessary, creatinine clearance
- avoid certain drugs:
  - aminoglycosides – inhibit vasodilatory PGs
  - nonsteroidal anti-inflammatory drugs – inhibit vasodilatory PGs (imidazole–salicylate may be acceptable because it inhibits thromboxane but not PGE_2 production, but further study is required)
  - metoclopramide – stimulates aldosterone

D Management of hepatic encephalopathy (see Ch. 13)

1 **Pathophysiology**: poorly understood state of disordered central nervous system function characterized by disturbances in consciousness, behavior, and personality; pathogenetic factors
- shunting of portal venous blood into the systemic circulation
- hepatic dysfunction and failure to detoxify neurotoxic agents
  - ammonia
  - mercaptans
  - fatty acids
  - altered levels of plasma aromatic and branched-chain amino acids → "false" neurotransmitters octopamine and serotonin
  - Gamma aminobutyric acid (GABA) – inhibitory neurotransmitter; possible role of endogenous benzodiazepines

2 **Diagnosis**
- obvious in patient with confusion or stupor, asterixis, and elevated blood ammonia level
- may be subtle: "day–night reversal," formal psychometric testing, EEG
- importance of preoperative recognition: high frequency in postoperative period of precipitating or exacerbating factors:
  - gastrointestinal bleeding
  - constipation
  - azotemia
  - hypokalemic alkalosis
  - sepsis
  - hypoxia
  - use of central nervous system depressant drugs

3 **Management**
- control clinically overt encephalopathy preoperatively (preventive therapy of unproven benefit)

- correction of precipitating factors, restriction of protein intake to 20–30 g daily initially, then 60–80 g; bowel cleansing (enemas, cathartics)
- lactulose: oral unabsorbable disaccharide in dose needed to achieve mild diarrhea:
  - converts intestinal NH_3 to unabsorbed NH_4^+
  - enhances growth of nonammoniagenic intestinal bacteria
- oral antibiotics (e.g., neomycin 1 g bid)

E   Miscellaneous issues

1 Risk of hypoglycemia in end-stage cirrhosis or fulminant hepatic failure: intravenous infusions of D10W

2 Gastroesophageal varices: endoscopic sclerotherapy or band ligation to prevent rebleeding; portal antihypertensive (propranolol) therapy to prevent initial variceal bleed in patients with large "high-risk" varices

3 Nutritional therapy in malnourished cirrhotic: use of standard or branched-chain amino acid solutions to satisfy patient's caloric requirements without worsening encephalopathy; perioperative nutritional support may reduce the rate of postoperative complications

5   Postoperative Jaundice

A   Three pathophysiologic mechanisms in postoperative period (often multiple causes: see Table 30.6)

Hepatic parenchymal disease

Anesthesia drugs: halothane, enflurane
Other drugs: phenothiazines, isoniazid, methyldopa, androgens, estrogens
Antibiotics: tetracycline, chloramphenicol, erythromycins, sulfonamides, nitrofurantoin
Hyperalimentation
Viral hepatitis
Ischemia
Sepsis
Benign postoperative intrahepatic cholestasis

Increased bilirubin load

Hemolysis after transfusion
Hematoma resorption
Underlying hemolytic anemia
Gilbert's syndrome[a]

Extrahepatic obstruction

Common bile duct stone
Cholecystitis
Biliary stricture, leak, tumor
Pancreatitis

[a]Unconjugated hyperbilirubinemia resulting from congenital defect in hepatic uptake of bilirubin

(Table 30.6: Causes of postoperative jaundice)

1 Increased pigment load
2 Impaired hepatocellular function
3 Extrahepatic obstruction

B Specific causes

1 **Increased pigment load** (indirect hyperbilirubinemia)
   - resorption of hematoma or hemoperitoneum
   - transfusion (especially of stored blood): 10% of erythrocytes in a unit of 14-day-old bank blood undergo hemolysis within 24 hours of transfusion; thus, 500 mL transfusion may liberate 7.5 g of hemoglobin or 250 mg of bilirubin
   - hemolysis (rare): usually in setting of congenital erythrocyte defect, such as G6PD deficiency or sickle cell anemia
   - postcardiac surgery: risk factors include preoperative elevations of serum bilirubin level and right atrial pressure, valve replacement (and number of valves replaced), and use of intra-aortic balloon counterpulsation; marker of increased mortality rate
   - inherited disorder of bilirubin metabolism (e.g., Gilbert's syndrome): may be coincidentally diagnosed after a surgical procedure

2 **Impaired hepatocellular function**
   - benign postoperative intrahepatic cholestasis: hepatocyte dysfunction from a variety of stresses, such as hypoxemia, anesthesia, hemorrhage, sepsis, extensive transfusions, often in setting of prolonged, difficult surgery with postoperative multiorgan failure:
     - peak serum bilirubin of up to 15–40 mg/dL on postoperative day 2–10 with variable elevation of alkaline phosphatase and no more than mild elevation of aminotransferases
     - may mimic extrahepatic obstruction
     - prognosis depends on overall condition of patient, not liver status; liver function returns to normal with recovery of patient
   - bacterial infections especially Gram-negative sepsis and pneumococcal pneumonia: cholestatic liver dysfunction
   a hepatitis:
   - viral:
     - hepatitis C historically has been most common cause of post-transfusion hepatitis (up to 90–95% of cases); frequency now less than 0.5%; acute hepatitis usually occurs 6–7 weeks after transfusion; diagnosis by detection of anti-HCV in serum – often appears after acute illness; 70–80% frequency of chronic hepatitis with cirrhosis ultimately developing in over 20%
     - hepatitis B uncommon with contemporary serologic screening of donated blood, but still accounts for 5–10% of transfusion-associated hepatitis; incubation period 12–14 weeks; <5–10% frequency of chronic infection
     - rarely Epstein–Barr viral, cytomegaloviral, or delta (with B) hepatitis
   - drugs:
     - halothane – rare with frequency of 1 in 10,000, increased risk with multiple

exposures; onset of fever within 2–10 days of exposure, occasionally with eosinophilia; may be fatal; pathophysiologic mechanism thought to involve immune sensitization to trifluoroacetylated liver proteins formed by oxidative metabolism of halothane by cytochrome P450 2E 1 in persons with a possible genetic predisposition

- enflurane – less commonly causes hepatitis
- isoflurane – only a few cases of hepatic toxicity reported (undergoes least metabolism by liver)
- other drugs (e.g., erythromycin, sulfonamides, phenytoin, isoniazid); other drugs cause intrahepatic cholestasis (e.g., chlorpromazine, anabolic steroids)

- ischemic (shock liver) – in setting of massive trauma, shock, hyperthermia, etc.; often associated with marked elevations of serum aminotransferase levels (to >5000 U/L with bilirubin of 5–20 mg/dL within 2–10 days of surgery and rapid return of aminotransferase levels to or toward normal within 5–7 days; liver usually recovers if patient survives

b Total parenteral nutrition: may be associated with hepatomegaly, minor elevations of serum aminotransferase levels, fatty infiltration (presumably due to high glucose load or possibly carnitine or choline deficiency), or intrahepatic cholestasis and nonspecific periportal inflammation (presumably due to intravenous amino acids or fat emulsions or toxic bile salts such as lithocholic acid). Fatty liver may reverse with lecithin or choline supplementation, while cholestasis may reverse with administration of metronidazole or ursodeoxycholic acid, though such therapies require further study

3 **Extrahepatic obstruction** (uncommon cause of jaundice in postoperative period)
- unrecognized bile duct injury with biloma (bile collection), usually during cholecystectomy
- cholangitis, subphrenic or subhepatic abscesses secondary to the above
- choledocholithiasis, biliary or pancreatic tumor
- if suspected, may require evaluation with ultrasound and/or CT and ERCP

References

1 Harville, Summerskill. *Surgery in acute hepatitis*. (JAMA 1963) 184: 257–61

2 Garrison RN, Cryer HM, Howard DA, et al. *Clarification of risk factors for abdominal operations in patients with hepatic cirrhosis*. (Ann Surg 1984) 199: 648–55

3 Bloch et al. *Cholecystectomy in patients with cirrhosis: a surgical challenge*. (Ann Surg 1985) 120: 669–72

4 Child CG, Turcotte. *Surgery and portal hyptertension*. In: Child CG, (ed.). *The Liver and Portal Hypertension*. (Philadelphia: Saunders, 1964)

5 Stone HH. *Preoperative and postoperative care*. (Surg Clin North Am 1977) 57: 409–19

6 Dixon JM, Armstrong CP, Duffy SW, et al. *Factors affecting morbidity and mortality after surgery for obstructive jaundice: a review of 373 patients*. (Gut 1983) 24: 845–52

7 Neoptolemos JP, Shaw DE, Carr-Locke DL. *A multivariate analysis of preoperative risk factors in patients with common bile duct stones: implications for treatment*. (Ann Surg 1989) 209: 157–61

8 Fan S-T, Lo C-M, Lai ECS, et al. *Perioperative nutritional support in patients undergoing hepatectomy for hepatocellular carcinoma*. (N Engl J Med 1994) 331: 1547–52

9 Friedman LS, Maddrey WC. *Surgery in the patient with liver disease.* (Med Clin N Am 1987) 71: 453–76

10 Lai ECS, Chu KM, Lo C-Y, et al. *Surgery for malignant obstructive jaundice: analysis of mortality.* (Surgery 1992) 112: 891–6

11 MacIntosh EL, Minuk GY. *Hepatic resection in patients with cirrhosis and hepatocellular carcinoma.* (Surg Gyn Obst 1992) 174: 245–54

12 Smith AC, Dowsett JF, Russell RCG, Hatfield ARW, Cotton PB. *Randomised trial of endoscopic stenting versus surgical bypass in malignant low bile duct obstruction.* (Lancet 1994) 344: 1655–60

13 Strunin L. *Anesthetic management of patients with liver disease.* In: Millward-Sadler GH, Wright R, Arthur MJP, (eds). *Wright's Liver and Biliary Disease.* (London: Saunders, 1992) 1381–93

14 Diamonds T, Parks RW. *Preoperative management of obstructive jaundice.* (Br J Surg 1997) 84: 147–9

15 Bruix J, Castells A, Bosch, et al. *Surgical resection of hepatocellular carcinoma in cirrhotic patients: prognostic value of preoperative portal pressure.* (Gastroenterology 1996) 111: 1018–22

16 Kharasch ED, Hankins D, Mautz D, Thummel KE. *Identification of the enzyme responsible for oxidative halothane metabolism: implications for prevention of halothane hepatitis.* (Lancet 1996) 347: 1367–71

Liver transplantation

JOANNE C. IMPERIAL, M.D.
EMMET B. KEEFFE, M.D.

Key Points

1 Liver transplantation was initiated in the 1950s and 1960s in experimental animals by Drs Thomas Starzl and Francis Moore. In 1963, the first human liver transplant was performed, but initial results were poor with most patients dying early after transplantation

2 In the early 1980s, the results of liver transplantation improved significantly because of better immunosuppression, standardization of surgical techniques, improved anesthesia, and better patient selection

3 Over the past decade, there have been further advances in organ preservation and immunosuppression that have enhanced the survival and quality of life of transplant recipients, resulting in 5-year graft and patient survival rates of 80–85%

4 Although the number of patients requiring liver transplantation continues to grow steadily, the number of available organ donors remains essentially unchanged; 15–20% of patients awaiting liver transplantation die prior to receiving an organ

5 Early recognition and referral of candidates who are appropriate for liver transplantation should improve survival rates further and reduce the cost of this complex procedure

1   Patient Selection for Liver Transplantation

A   Overview

1   Liver transplant evaluation encompasses a complete medical history and physical examination, laboratory tests, assessment of psychosocial factors, and consideration of financial issues

2   The extent and pace of evaluation depend on the etiology of the liver disease, whether it is acute or chronic, and the presence of comorbid conditions

B   Principal indications for liver transplantation

1   Pediatric patients

- biliary atresia
- inborn errors of metabolism
- chronic hepatitis
- fulminant liver failure
- benign and malignant hepatic tumors
- cryptogenic cirrhosis
- miscellaneous disorders

2   Adult patients

- postnecrotic cirrhosis, including chronic hepatitis B and C
- cholestatic liver diseases
- alcoholic liver disease
- metabolic disorders
- acute liver failure
- metabolic liver diseases
- benign and malignant hepatic tumors
- miscellaneous disorders

C   Timing of referral for liver transplantation evaluation

1   When chronic liver disease decompensates:

- ascites
- spontaneous bacterial peritonitis
- variceal hemorrhage
- protein–calorie malnutrition
- portosystemic encephalopathy
- severe metabolic bone disease (hepatic osteodystrophy)
- persistent and severe coagulopathy
- uncontrolled biliary sepsis
- certain hepatobiliary malignancies

2   When biochemical tests of liver function worsen:

- new-onset jaundice in a stable cirrhotic (bilirubin >3.0 mg/dL)

- hypoalbuminemia (serum albumin <3.0 g/dL)
- coagulopathy (prothrombin time >3 s over control or international normalized ratio (INR) >1.8

- referral for evaluation does not imply immediate transplantation; the majority of patients wait 6 months to 1 year for a donor liver. In some regions in the USA, the waiting time for an organ exceeds 2 years

D   Evaluation and selection criteria

1 Liver transplant evaluation should be performed as soon as a patient is diagnosed with biochemical impairment of liver function or experiences a complication of end-stage liver disease

2 The evaluation process is usually completed as an outpatient. The following information is determined:
- diagnosis for which liver transplantation is being considered
- severity of underlying liver disease
- complications of liver disease that may require additional medical evaluation and/or treatment
- co-morbid conditions that may require additional evaluation and/or treatment
- psychosocial aspects that may require intervention before transplantation
- financial and insurance status

3 The following criteria are used to determine when a patient approved for transplantation might receive a donor organ:
- United Network for Organ Sharing (UNOS) status (Table 31.1)

Status	Definition	Points
4	At home	6
3	Requires continuous care	12
2	Continuously hospitalized	18
1	ICU bound	24
	Blood type	Up to 10
	Waiting time	Up to 10
	Logistic factors	Up to 10

From: *UNOS Annual Report of the US Scientific Registry of Transplant Recipients and the Organ Procurement and Transplantation Network*, 1995

(Table 31.1: UNOS liver allocation point system)

- patient blood type
- patient weight
- waiting time

2 Donor Selection Criteria

A Overview

1 The increasing number of liver transplant candidates on the waiting list and an increasing number of deaths while waiting for an organ have led to liberalization of donor criteria, which has led in turn to an increase in the number of transplants performed annually over the last several years

2 The use of hepatitis C antibody-positive or hepatitis B core antibody-positive donors remains controversial. Liver from such donors have been used in critically ill patients needing urgent transplantation or in patients already infected with the respective virus. Recent data indicate that the risk of transmission of hepatitis B virus from a hepatitis B core antibody-positive donor to a recipient may be as high as 70%

3 Use of donors over the age of 65 years is controversial, but recent data suggest that the use of livers from these donors is not associated with increased complications or mortality rates after liver transplantation

4 Other efforts directed at increasing the donor pool include the use of living-related liver transplantation (from adult to child) and split liver transplants (using the right lobe of the donor liver for an adult and the smaller left lobe for a pediatric patient).

Nevertheless, the organ donor shortage is the primary challenge faced by liver transplant centers today

B Organ donation

1 General criteria for liver donation:
  - brain death confirmed
  - consent for donation signed by family
  - no transmissible systemic disease:
    - infectious (HIV, HBV, HCV, bacterial, fungal)
    - neoplastic (except skin or brain)
  - normal or near-normal liver function tests
  - correctable prothrombin time
  - absence of disseminated intravascular coagulopathy
  - no donor and recipient body size incompatibility
  - ABO identical or compatible

2 Donor factors associated with poor graft function:
  - moderate steatosis (>30% fat) in the graft
  - prolonged cold preservation time (>12 hours)
  - donor age >50 years
  - initial poor function of graft ofter transplantation

3 Recipient factors associated with poor graft function:
  - UNOS status 1
  - renal failure

4 Intraoperative factors associated with poor graft function:

- prolonged warm ischemia time (>150 minutes)

5 All of the above risk factors contribute to the development of initial poor function (IPF) and primary nonfunction (PNF) of the graft

3   Contraindications to Liver Transplantation

A   Overview

1 Contraindications to liver transplantation may be absolute or relative. Absolute contraindications include conditions for which the outcome of liver transplantation is so poor that the procedure should not be done. Relative contraindications include conditions that increase morbidity and mortality, but do not disqualify a patient from undergoing the procedure

2 Absolute contraindications:

- acquired immunodeficiency syndrome
- extrahepatic malignancy
- advanced cardiopulmonary disease
- active substance abuse
- social or family problems that preclude transplantation
- multiorgan failure

3 Relative contraindications:

- hepatocellular carcinoma
- renal insufficiency
- advanced protein–calorie malnutrition
- active infection outside the biliary tract
- portal vein thrombosis
- hepatitis B infection

Many of the relative contraindications to liver transplantation are center-dependent and reflect the philosophies and experience of the transplant team. Renal insufficiency (serum creatinine of greater than 1.6 mg/dL) has been associated with:

- increased morbidity and mortality after liver transplantation
- increased ICU length of stay
- increased immunosuppression-related side effects
- increased need for postoperative hemodialysis or continuous venovenous hemoperfusion
- increased cost of transplantation
- decreased survival, especially in patients undergoing hemodialysis after liver transplantation (75% compared with >90% in patients who do not require hemodialysis)

Protein–calorie malnutrition:

- contributes to morbidity and, in severe cases, to mortality of patients undergoing liver transplantation
- prolongs ICU length of stay
- increases the need for ventilatory support
- increases difficulty in weaning patients from the respirator
- increases the rate of postoperative wound infections and active infection outside the biliary tract, e.g., spontaneous bacterial peritonitis (SBP):
- can be a recurrent problem in cirrhotic patients
- can be eradicated within 48–72 hours of antibiotic therapy
- should not be a contraindication to transplantation, unless systemic side effects such as hypotension and renal insufficiency persist despite 48 hours of intravenous antibiotics

Portal vein thrombosis:

- occurs in 15% of cirrhotic patients
- not a contraindication to liver transplantation, but necessitates either magnetic resonance imaging or angiography to define vascular anatomy before transplantation
- may be associated with thromboses of the superior mesenteric vein (SMV) and splenic vein (SV), which may also occur in patients with deficiency of antithrombin III, protein C, or protein S
- when associated with thromboses of the SMV and SV, portal vein thrombosis is an absolute contraindication to liver transplantation

Hepatitis B (see below)
Hepatocellular carcinoma (see below)

4 Liver Transplantation in Patients with Chronic Hepatitis B and C

A Overview

1 Chronic viral hepatitis is one of the most common causes of end-stage liver disease for which liver transplantation is performed (see also Ch. 4)

2 Efforts to prevent recurrence of hepatitis B in the allograft have been successful in improving the survival in patients undergoing liver transplantation for this indication

3 There is no effective antiviral regimen for preventing recurrence of hepatitis C in the allograft, but fortunately reinfection infrequently leads to graft failure and death within the first 3–5 years (~5–10% of cases)

B Liver transplantation for chronic hepatitis B

1 Early studies from the University of Pittsburgh showed that long-term survival after

liver transplantation was markedly diminished for patients who were hepatitis B surface antigen (HBsAg)-positive as compared with those that were HBsAg-negative (40% vs. >65% at 5 years)

2 Death from recurrent HBV infection is ususally related to chronic hepatitis B with cirrhosis but may also result from a rare but usually rapidly fatal cholestatic post-transplant syndrome called **fibrosing cholestatic hepatitis**

3 Factors associated with improved survival in HBV-infected patients undergoing liver transplantation include:

- absent/low viral replication (absence in serum of HBV DNA and/or hepatitis B e antigen (HBeAg))
- use of prophylactic hepatitis B immune globulin (HBIG)
- fulminant HBV infection
- hepatitis D (delta) virus coinfection

4 Prior to use of HBIG, the rate of recurrent HBV infection in graft was approximately 70–90%. Use of HBIG therapy peri- and postoperatively has reduced the HBV recurrence rate to 10–40% and improved long-term survival (Table 31.2)

HBIG 10,000 IU i.v. intraoperatively
HBIG 10,000 IU i.v. daily ×6, then
HBIG 10,000 IU i.v monthly thereafter to maintain HBsAg titer >150 IU/L

(Table 31.2: Usual hepatitis B immune globulin (HBIG) protocol)

5 Pretransplant antiviral therapy with interferon alpha, lamuvidine, or famciclovir to reduce or eliminate serum HBV DNA and HBeAg is undergoing study, since patients with low or absent viral replication have lower recurrence rates of HBV after transplantation

6 Recurrent HBV infection after liver transplantation may improve with reduction of immune suppression and antiviral therapy

7 Retransplantation of patients with recurrent HBV may be successful with the use of higher doses of HBIG therapy

8 **With use of HBIG, the 5-year survival of patients undergoing transplantation for HBV infection is now equivalent to that of patients undergoing liver transplantation for other etiologies of postnecrotic cirrhosis**

C   Liver transplantation for chronic hepatitis C

1 Chronic hepatitis C is the most common type of chronic viral hepatitis in the USA, with approximately 30,000 new cases diagnosed annually and a prevalence rate of 1.8%

2 Postnecrotic cirrhosis secondary to chronic hepatitis C is one of the most common indications for liver transplantation in adults, accounting for up to 40% of patients transplanted in some centers.

3 The overall 3–5-year survival rate after liver transplantation for chronic hepatitis C is 80–85%

4 Prognosis after transplantation is affected by co-morbid conditions of renal insufficiency secondary to chronic glomerulonephritis, cryoglobulinemia, or hepatocellular carcinoma

5 Accounting for 20 to 25% of all transplants are cases in which patients have hepatocellular carcinoma in the explant liver, often undetectable by pretransplant hepatic imaging studies

6 The post-transplant recurrence rate of HCV in the allograft is 90–100%

7 50% or more of patients with chronic HCV infection pretransplantation develop clinical and histologic hepatitis in the graft, which may respond to reduction of immune suppression, antiviral therapy, or both

8 Recurrence of HCV in the allograft is only rarely associated with an aggressive form of hepatitis, rapid graft loss, and death; in some patients cirrhosis and end-stage liver disease develop over 2–4 years post transplantation

9 Retransplantation for patients with graft failure secondary to recurrent HCV infection appears to be associated with poor survival (approximately 40% 1-year survival)

5 Liver Transplantation for Cholestatic Liver Diseases

A Overview

1 Biliary atresia and Alagille's syndrome are the most common diagnoses for which liver transplantation is performed in children

2 In adults, primary biliary cirrhosis and primary sclerosing cholangitis are the most common cholestatic diseases for which transplantation is performed and together account for about 20% of patients who undergo transplantation

3 Because these diseases primarily affect the small- and medium-sized bile ducts, jaundice may occur early in the course of the disease, with synthetic dysfunction occurring later

4 Prognostic models based on the natural history of cholestatic liver diseases have made it possible to estimate the appropriate time to refer patients for liver transplantation and to predict survival

B Primary biliary cirrhosis (PBC)

1 PBC is a cholestatic disease of middle-aged women, affecting small and medium-sized bile ducts. Presenting clinical features include fatigue and pruritus with associated elevation of alkaline phosphatase and a positive antimitochondrial antibody (AMA) in high titer (>1:80) (see Ch. 14)

2 Investigators from the Mayo Clinic have formulated a PBC risk score (R), based on the above variables, to predict short-term survival and to optimize the timing of liver transplantation (Fig. 31.1)

3 The cost of liver transplantation increases with the pretransplant severity of PBC

4 Patients should be referred when serum bilirubin is ≥10 mg/dL or before the patient

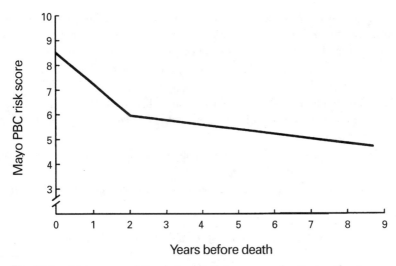

Fig. 31.1   Risk score and time before death in a group of patients with primary biliary cirrhosis. From Klion et al. (1992)[1]

experiences uncontrollable ascites, recurrent variceal bleeding, severe osteodystrophy, or intolerable pruritus

5   Post-transplant recurrence of PBC is reported but is rare and not usually associated with graft dysfunction

Yale	European	Mayo	Oslo	Glasgow	Australia
	Age	Age	Variceal bleeding	Age	Age
Bilirubin	Bilirubin	Bilirubin	Bilirubin	Bilirubin	Bilirubin
Hepatosplenomegaly	Albumin	Albumin		Ascites	Albumin
Cirrhosis	Cirrhosis	Prothrombin time	Variceal bleeding		
	Cholestasis	Edema		Fibrosis Cholestasis Mallory's bodies	

From Maddrey & Sorrell (1995)[2]

(Table 31.3: Independent clinical variables predictive of survival in primary biliary cirrhosis)

6   Table 31.3 shows independent clinical variables used in different centers to predict survival in PBC

C   Primary sclerosing cholangitis (PSC)

1   PSC is a cholestatic liver disease associated with inflammatory bowel disease (in approximately 75% of cases) and diagnosed more frequently in men than women (see Ch. 15)

2 PSC is characterized by progressive destruction of both medium and large-sized bile ducts, resulting in chronic cholestasis, biliary obstruction, frequent episodes of biliary sepsis, liver failure, and an increased risk of cholangiocarcinoma

3 Bacterial infections in the biliary tree result from chronic inflammation and strictures of bile ducts

- patients should be referred when the serum bilirubin is ≥10 mg/dL or after the development of recurrent biliary sepsis, intractable ascites, or protein–calorie malnutrition
- a Mayo model, similar to that for patients with PBC, may provide more accurate prognostic information

4 Post-transplant disease recurrence is reported in a small percentage of patients

6 Liver Transplantation for Alcoholic Liver Disease

A Overview

1 Although alcoholic liver disease is the most common cause of end-stage liver disease in the USA, accounting for nearly 13,000 deaths annually, the majority of patients with alcoholic cirrhosis do not qualify for liver transplantation for various medical or psychosocial reasons

2 Strict selection criteria are necessary to identify candidates with alcohol abuse who are appropriate for liver transplantation. The burden of the pretransplant evaluation rests on the psychiatrist and social worker on the liver transplant team

3 Although most transplant centers require a period of sobriety prior to transplantation (usually >6 months), most data have shown that this factor alone is not predictive of post-transplant use of alcohol (recidivism). Psychosocial factors that predict maintenance of sobriety post-transplantation appear to be equally important. Alcoholic patients who maintain sobriety are usually expected to participate in alcohol rehabilitation programs and submit to random blood and urine alcohol screening

4 Many alcoholic patients are very ill pre-transplant with multiple organ system dysfunction (e.g., heart, kidneys) and severe protein–calorie malnutrition that requires aggressive preoperative management

5 Alcoholic patients may also have coexistent liver diseases that need to be identified pre-transplant, including hemochromatosis, chronic viral hepatitis, or hepatocellular carcinoma

6 The survival of alcoholic patients who undergo transplantation does not differ significantly from that of nonalcoholic patients, nor does their utilization of resources

7 Liver Transplantation for Hepatic Tumors

A Overview

1 Liver transplantation is a therapeutic option for many patients with primary liver tumors who are not able to undergo liver resection because of the severity of underlying liver disease or anatomic location of tumor

2 In general, benign liver tumors and slow-growing malignant liver tumors are best treated by liver resection, since the majority of patients with these tumors are not associated with cirrhosis. Liver transplantation should be reserved for patients with malignant tumors arising in a cirrhotic liver or in whom tumor size or location prevents resection (see Ch. 27)

3 Tumors of the liver for which liver transplantation should be considered include:
   • hepatocellular carcinoma (HCC)
   • fibrolamellar HCC
   • epithelioid hemangioendothelioma
   • hepatoblastoma
   • certain metastatic neuroendocrine tumors
   • multiple hepatic adenomas
   • certain giant hemangiomas or adenomas

B   Liver transplantation for hepatocellular carcinoma

1 In the USA, most cases of HCC occur in patients with concomitant cirrhosis, particularly chronic hepatitis B or C, alcoholic liver disease, or hemochromatosis

2 Adequate screening programs for HCC have not been instituted in the USA, and the majority of patients with HCC present with symptoms – abdominal pain, weight loss, anorexia, and ascites – features associated with advanced disease and extension outside of the liver. At this late stage, there is no effective palliative medical or surgical treatment

3 Treatment of HCC is directed towards patients with small, asymptomatic tumors identified on routine hepatic imaging or on the basis of an elevated serum alpha fetoprotein (AFP) level

4 Because the majority of patients with HCC have cirrhosis, only a small percentage are able to undergo hepatic resection safely. Liver transplantation is the treatment of choice for patients that fulfill the following criteria:
   • tumor confined to liver, as documented by CT of the abdomen, chest, and brain
   • negative bone scan
   • no evidence of thrombosis of portal vein on Doppler ultrasound, magnetic resonance imaging, or arteriography

5 Prognostic factors associated with good survival for patients with HCC who undergo liver transplantation include:
   • single tumor <5 cm in diameter
   • fewer than three tumours, each <3 cm in diameter
   • absence of tumor invasion of the portal vein (macroscopic or microscopic)
   • unilobar disease
   • absence of local lymph node involvement

6 For patients fulfilling the above criteria, the long-term survival may approach that seen in patients without HCC who undergo liver transplantation.

8 Liver Transplantation for Fulminant Hepatic Failure

A Overview

1 Fulminant hepatic failure (FHF) is typically defined as the onset of hepatic encephalopathy within 8 weeks of the onset of acute hepatitis (see Ch. 2)

2 The etiology of FHF is usually viral, drugs, or toxins, but in 15–30% of cases no demonstrable etiology is found

3 Early referral to a transplant center is critical; recent advances in the development of prognostic indicators for FHF allow early determination of patients likely to die and thus in need of liver transplantation (Table 31.4)

Patients with acetaminophen toxicity 　pH <7.3 　or Prothrombin time >6.5 INR and serum creatinine >3.4 mg/dL
Patients with other causes of fulminant hepatic failure Prothrombin time >6.5 INR or Any three of the following variables: 　Age <10 or >40 years 　Etiology: non-A, non-B hepatitis, halothane hepatitis, idiosyncratic drug reaction 　Duration of jaundice before encephalopathy >7 days 　Prothrombin time >3.5 INR 　Serum bilirubin >17.6 mg/dL

INR, international normalized ratio
From: O'Grady et al. (1989)[3]

(Table 31.4: Prognostic criteria guiding the need for liver transplantation in patients with fulminant hepatic failure)

4 Identifying the cause of FHF prior to transplantation may assist in determining the prognosis, but referral to a transplant center should not be delayed in order to confirm of the etiology of FHF

5 Most patients with FHF are < age 40 years, otherwise healthy, and usually good candidates for liver transplantation; survival of patients with FHF should be excellent, as long as patients are referred early

6 **Death of patients with FHF is usually due to late referral and inability to find an appropriate donor within the allotted time. Survival of patients with FHF referred early for liver transplantation should be 70–80% (see Ch. 2)**

9 Postoperative Complications of Liver Transplantation

A Overview

1 Postoperative complications of liver transplantation may be immediate or late

2 Immediate complications include those related to the operation, rejection, infection, or drug-related toxicity (Table 31.5). The most common complications related to the operation include vascular thrombosis of the hepatic artery (seen primarily in pediatric liver transplantation) or portal vein and biliary strictures

Diagnosis	Liver enzymes			Hepatic imaging		Liver
	Alk. Phos.	GGT	AST/ALT	Ultrasound	Cholangiogram	biopsy
Acute rejection	↑	↑	± ↑	Normal	Normal	Abnormal
Biliary obstruction	↑	↑	± ↑	Abnormal	Abnormal	Abnormal
Infection	Occ. ↑	Occ. ↑	± ↑	Normal	Normal	Occ. abnormal
Drug-induced hepatitis	Occ. ↑	Occ. ↑	± ↑	Normal	Normal	Abnormal
Hepatic artery thrombosis	Occ. ↑	Occ. ↑	↑	Abnormal	Abnormal	Abnormal
Disease recurrence	Occ. ↑	Occ. ↑	Occ. ↑	± normal	± normal	Abnormal

(Table 31.5: Differential diagnosis of post-transplant liver dysfunction)

3 The most common late complications after liver transplantation include chronic rejection, infection, complications of immunosuppressive drug therapy, and recurrence of the original disease

B Acute allograft rejection

1 Acute rejection occurs in 40–70% of patients in the first 1–2 months after liver transplantation, but the overall frequency has declined since the introduction of the immunosuppressive agent tacrolimus (Prograf®)

2 Because the frequency of acute rejection has decreased, the hospital length of stay has also been reduced, contributing to a decreased cost of liver transplantation

C Infections in the liver transplant patient (Table 31.6)

1 Infections in the early postoperative period are most often bacterial or viral, usually cytomegalovirus hepatitis (CMV), although Epstein–Barr virus (EBV), and HBV and HCV infection can also occur

2 Diagnosis of these infections can be confirmed with the use of polymerase chain reaction (PCR) tests for the suspected virus and liver biopsy with appropriate stains, when applicable

D Immunosuppression-related drug toxicity

1 Drug toxicity (due to cyclosporine or tacrolimus) usually results in neurologic or renal toxicity and is reversible with adjustment of the doses of immunosuppression

Early infections related to immunosuppression:
  Cytomegalovirus
  Epstein–Barr virus (lymphoproliferative disease)
  Pneumocystis pneumonia
  Cryptococcal meningitis
  Coccidiodomycosis
  Listerial meningitis
  Tuberculous

Community acquired:
  Bacterial infections
  Influenza A or B
  Related to disease recurrence
    Hepatitis B
    Hepatitis C

(Table 31.6: Infections in liver transplant patients)

2 Other toxicity includes hypertension, hyperlipidemia, metabolic bone disease, and diabetes

3 Immunosuppressive drug therapy is gradually reduced during the first year post-transplantation, minimizing drug-related toxicity

E Post-transplant biliary complications

1 Anastomotic strictures are often progressive over time and difficult to dilate under radiologic guidance; they often require surgical revision of the biliary anastomosis

2 Intrahepatic biliary strictures are often secondary to ischemia, prolonged preservation time, ABO mismatch, or chronic rejection. These strictures are progressive over time and may be amenable to dilation and stenting, depending on their location. They may lead to retransplantation because of chronic cholestasis and progressive ductopenia. A small percentage of patients improve on switching immunosuppressive therapy from cyclosporine to tacrolimus

3 T-tube complications occur when the tube is removed (typically 3 months post-transplantation) and include bile leaks and peritonitis. These may respond to antibiotics, endoscopic management, or surgical intervention. Currently, surgeons favor primary biliary anastomosis without the use of a T-tube

10 Long-term Management of the Liver Transplant Patient

A Overview

1 Patients who have undergone liver transplantation typically have a hospital length of stay of 7–14 days for adults and 10–20 days for pediatric patients

2 Once the patient has been discharged from hospital, extended care may be necessary in the outpatient setting; some patients may require additional nutritional support, antibiotics, antiviral therapies, or intravenous antibiotics

3 Patients are often required to remain near the transplant center for 2–6 weeks after transplantation for intensive monitoring of liver function and immunosuppression

B   Outpatient visits and laboratory testing

1 Outpatient clinic visits occur approximately twice weekly initially then weekly for the first month and less frequently thereafter. Laboratory tests are usually performed monthly indefinitely.

2 For patients followed at home, the focus of the outpatient visits to their local physicians includes:

- symptom survey
- assessment of compliance with medications
- physical examination
- laboratory testing (CBC, chemistry panel, trough cyclosporine or tacrolimus levels)

C   Immunosuppressive drug regimen and monitoring

1 Monitoring of immunosuppressive drug levels is typically coordinated by the transplant center, but the primary physician is instrumental in following patients and in monitoring for side effects

2 Guidelines for monitoring and adjusting immunosuppressive therapy may differ slightly among centers, but the general principles are similar and include gradual reduction of immunosuppression and other medications

3 The two primary immunosuppressive agents widely used in liver transplantation include cyclosporine or tacrolimus, in combination with prednisone

- tacrolimus is available in 1 mg or 5 mg capsules and as a solution (5 mg/mL) for intravenous use
- although different from cyclosporine, tacrolimus shares many similar pharmacologic properties, primarily inhibiting T lymphocyte activation
- two large studies, conducted in the USA and Europe, have demonstrated that when tacrolimus is compared with cyclosporine (Sandimmune®), patient and graft survival is equivalent in the two groups
- the principal side effects of tacrolimus are neurotoxicity and nephrotoxicity; others include hyperkalemia, hyperglycemia, hypertension, and gastrointestinal dysfunction with nausea, vomiting, or diarrhea
- lymphoproliferative disorders, which also occur in patients receiving cyclosporine and other immunosuppressive agents, have been reported in patients treated with tacrolimus

4 Azathioprine (Imuran®) is used when cyclosporine or prednisone doses are reduced to decrease side effects, such as nephrotoxicity

5 Prednisone can ultimately be discontinued in many patients treated with tacrolimus. However, withdrawal of prednisone in patients treated with cyclosporine has not been well studied and has led to rejection

6 Patients undergoing liver transplantation for chronic hepatitis B or C generally undergo a more rapid prednisone taper and may even discontinue prednisone when they are receiving a cyclosporine-based immunosuppressive agent, primarily to reduce viral replication

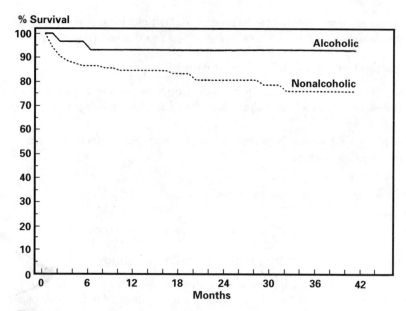

Fig. 31.2   Actuarial survival of alcoholic versus nonalcoholic patients undergoing liver transplantation. From Gish et al. (1993)[4]

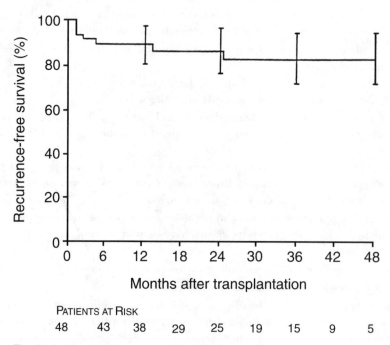

Fig. 31.3   Survival of patients with small hepatocellular carcinomas and cirrhosis. From Mazzaferro et al. (1996)[5]

D Daily activities and quality of life

1 Although some patients are able to return to work as soon as 3–6 months post-transplantation, most return to work later than this time

2 Quality of life is very good for the majority of individuals, although lack of concentration and reduced physical endurance occur in many

3 Active physical fitness programs and psychotherapeutic support facilitate return to normal or near-normal daily activities

4 Long-term survival after liver transplantation is excellent. Figures 31.2 and 31.3 show survival rates in alcoholic vs. nonalcoholic patients, and in patients with small hepatocellular carcinomas and cirrhosis, respectively

References

1 Klion FM, Fabry TL, Palmer M, Schaffner F. *Prediction of survival of patients with primary biliary cirrhosis.* (Gastroenterology 1992) 102: 310–13

2 Maddrey WC, Sorrell MF. *Transplantation of the Liver,* 2nd edn. (Norwalk: Appleton & Lange, 1995)

3 O'Grady JG, Alexander GJM, Hayllar KM, et al. *Early indications of prognosis in fulminant hepatic failure.* (Gastroenterology 1989) 97: 439–45

4 Gish RG, Lee, AH, Keeffe EB, et al. *Liver transplantation for patients with alcoholism and end-stage liver disease.* (Am J Gastroenterol 1993) 88: 1337–42

5 Mazzaferro V, Regalia E, Doci R, et al. *Liver transplantation for the treatment of small hepatocellular carcinomas in patients with cirrhosis.* (N Engl J Med 1996) 334: 693–9

6 Esquivel CO, Martinez O, Krams S, et al. *Liver transplantation at California Pacific Medical Center, San Francisco, California. Clinical Transplants 1994.* (Los Angeles: UCLA Tissue Typing Laboratory, 1994) 163–71

7 Lucey MR, Merion RM, Henley KS, et al. *Selection for and outcome of liver transplantation in alcoholic liver disease.* (Gastroenterology 1992) 102: 1736–41

8 Strasberg SM, Howard TK, Molmenti EP, et al. *Selecting of donor liver: risk factors for poor function after orthotopic liver transplantation.* (Hepatology 1994) 20: 829–38

9 Wood RP, Ozaki CF, Katz SM, et al. *Liver transplantation: the last ten years.* (Liver Transplant 1994) 74: 1133–54

10 Zetterman RK. *Primary care management of the liver transplant patient.* (Am J Med 1994) 96: 1A–10S

Cholelithiasis and cholecystitis

PETER F. MALET, M.D.

Key Points

1 There are two main types of gallstones: cholesterol and pigment. Pigment gallstones are further subdivided into black and brown varieties. The pathogenesis of cholesterol and pigment stones is different, but the clinical syndromes they cause are similar

2 Most gallbladder stones are asymptomatic. When they become symptomatic, biliary pain is the most common manifestation. Hallmarks of biliary pain are its episodic nature and location in the upper abdomen, usually in the right upper quadrant. Other conditions may coexist with gallstones and account for symptoms attributed initially to the stones

3 The treatment of choice for symptomatic gallbladder stones is laparoscopic cholecystectomy; when this approach is not feasible, open cholecystectomy is the alternative

4 Acute cholecystitis is the most common complication of gallstones. Cholescystectomy is the treatment of choice. Consultation among the internist, gastroenterologist, surgeon, and radiologist is frequently warranted in order to arrive at the most efficient plan for care

5 Acute acalculous cholecystitis requires a high index of suspicion for diagnosis; patients are usually quite ill, and rapid therapy is necessary

1 Gallstones: classification

- gallstones are common worldwide and, although mostly asymptomatic, can result in a wide spectrum of symptoms and presentations
- **there are two main types of gallstones: cholesterol and pigment**
- cholesterol and pigment stones have distinctly different compositions, pathogenesis, and clinical associations. Some gallstones do not readily fit into this classification
- in the USA and other Western countries, cholesterol stones comprise the great majority of stones in the gallbladder, generally 80–90% pigment stones comprise the remainder. In some South American countries, pigment stones are rare. In Japan, cholesterol stones are more common than pigment stones, while in other East Asian countries the proportion of pigment stones is significantly higher than in Western countries

A Cholesterol stones

- these are comprised primarily of cholesterol (proportion varies, generally >60%) and mucin, calcium salts of bilirubin, phosphate, carbonate and palmitate, and small amounts of various other substances. "Pure" (100%) cholesterol stones account for about 10–15% of all cholesterol stones
- some stones contain less than 60% cholesterol but have the morphologic and microstructural features of typical cholesterol stones; these are usually termed **mixed stones**

- major clinical associations with cholesterol stones:
  - aging
  - female gender
  - obesity
  - pregnancy
  - rapid weight loss
  - native American ethnicity

B Pigment stones

- these are comprised mostly of pigment and calcium salts
- **two types of pigment stones: black, brown**

1 **Black pigment stones**: black colored, comprised primarily of calcium bilirubinate and other pigment, mucin, calcium salts of phosphate and carbonate, and small amounts of various other substances. Found almost exclusively in the gallbladder and only rarely in the bile ducts
  - major clinical associations with black stones: the great majority of patients have no identifiable predisposing condition. The major known associated conditions are:
    - old age

- cirrhosis
- hemolysis (particularly sickle cell anemia and hereditary spherocytosis)
- possibly total parenteral nutrition (TPN)

2 **Brown pigment stones**: typically brown colored and comprised primarily of calcium bilirubinate, cholesterol, calcium palmitate, and small amounts of various other substances. Found mostly in the bile ducts and, in East Asia, frequently in the gallbladder as well; in Western countries, brown stones in the gallbladder are unusual

- most patients with brown stones in the bile ducts have stasis and/or infection as a predisposing condition. This type of stone may occur in patients many years post-cholecystectomy

The clinical syndromes caused by gallstones in the gallbladder are similar regardless of the type of stone involved

2 Formation of gallstones

A Cholesterol gallstones

1 Supersaturation of bile with cholesterol (cholesterol saturation index (CSI) >1.00) is a necessary but not sufficient condition. Also thought to be important are an absolute or relative increase in gallbladder mucin, other nucleating factors, and calcium ions and possibly a decrease in antinucleating factors. Gallbladder stasis plays a role in some cases

2 Initial events in cholesterol stone formation involve the nucleation of cholesterol monohydrate crystals from biliary cholesterol–phospholipid vesicles and formation of a stone nidus by an aggregation of calcium salts, pigment and/or mucin. The nucleation time of gallbladder bile (time to formation of cholesterol crystals) of patients with cholesterol stones is significantly shorter than that of normal controls

B Pigment gallstones

1 **Black pigment**: precipitation of calcium salts and pigment is the major pathophysiologic event. Failure to maintain calcium ions in solution is considered important, resulting in the precipitation of calcium bilirubinate, phosphate, and carbonate. Gallbladder mucin is thought to act as a nucleating factor, and other nucleating factors are postulated to be involved

2 **Brown pigment**: precipitation of calcium bilirubinate and calcium salts of fatty acids are the major pathophysiologic events. Studies in East Asians have shown that beta glucuronidase from bacterial or tissue sources is important in deconjugating bilirubin, resulting in its precipitation with calcium; an analogous process is thought to result in fatty acid precipitation. Biliary stasis and bacteria in bile are thought to be important for stone formation

3 Diagnosis

1 Ultrasonography is the primary method of diagnosis of gallbladder stones (sensitivity

approximately 95%). Ultrasonography can also visualize the bile ducts, liver, and pancreas and can thus provide valuable additional information

- while stones in the bile ducts may sometimes be demonstrated on ultrasonography (approximately 30% sensitivity) the principal method of demonstrating ductal stones is direct cholangiography, usually via endoscopic retrograde cholangiopancreatography (ERCP)
- less frequently, percutaneous transhepatic cholangiography (PTC) or intraoperative cholangiography, usually performed selectively during cholecystectomy, may also demonstrate ductal stones. Endoscopic ultrasonography (EUS) can demonstrate ductal stones with a sensitivity level approximating that of ERCP (≥90%)

2 Other radiologic studies may demonstrate gallstones and are useful in selected circumstances:
- about 15% of gallstones are radioopaque on plain abdominal X-rays
- computed tomographic (CT) scanning can often provide more extensive information than ultrasonography, but its sensitivity for detecting gallstones is significantly lower
- oral cholecystography is uncommonly used but can provide information on cystic duct patency and stone lucency or opacity in assessing patients for medical dissolution therapy with bile salts
- magnetic resonance cholangiography (MRC) is being investigated as a method of demonstrating ductal anatomy and stones

3 Diagnosis of "occult" lithiasis: infrequently, symptoms suggestive of gallstones are present, but ultrasonography is negative for stones. If the index of suspicion is high enough, microscopic examination of a bile sample collected via endoscopy for cholesterol crystals may be useful; finding such crystals is highly suggestive of the presence of stones. The significance of finding pigment crystals (granules) is less certain. EUS may provide useful information about sludge or stones in the gallbladder

4 Natural History

A Asymptomatic gallstones

The majority of patients with gallstones are asymptomatic and remain asymptomatic after decades of follow-up. The incidence rate at which asymptomatic patients develop biliary pain is approximately 1–2% annually. The risk of presenting initially with a complication rather than just biliary pain is very low. Because the rate of developing symptoms is low, the consensus is that asymptomatic patients with gallstones should not undergo prophylactic cholecystectomy

B Biliary pain

The term biliary pain is preferred to biliary colic, because biliary pain is not true colic. It is thought to arise from transient obstruction of the cystic duct by stones or sludge

1 Features
- typically characterized by its location in the right upper quadrant or epigastrium.

May radiate around to the right lower–mid back or occasionally to the right shoulder. Sometimes, the pain may be felt in the mid–lower chest

- the pain may range from mild to severe and may be described in various ways, for example, as crampy, pressure-like, toothachy, stabbing-like, like childbirth, or like a heavy weight. Patients often state that they cannot get comfortable during an attack and may walk around waiting for it to end. Some patients may experience nausea during an episode, but vomiting is uncommon. There are no systemic signs of toxicity

- usually has a definite onset, a duration of 15–30 minutes up to (most typically) 3–4 hours. Sometimes the duration may be 6–8 hours or more, but a duration over 12 hours is unusual unless acute cholecystitis is developing. After the pain abates, the patient may feel residual abdominal soreness for a while

- **typically episodic**
  the interval between episodes varies from daily to once every few months or even longer; some patients have only one episode every year or more. It is unusual for a patient to have only a single episode of biliary pain. In an individual patient, the interval between episodes tends to remain about the same over time

- **in many cases, biliary pain may not be as typical as that just described; it may be atypical in one or more features such as location, duration, or character**

- the term "chronic cholecystitis" is still used by clinicians to describe the condition in which a patient experiences repeated bouts of biliary pain. Strictly speaking, however, the term should be used to describe histologic changes in the gallbladder. There is frequently an inexact correlation between the pathologic changes in the gallbladder and clinical symptoms

- it is not unusual for a patient to present with vague abdominal or lower chest symptoms and gallstones, but the relationship, if any, between the stones and the symptoms is often not clear. In these cases, clinical judgment, further diagnostic testing, follow-up over time, and perhaps empiric treatment for gastroesophageal reflux or irritable bowel syndrome may clarify the clinical picture. In such cases decisions regarding cholecystectomy need to be considered carefully based on the patient's wishes and surgical consultation. If the stones are small enough, it may be judicious to consider an attempt at medical dissolution with ursodeoxycholic acid (see below)

2 Differential diagnosis

- Many conditions need to be considered in the differential diagnosis of right-upper-quadrant and epigastric abdominal pain:
  - peptic ulcer disease
  - choledocholithiasis
  - pancreatitis
  - gastroesophageal reflux
  - angina
  - bowel obstruction
  - liver-related conditions
  - lower rib pain

- irritable bowel syndrome
- nephrolithiasis
- usually, after a detailed history and physical examination, the differential diagnosis can be narrowed to a few leading possibilities

3 Natural history

- once a patient experiences the first episode of biliary pain, it is likely that subsequent episodes will occur. Approximately 75% of patients will have at least one additional attack within a 2-year period
- the risk of developing a serious complication (acute cholecystitis, pancreatitis, or cholangitis) in a patient who has experienced a first episode of biliary pain is approximately 1% per year of follow-up. This rate is approximately 2% per year if the patient has an occluded cystic duct on oral cholecystography

5 Elective Treatment of Gallbladder Stones: Surgical

- it is now generally agreed that cholecystectomy for asymptomatic gallstones is not warranted, with very few exceptions, subject to individual patient and physician preference. One exception is porcelain gallbladder (see below) because of the risk of cancer
- the threshold for performing cholecystectomy for abdominal symptoms atypical of biliary pain varies considerably among surgeons

A Elective surgery for biliary pain

- laparoscopic cholecystectomy (LC) is the treatment of choice for symptomatic gallstones. The timing of surgery is highly influenced by patient preference. In fact, many patients postpone surgery for months or even years
- consideration may have to be given to investigation for common bile duct (CBD) stones before elective cholecystectomy based on clinical, radiologic, and laboratory findings (see below)
- about 5% of planned laparoscopic cholecystectomies are converted to an open cholecystectomy at the surgeon's discretion, usually because of dense adhesions or other technical factors. Occasionally, an initial attempt at LC may be deemed inappropriate because of expected extensive right-upper-quadrant scarring due to previous surgery

B Investigation for stones in the bile duct in association with cholecystectomy

- about 5–10% of patients undergoing cholecystectomy will have stones in the bile duct, often asymptomatic. The decision to evaluate the patient preoperatively, intraoperatively, or postoperatively is based on a number of clinical factors. Currently, the standard approach to diagnosis is preoperative ERCP, although there are several alternative approaches

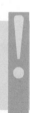

- the decision to investigate for CBD stones is straightforward when the patient has jaundice and a dilated CBD, on ultrasonography
- firm criteria that can be used to decide whether to evaluate the CBD in less straightforward cases have not been arrived at. The decision is influenced by the clinician's judgment, availability of ERCP, preference of the surgeon, and acceptance of the patient
- commonly accepted indications for CBD investigation pre LC are:
  - jaundice, significant elevations ($>3 \times$ the upper limit of normal) of serum alkaline phosphatase, aspartate aminotransferase, or alanine aminotransferase
  - dilated bile duct on ultrasonography
  - cholangitis
- the threshold for investigating for CBD stones before elective LC varies greatly among clinicians. Some clinicians favor an aggressive diagnostic approach and accept a high rate of negative results. Others favor a "wait-and-see" approach with rapid postoperative investigation if a CBD stone is suspected
- similarly, approaches vary among surgeons. Some prefer preoperative ERCP for suspected stones. Others favor routine or selective intraoperative cholangiography (IOC) via a catheter placed in the cystic duct. If IOC is positive for stones, ERCP postoperatively to remove the stones is the usual approach
- some surgeons can perform intraoperative cholangioscopy with a choledochoscope inserted through the cystic duct to find and remove CBD stones This approach is uncommon, however
- with open cholecystectomy, access to the common duct for direct cholangiography is simple and preoperative ERCP does not play much of a role

6 Elective Treatment of Gallbladder Stones: Medical

A Bile salts (ursodeoxycholicacid, or ursodiol, or chenodeoxycholic acid, or chenodiol)

- administered orally, these may be considered in patients who are at high surgical risk or who refuse surgery
- the cystic duct must be patent (usually determined by oral cholecystogram (OCG)) and the stones radiolucent. The complete dissolution rate for all patients is only 20–30%. The highest success rates (approximately 60–70%) are in patients with stones smaller than 5 mm in diameter. If the stones are floating on OCG, the dissolution rate is even higher. Oral dissolution therapy is not recommended for stones over 20 mm
- Patients with frequent or relatively severe biliary pain are not good candidates because 12–24 months are required for dissolution in most cases
- ursodiol is the agent of choice. Chenodiol is rarely used because of its side effects. The dose of ursodiol is 10 mg/kg/day; the usual total dose is either 600 or 900 mg daily. Side effects are uncommon; transient diarrhea may occur in <5%. Dissolution is monitored with periodic ultrasonography, generally every 6 months
- after complete dissolution, stones recur in about 50% of patients within 5 years

B Extracorporeal shock wave lithotripsy

- this is not performed in the USA but is available elsewhere. After lithotripsy, stone fragments are dissolved with oral bile salts. The main utility of lithotripsy is for single stones <20 mm in diameter, which have a dissolution rate of approximately 80%

C Percutaneous radiologic-guided extraction of gallbladder stones

- this is rarely used

7 Acute Complications of Gallstones

In managing acute gallstone complications, the pace of the diagnostic evaluation, the number and type of diagnostic studies, and the threshold for therapeutic intervention are dictated by the patient's overall condition.

A Acute cholecystitis

Acute cholecystitis is the most common acute complication of gallbladder stones and the leading indication for emergency cholecystectomy. Usually, the diagnosis is straightforward, but in some cases the presentation is atypical. The clinician should have a high index of suspicion for acute cholecystitis in any patient with abdominal pain

1 **Pathogenesis:** cystic duct obstruction is the precipitating event and usually caused by a stone; mucus, sludge, and viscous bile may also play a role. Bacteria are not involved in the initial events, although the inflamed gallbladder may later become secondarily infected. Lysolecithin, prostaglandins, and other substances that form as a result of stasis in the obstructed gallbladder lead to inflammation of the gallbladder wall; in addition, the normally protective mucus layer over the mucosal surface is disrupted, allowing relatively toxic bile salts to come in contact with the mucosa

2 **Presentation:** may range from deceptively mild to quite severe with systemic toxicity

- most patients present with moderate pain in the epigastrium or right upper quadrant, which may radiate to the right shoulder or scapula. The pain usually has been present for several hours, commonly 3–6 hours, before the patient presents to a physician. Many patients have nausea and some have vomiting, although rarely severe. They may be febrile, but usually not above 102° F; a higher fever suggests bacteremia or an abscess. There is right-upper-quadrant tenderness and often a Murphy's sign (accentuated tenderness to palpation during inspiration)

- in some cases, it may be difficult to determine if the patient has mild acute cholecystitis or a bout of prolonged biliary pain. Several hours of observation usually resolve the issue and, if there is still doubt, admission to the hospital for continued observation and testing is justified. In cases of prolonged biliary pain, cholecystectomy is still the treatment of choice

- Variations in the presentation of acute cholecystitis:
  - there may be no or minimal pain and tenderness, particularly in the elderly or an obtunded patient. Acute cholecystitis should be considered in all patients with unexplained bacteremia or sepsis, intra-abdominal abscess, and peritonitis
  - some patients present in a toxic manner with high fever, severe abdominal pain and tenderness, bacteremia, and marked leukocytosis. In such patients, the diagnosis may be made on clinical grounds. A confirmatory hepatobiliary scan or ultrasound examination may be warranted, unless surgery must be done urgently. When a suppurative complication such as an abscess is suspected, a CT scan is often useful
  - some patients present with signs and symptoms typical of biliary disease and decompensation of one or more organ systems or multisystem organ failure. In such cases, stabilization of the patient's overall medical condition takes precedence over cholecystectomy. In these cases, drainage of the gallbladder via cholecystostomy should be considered
  - patients with mild gangrene or necrosis of part of the gallbladder wall may not present differently from those with uncomplicated disease. With more extensive complications, such as empyema, gangrene, localized or free perforation, peritonitis, or emphysematous cholecystitis, the clinical presentation is usually severe with systemic toxicity. Such presentations represent a surgical emergency

3 Laboratory findings

- WBC count of 10–15,000/mm^3 is typical
- AST, ALT alkaline phosphatase, and bilirubin levels may be normal or just slightly elevated
- if the alkaline phosphatase is disproportionately elevated relative to the aminotransferases, choledocholithiasis should be considered and the diameter of the bile ducts should be determined by ultrasonography
- in about 10% of patients with obstructive CBD stones, the duct may not be dilated on ultrasonography, particularly early in the process or if obstruction is only partial. ERCP should be considered if the index of suspicion for obstruction is high, regardless of the ultrasound results
- some patients have serum amylase elevations, sometimes quite high (> 1000 units), without evidence of pancreatitis, although the latter should be considered

4 Diagnosis

- diagnosis of acute cholecystitis is based on the combination of characteristic clinical findings and confirmatory radiologic studies
- either ultrasonography or radionuclide hepatobiliary scanning with iminodiacetic acid derivatives (HIDA or DISIDA) may be used. Ultrasonography is preferred as the first test by most clinicians, since it provides additional information regarding the liver, bile ducts, pancreas, and other organs

a Hepatobiliary scanning

- performed by injecting a fasting patient with radiolabeled HIDA or DISIDA which is taken up by the liver and excreted into bile. Normally, the radionuclide enters the gallbladder and is excreted into the duodenum within 1–2 hours. With acute cholecystitis, the radionuclide fails to enter the gallbladder but does enter the duodenum (except with high-grade CBD obstruction)

- a "positive" scan (read after 3–4 hours after injection) reveals nonfilling of the gallbladder with excretion of the radionuclide into the small bowel
- if the gallbladder does not visualize by 1 hour, intravenous morphine may be administered in order to enhance gallbladder filling ("morphine-augmented hepatobiliary scanning")
- the sensitivity of hepatobiliary scanning for acute cholecystitis is approximately 95% and specificity 90%
- false-positive scans may occur in patients with gallbladder stasis; this can present a diagnostic problem in patients suspected of acute acalculous cholecystitis (see below)

b **Ultrasonography**

- signs of acute cholecystitis include gallstones, dilated gallbladder, thickened gallbladder wall, edema within the gallbladder wall, or pericholecystic fluid; sludge in the gallbladder may also be seen
- ultrasonography is more operator dependent than hepatobiliary scanning but provides more information, is more rapidly performed, and is generally available throughout the day and night. Dilatation of the bile duct can be detected on ultrasonography
- the sensitivity of ultrasonography for acute cholecystitis is approximately 90–95% and the specificity is 80%

5 **Management**

Measures to take within the first few hours after admission in patients with suspected acute cholecystitis	WBC count US or HIDA scan Surgical consultation

a **Initial treatment measures**

- usual practice is to administer antibiotics to all patients with acute cholecystitis. Coverage for enterococci and Gram-negative aerobic organisms is usually sufficient. In patients who are extremely toxic, coverage for anaerobic organisms is also judicious
- intravenous fluids must be started immediately. The patient may be dehydrated due to fever, lack of oral intake for a number of hours before admission, vomiting, vasodilation, etc.
- correct any electrolyte (particularly K, Mg, Ca and P) abnormality or acid/base imbalance
- keep patients nil by mouth; occasionally a nasogastric tube may be required if vomiting is severe
- mild analgesia may be necessary for pain, but symptoms and signs should not be masked

- medical treatment of associated medical conditions should be prompt and thorough, in anticipation of surgery

b **Course after hospital admission**

- most patients improve over 24–72 hours without surgical intervention. This allows time to optimize their fluid and electrolyte status and treat any other coexisting medical conditions before planned surgery
- some patients either do not improve after admission or worsen. In such cases, urgent surgery must be strongly considered. This decision is highly influenced by the patient's overall medical condition, particularly their cardiovascular, pulmonary, neurologic, and renal status
- if the patient has a seriously decompensated medical condition, such as congestive heart failure or pulmonary insufficiency, attention must be directed to this condition prior to surgery or another intervention. In such patients serious consideration must be given to either surgical or radiologic-guided cholecystostomy as a temporizing measure for relieving cholecystitis

6 Timing of surgery

- immediate surgical consultation should be obtained for patients with suspected acute cholecystitis. The diagnosis and decision to operate or not depend on the judgment of an experienced clinician

Treatment options for acute cholecystitis	laparoscopic cholecystectomy open cholecystectomy cholecystostomy – surgical or radiologic-guided

- Cholecystectomy may be performed as soon as the diagnosis is reasonably secure and the patient is stable enough to undergo the surgery. Generally, this is within the first 2–4 days after admission. In the great majority of cases, laparoscopic cholecystectomy is appropriate
- in cases in which a complication, such as an abscess, gangrenous wall, or perforation, has occurred or is suspected, an open cholecystectomy is warranted
- Patients with cirrhosis are at particularly high risk for surgery, and great attention to detail is required to optimize their medical status preoperatively. Transfusion of fresh frozen plasma may be necessary in order to correct severe coagulation defects (see Ch. 30)

B   Acute acalculous cholecystitis (AAC)

Acute cholecystitis may occur in the absence of gallstones in the gallbladder, in which case it is termed acalculous. AAC accounts for <5% of all cases of acute cholecystitis and is most frequently encountered in already hospitalized patients but is also seen in outpatients and those with AIDS

1 Pathogenesis: as with calculous disease, cystic duct occlusion is thought to be the principal pathophysiologic event. Ductal occlusion may be due to sludge, microlithiasis, viscous bile, or mucus and mural inflammation and edema. Gallbladder stasis is also a factor. Gallbladder ischemia is considered to play a significant role

- in patients with AIDS, infectious causes, especially viral, are common

2 **Clinical associations**: most common following nonbiliary tract surgery, severe burns, severe trauma, sepsis, use of TPN. Other associations include AIDS, vasculitis, allergic arteritis, and *Salmonella* infection

- sometimes no identifiable underlying condition is present

3 **Diagnosis**

- a high index of suspicion for AAC is warranted, since symptoms and signs may be less apparent than in calculous disease. This is particularly so in hospitalized patients with serious underlying disorders and on mechanical ventilation. Some patients may present with fever and bacteremia alone

- The diagnostic approach is similar to that for calculous cholecystitis but complicated by the fact that many patients with AAC are already seriously ill and may have atypical, masked, or minimal symptoms and signs. If AAC is suspected, diagnostic evaluation should be expeditious

- ultrasonography or HIDA scanning should be performed immediately if AAC is suspected. Ultrasonography may show sludge in the gallbladder lumen, in addition to the ultrasonographic signs of cholecystitis seen with calculous disease. HIDA scanning is positive in over 90% of patients with AAC

- a significant problem with the radiologic diagnosis of AAC is false-positive HIDA scanning. Nonfilling of the gallbladder occurs in many hospitalized patients as a result of gallbladder stasis. In such patients, a normal (filling) scan excludes AAC, but a positive scan needs to be interpreted in light of the clinical findings

- In cases in which diagnostic uncertainty exists despite HIDA scanning and ultrasonography, particularly if the patient is septic, a **diagnostic ultrasound-guided percutaneous puncture of the gallbladder** should be considered. If the aspirated bile suggests infection, a catheter can be left in place for gallbladder drainage, thus providing therapy as well

- AAC has a high mortality especially if treatment is delayed. Gangrene, perforation, and abscess of the gallbladder are more frequent than in calculous cholecystitis

4 **Treatment**

- medical measures are the same as for calculous cholecystitis; broad antibiotic coverage is indicated

- optimally, cholecystectomy should be performed without undue delay. An open approach is required more often than for calculous disease

- in patients too ill to undergo cholecystectomy, either surgical or radiologic-guided cholecystostomy for gallbladder drainage may be performed

- associated pericholecystic abscesses should be drained

8   Post-cholecystectomy Problems

- the term "post-cholecystectomy syndrome" has been used to describe persisting symptoms after cholecystectomy; it usually applies to patients who are past the immediate postsurgical period, so as not to be confused with immediate postsurgical incisional pain. The term is nonspecific and does not adequately convey the differential diagnosis in this setting; its continued use is to be discouraged
- most commonly persisting symptoms post-cholecystectomy are caused by a condition that the patient had prior to surgery that is not related to gallstones, such as gastroesophageal reflux, peptic ulcer, or irritable bowel syndrome
- other causes of symptoms after cholecystectomy include bile duct stones or stricture, pancreatitis, or other diagnoses missed at surgery such as colon or pancreatic cancer. Non-gastrointestinal causes may also be responsible. Gallstones spilled into the peritoneal cavity at LC may occasionally cause complications, most seriously abscess formation
- a careful history and physical examination can often narrow the differential diagnosis. It is important to ascertain whether the pain was present prior to surgery or not. Additional radiologic, endoscopic, or other studies may be necessary

9   Biliary Sludge

The same symptoms and complications that can occur with gallstones may also occur with biliary sludge, although probably less frequently

A   Definition

- the term sludge is used to describe microscopic agglomerations of cholesterol crystals, mucin, calcium bilirubinate, and other pigment crystals. Sometimes, microsepheroliths (microscopic gallstones) are also present
- the term **microlithiasis** is used to describe visible gallstones that are generally <2–3 mm in diameter and often not detectable by transabdominal ultrasonography or that may be interpreted as sludge (since stones this small usually do not demonstrate acoustic shadowing). Microlithiasis is often associated with sludge in the gallbladder
- sludge may also be found in the intra- or extrahepatic bile ducts, particularly when stasis is present

B   Formation

- little is known about the formation of gallbladder sludge; whether sludge is a prerequisite for the formation of stones is not clear. Once sludge has formed, it does not inevitably progress to stone formation
- in most cases of sludge, no definable clinical association is apparent. One predisposing condition is prolonged TPN. Pregnancy may also contribute to sludge formation, as may use of the antibiotic ceftriaxone

- the presumed mechanism for sludge formation is nucleation (precipitation) of cholesterol crystals in bile; gallbladder stasis probably plays a significant role in many cases. Factors that maintain calcium in solution may be disrupted in bile probably contributing to the precipitation of calcium bilirubinate

C Diagnosis

- the standard method is ultrasonography. Sludge appears as mobile echogenic material within the lumen without acoustic shadowing. A newer means for diagnosing sludge is with endoscopic ultrasonography, although the utility of this technique has not been thoroughly evaluated
- in selected cases, bile can be collected from the duodenum via endoscopy and examined for cholesterol or pigment crystals by light microscopy

D Natural history

- not well established. Spontaneous resolution and reappearance of sludge may occur over time
- gallbladder sludge may be associated with acute cholecystitis, acute cholangitis, and probably acute pancreatitis.

E Treatment

- depends on the clinical setting; is similar to the treatment of gallstones. In asymptomatic cases, observation alone is sufficient

10 Other less Common Syndromes Associated with Gallstones

- **hydrops** is noninflammatory distention of the gallbladder resulting from occlusion of the cystic duct by a stone or sludge. The clinical presentation of hydrops may vary from mildly symptomatic to severe pain caused by acute distention.
- calcification in the gallbladder wall (**porcelain gallbladder**) may develop over many years and, if dense enough, may be detected on plain abdominal X-rays or, if less dense, by CT scanning. Gallbladder carcinoma is found in a variable proportion of gallbladders with wall calcification. Prophylactic cholecystectomy has been recommended for patients with porcelain gallbladder
- **milk of calcium bile** is an unusual condition resulting from chronic occlusion of the cystic duct with subsequent increase in the calcium concentration in bile; the gallbladder becomes radioopaque on plain abdominal X-rays
- **Mirizzi syndrome** is the obstruction of the common hepatic duct as a result of extrinisic pressure by a gallstone in the cystic duct or the gallbladder neck. The clinical presentation is usually that of acute cholangitis. A high index of suspicion is essential to make the diagnosis
  - treatment is by cholecystectomy; as a temporizing measure in patients with severe cholangitis, drainage of the bile duct may be accomplished via either ERCP or PTC

- **fistulae between the gallbladder and other organs** may develop as a result of erosion of a gallstone through the gallbladder wall. The most common sites of fistulization are into the duodenum or colon; the pleura, bronchus, or other sites may also be involved. Occasionally, the fistula may develop between the common bile duct and another organ, usually the duodenum. The majority of gallbladder fistulae are not associated with a preceding history of acute cholecystitis. Cholecystoenteric fistulae may or may not require specific intervention depending on the patient's symptoms; for example, an asymptomatic fistula between the gallbladder and the duodenum does not necessitate further treatment

- **Gallstone ileus** is a bowel obstruction resulting from a stone, typically a fairly large one, which has eroded into (usually) the duodenum and has become impacted at the ileocecal valve or some other strictured area in the gastrointestinal tract leading to a mechanical obstruction. Gallstone ileus is not rare and most often affects older patients. The diagnosis should be suspected when air is found in the biliary tract, although absence of biliary air does not exclude the diagnosis. Treatment is as for other causes of bowel obstruction; underlying biliary disease may be managed electively or else need no further management

References

1   Malet PF. *Complications of cholelithiasis*. In: Kaplowitz N, (ed.). *Liver and Biliary Diseases*, 2nd edn. (Baltimore: Williams & Wilkins, 1996) 673–91

2   Diehl AK. *Epidemiology and natural history of gallstone disease*. (Gastroenterol Clin North Am 1991) 20: 1–19

3   Holzbach RT. *Cholesterol nucleation in bile*. (Ital J Gastroenterol 1995) 27: 101–5

4   Dahan P, Andant C, Lévy P, et al. *Prospective evaluation of endoscopic and microscopic examination of duodenal bile in the diagnosis of cholecystolithiasis in 45 patients with normal conventional ultrasonography*. (Gut 1996) 8: 277–81

5   Kadakia SC. *Biliary tract emergencies: acute cholecystitis, acute cholangitis and acute pancreatitis*. (Med Clin N Am 1993) 77: 1015–36

6   Erickson RA, Carlson B. *The role of endoscopic retrograde cholangiopancreatography in patients with laparoscopic cholecystectomies*. (Gastroenterology 1995) 109: 252–63

7   Shea JA, Berlin JA, Escarce JJ, et al. *Revised estimates of diagnostic test sensitivity and specificity in suspected biliary tract disease*. (Arch Int Med 1994) 154: 2573–81

8   French AL, Beaudet LM, Benator DA, Levy CS, Kass M, Orenstein JM. *Cholecystectomy in patients with AIDS: clinicopathologic correlations in 107 cases*. (Clin Infect Dis 1995) 21: 852–8

9   Tait N, Little JM. *The treatment of gall stones*. (Br Med J 1995) 311: 99–105

10 Lee SP, Maher K, Nicholls JF. *Origin and fate of biliary sludge*. (Gastroenterology 1988) 94: 170–6

Diseases of the bile ducts

IRA JACOBSON, M.D., F.A.C.P.
SRINIVAS CHANNAPRAGADA, M.D.

▼

Key Points

1 In recent years there has been a notable increase in the use of nonoperative techniques to treat diseases of the bile ducts. Foremost among these is endoscopic retrograde cholangio-pancreatography (ERCP) and its therapeutic applications, which include sphincterotomy and stent placement

2 Biliary diseases usually present with symptoms and signs related to ductal obstruction. These include pain, jaundice, pruritus, fever, and elevations in serum levels of liver function tests

3 Choledocholithiasis is the most common benign disorder of the biliary tree. Stones in the bile duct may be recognized on noninvasive imaging studies, or may require direct cholangiography for diagnosis. Endoscopic sphincterotomy is the most common technique used for removal for bile duct stones, either before or after cholecystectomy

4 Endoscopic intervention plays an important role in the diagnosis and treatment of complications of cholecystectomy, such as biliary leaks and strictures

5 Anatomic and congenital anomalies, such as choledochal cysts, can lead to jaundice, pancreatitis, and even biliary carcinoma if not recognized and treated properly

1 Bile Duct Stones

A Composition

1 **Stones originating from the gallbladder and migrating into the bile duct reflect the chemical composition of gallbladder stones, which are usually cholesterol rich. In contrast, stones forming primarily within the bile duct are usually pigment stones, composed predominantly of calcium bilirubinate**

2 Stones forming in the setting of chronic biliary stasis, such as those proximal to a stricture, are pigment stones, as are stones in patients with Oriental cholangiohepatitis (see below)

B Clinical presentation

1 In patients with intact gallbladders, the clinical presentation of gallstone disease may be dominated by symptoms and signs produced by stones in the bile duct

2 Patients who have undergone cholecystectomy may present within days after their operation, in which case bile duct stones were either unrecognized at the time of surgery or resulted from intraoperative migration of a stone from the gallbladder into the bile duct via the cystic duct

3 Patients may present with symptomatic choledocholithiasis decades after cholecystectomy (often to their disbelief). Stones in such patients may be numerous or large (up to 3–4 cm)

4 Presenting manifestations of bile duct stones include pain, fever, and chills, obstructive jaundice, and pancreatitis. **In general, obstructive jaundice from stones is accompanied by pain, while jaundice associated with malignancy is more likely to be painless.** However, patients with bile duct stones may occasionally present with painless jaundice, which is indistinguishable from the clinical presentation of patients with malignant biliary obstruction

5 Small gallstones pose a greater risk of pancreatitis than large stones because of easier migration through the cystic duct and greater likelihood of impaction near the pancreatic ductal orifice

6 Pain from bile duct stones often resembles pain of gallbladder origin, predominating either in the epigastrium or right upper quadrant. However, abdominal tenderness tends to be greater with cholecystitis because of the proximity of the gallbladder to the abdominal wall

7 The presentation of bile duct stones may be dominated by signs of infection. **Cholangitis** is much more frequent with bile duct stones than with malignant obstruction. The classic features of Charcot's triad – abdominal pain, fever and jaundice – may not all be present in patients with cholangitis. Overtly septic patients may present with marked hyperpyrexia with leukocytosis, rigors, shock, and obtundation. Such a picture is a life-threatening situation requiring immediate intervention

C Laboratory features

1 Most patients with symptomatic choledocholithiasis present with elevations in serum

liver function test levels. The course of these serum enzyme abnormalities depends to some extent on whether the stones remain impacted or whether they disimpact, either remaining in the duct without significantly obstructing bile flow or passing through the ampulla of Vater into the duodenum

2   Biochemical abnormalities include elevated alanine and aspartate aminotransferase (ALT and AST), alkaline phosphatase, and gamma glutamyltranspeptidase (GGTP) levels. Hyperbilirubinemia may be absent. Significant elevations in serum amylase signal the presence of concomitant pancreatitis (see below)

3   Early in the course of acute biliary obstruction, marked elevations in the serum ALT and AST may predominate over alkaline phosphatase and GGTP, particularly when cholangitis is present. Such elevations may cause diagnostic confusion with hepatocellular disease, such as viral hepatitis. Marked elevations in lactate dehydrogenase (LDH) occur concomitantly, but the alkaline phosphatase may initially be normal or nearly normal

4   A characteristic feature of the marked elevations in ALT and AST in acute biliary obstruction, in contrast to hepatitis, is their rapid rate of fall even in the face of persistent biliary obstruction. The aminotransferase levels fall as alkaline phosphatase and GGTP levels rise

5   Blood cultures must be obtained when signs of infection are present (fever, rigors, leukocytosis, etc.). Enteric Gram-negative bacteria or enterococci are the organisms usually implicated in cholangitis

D   Imaging studies

1   Ultrasonography and computed tomography (CT) may reveal dilated bile ducts, but the absence of ductal dilatation does not exclude choledocholithiasis

2   The yield of CT in visualizing common bile duct (CBD) stones directly is higher than that of ultrasonography.[1] The major limitation of ultrasonography is in visualization of the distal CBD. With both modalities, visualization of stones is better when the CBD is dilated. When CT is performed in patients in whom there is a high index of suspicion of bile duct stones, oral contrast should be avoided initially because it can obscure stones in the distal duct

3   Magnetic resonance cholangiopancreatography (MRCP), an adaptation of magnetic resonance imaging, has the potential to increase diagnostic yield over CT.[2] Imaging quality with this technique may prove sufficiently high that eventually MRCP may compete with ERCP as a diagnostic procedure of choice. Other than limited experience thus far, disadvantages of MRCP include its cost and lack of therapeutic capability

4   Endoscopic ultrasound (EUS) has demonstrated impressive sensitivity, rivaling that of ERCP.[3] Experience thus far is more extensive with radial sector than linear array instruments

5   **Direct cholangiography remains the definitive modality to diagnose bile duct stones.** The merger of diagnostic and therapeutic ERCP has led to the frequent performance of ERCP even when the existence of stones is already known or suspected from other imaging studies. At ERCP the size and number of stones can be clearly defined. Even when ultrasonography and CT reveal bile duct stones, they often underestimate their number

E   Treatment

1   In the past, standard treatment of bile duct stones was removal by open choledochotomy, either at the time of cholecystectomy or after the patient presented with symptomatic choledocholithiasis

2   **Since its introduction in the 1970s, endoscopic sphincterotomy has become the treatment of choice in most centers.** Advantages in postcholecystectomy patients include:
   - more rapid recovery and discharge from the hospital
   - less scarring
   - lower morbidity and mortality rates in old or high-risk patients

3   Before the advent of laparoscopic cholecystectomy in the late 1980s, a common practice was to extract symptomatic bile duct stones by ERCP before open cholecystectomy. The rationale was to spare the patient the additional surgical risk and potentially longer hospitalization associated with common duct exploration. Data from nonrandomized trials supported this practice.[4] However, randomized, controlled trials of ERCP followed by open cholecystectomy versus cholecystectomy plus common duct exploration did not reveal reductions in morbidity with the former approach, although in the largest study the length of hospitalization was reduced[5]

4   With the rapid dissemination of laparoscopic cholecystectomy, the two-step approach has been widely adopted because of the nearly universal preference for laparoscopic to open cholecystectomy (see Ch. 32)

5   Another common practice before the advent of laparoscopic cholecystectomy was to leave the gallbladder intact in high-risk patients when presenting symptoms were attributed to bile duct stones alone. Numerous studies of such patients indicated that the risk of requiring subsequent cholecystectomy was only 10–20% within 5–10 years. However, with the advent of laparoscopic cholecystectomy, the gallbladder is now removed more often than previously in such patients

6   Endoscopic sphincterotomy and stone extraction clear the bile duct successfully of stones in over 90% of patients. Several technical variations are employed by endoscopists:
   - when choledocholithiasis is known to be present, many endoscopists perform the initial cannulation with a sphincterotome
   - an increasingly popular approach has been to place a guidewire into the bile duct and advance a double-lumen sphincterotome over the wire. If the wire is insulated, sphincterotomy can be performed with the wire in place; otherwise, it must first be removed in order to avoid conducting current through the wire
   - when cannulation of the bile duct is difficult, many endoscopists resort to needle-knife sphincterotomy to open the duct. Success rates are high, although occasionally a second session may be required

7   Complications of ERCP and sphincterotomy:
   - **pancreatitis**: in 5%; may result from either the diagnostic portion of the procedure or from cautery-induced injury to the pancreatic ductal orifice. Symptoms may not occur until 8–12 hours following the procedure. Management is similar to that of other forms of pancreatitis
   - **bleeding**: in 2–3%; often self-limited but occasionally requiring blood

transfusions and even angiographic embolization or surgery. Local measures such as injection of epinephrine, balloon tamponade, or electrocautery may stop bleeding

- **perforation**: in 1%; results in retroperitoneal contamination. May be recognized during the procedure or hours later. Its presentation may be more subtle than pancreatitis, with less abdominal tenderness and more back pain. Retroperitoneal air may be recognized on plain films but CT may be required for diagnosis. Perforation often responds to nonsurgical management with nasogastric decompression, nasobiliary drainage (if the complication has been recognized during the ERCP), and broad-spectrum antibiotics. Surgery is required if signs of infection cannot be controlled with antibiotics

- **infection**: occurs only when adequate drainage is not provided following ERCP. If stones cannot be cleared after sphincterotomy, a nasobiliary tube or endoprosthesis should be placed to provide drainage until the duct can be cleared

8 Techniques to remove large common duct stones:
- mechanical lithotripsy
- extracorporeal shock wave lithotripsy
- laser lithotripsy
- electrohydraulic lithotripsy

Mechanical lithotripsy, which utilizes strong crushing baskets, may fail if the stone cannot be entrapped within the basket. Shock wave lithotripsy, which has fallen out of favor for gallbladder stones since the advent of laparoscopic surgery, is seldom used for CBD stones in the USA. Laser and electrohydraulic lithotripsy optimally use a "mother–baby" scope system, in which the fiber used for stone fragmentation is placed in direct proximity to the stone through a cholangioscope under direct visualization.

When these techniques fail or are unavailable, patients who are poor operative candidates can be managed with long-term placement of a stent in the bile duct. This approach carries a risk of complications, usually cholangitis, of 10–40% over the next 5–10 years.[6] It has been suggested that oral therapy of stented patients with the bile salt ursodeoxycholic acid for 6–12 months results in significant shrinkage or even dissolution of retained ductal stones, facilitating subsequent attempts to clear the duct after stents have been placed[7]

9 In good operative candidates, surgery should be performed for otherwise unextractable common duct stones

10 Oral dissolution therapy with bile salts is generally unacceptable for patients with common duct stones in the absence of sphincterotomy and stenting, because of poor efficacy and the time that would be required for dissolution to be achieved

11 There is now an overwhelming consensus that universal ERCP before cholecystectomy is inappropriate. Investigators have applied a variety of **criteria to select patients with a high likelihood of harboring bile duct stones**. These include:
- **persistent elevations of serum levels of liver function tests**. The course of liver test abnormalities over time is more useful than elevation above a cut-off value on a single occasion. Rapid normalization is associated with a low

likelihood of residual stones, while persistent elevations, particularly without a sharp trend toward normal, are often predictive of stones

- **dilatation of the bile duct on ultrasonography or CT**: more likely to be associated with choledocholithiasis than a duct of normal caliber; however, a dilated duct may lack stones and a nondilated duct may contain them
- **common bile duct stones seen on ultrasonography or CT**: a strong indication for pre-laparoscopy ERCP. Occasionally, however, cholangiography may fail to reveal stones that were visualized on a noninvasive study. In this situation, judgment is required in deciding whether to perform a sphincterotomy despite the negative cholangiogram. Occasionally, sweeping the duct with a balloon after sphincterotomy does result in extraction of small stones that were not appreciated on cholangiography.
- **mode of presentation**: patients presenting with cholangitis are more likely to have persistent ductal stones than those who present with transient pain

12 **Severe cholangitis is an indication for urgent ERCP**, which has been shown to be superior to emergency surgery in a randomized trial[8]

F Gallstone pancreatitis

1 Related to impaction of a stone in the ampulla of Vater with occlusion of the pancreatic ductal orifice

2 Clinical features at presentation:
- epigastric pain which may be severe and radiates directly into the back
- nausea and vomiting
- low-grade fever
- tachycardia
- hypotension, if there has been significant "third-spacing" of fluid

3 Laboratory features:
- leukocytosis
- elevated liver function tests (usually to a greater degree than in alcoholic and other causes of pancreatitis)
- elevated serum amylase and lipase levels
- elevated blood urea nitrogen and creatinine if there is sufficient third-spacing to compromise renal blood flow
- hypocalcemia in moderate to severe cases
- hypoxemia in more severe cases; due to pulmonary capillary leak, which may result in adult respiratory distress syndrome

4 Various criteria have been proposed to predict the severity of an episode of pancreatitis. The most widely used classification system, either in original or modified form, is that based on "the Ranson criteria"[9]

5 Medical treatment of gallstone pancreatitis is similar to that for other forms of pancreatitis:
- strict nil by mouth status
- intravenous hydration
- careful recording of intake and output

- intravenous antibiotics are recommended to prevent cholangitis or pancreatic abscess, although their efficacy to prevent abscesses has been the subject of debate for years. Their use is supported by a recent study demonstrating the benefit of imipenem[10]
- monitoring of laboratory data, including blood counts and electrolytes
- serial CT scans to monitor patients with moderate or severe pancreatitis for the development of pancreatic necrosis, pseudocysts, or abscesses

6 **Patients with mild gallstone pancreatitis do not benefit from emergent ERCP. However, patients with gallstone pancreatitis that is predicted to be severe have an increased rate of retained ductal stones. They have a reduced risk of local and systemic complications, and shorter hospitalizations, when ERCP and stone extraction are performed early in their course.**[11] They also have a reduced risk of developing cholangitis[12]

7 Because stones that cause pancreatitis are usually small and impacted in the distal bile duct, they have a better chance of migrating into the duodenum than larger stones that have become impacted more proximally in the bile duct. In fact, most patients (80–90%) with self-limited gallstone pancreatitis pass their gallstones and do not require ERCP before cholecystectomy

8 Concomitant pancreatitis and cholangitis is a strong indication for urgent ERCP and sphincterotomy

2   Postcholecystectomy Syndrome

A   Definition

Biliary-type pain in a patient who has undergone cholecystectomy

B   Differential diagnosis

1 In addition to common bile duct stones, several nonbiliary entities require consideration in such patients:
- irritable bowel syndrome
- gastroesophageal reflux
- esophageal spasm
- peptic ulcer disease
- chronic pancreatitis

C   Sphincter of Oddi dysfunction

1 When the above conditions are excluded, attention focuses on the sphincter of Oddi, which may be affected by either stenosis or spasm, resulting in episodic or constant partial biliary obstruction. Since the papilla of Vater is visually normal in most patients with sphincter of Oddi dysfunction, three criteria have been applied to postcholecystectomy patients:
- bile duct dilation on ultrasonography, CT, or direct cholangiography
- delayed drainage of contrast from the bile duct beyond 45 minutes after ERCP
- elevated liver enzymes, especially on repeated occasions

2 When all three of the above criteria are met in postcholecystectomy patients with biliary-type pain, sphincter of Oddi dysfunction as defined by manometric studies is usually present and these patients respond well to endoscopic sphincterotomy[13] Thus, manometry is not required in such patients

3 When patients with pain have only one or two of the above criteria, only about half have manometric abnormalities (i.e., elevated basal sphincter pressure above 40 mmHg). When manometric abnormalities are present, patients have a good long-term response to sphincterotomy. Thus, manometry is considered important in planning management

4 Postcholecystectomy patients with biliary pain alone also have manometric abnormalities in up to 50% of cases, but their response to sphincterotomy has not been studied as rigorously. Treatment decisions in such patients must be individualized

5 Sphincter of Oddi manometry is unavailable in many centers where ERCP is performed and carries a higher risk of pancreatitis than does diagnostic ERCP alone. This has stimulated interest in the development of noninvasive imaging techniques. Nuclear hepatobiliary (e.g., DISIDA) scanning has been reported to be useful by some investigators, but is generally an insufficient test on which to base major therapeutic decisions

6 Manometric sphincter of Oddi dysfunction has been described in patients with intact gallbladders. When patients with intolerable right-upper-quadrant pain and no gallstones or other identifiable pathology require intervention, the dilemma faced by the physician is whether to remove the gallbladder, perform sphincterotomy if sphincter of Oddi pressures are abnormal, or do nothing. More long-term data on the efficacy of sphincterotomy in this group of patients are required before this approach can be adopted on a widespread scale

3 Postoperative Bile Duct Injuries

A Introduction

1 Perhaps the only negative aspect of the increased use of laparoscopic cholecystectomy is the concomitant increase in the incidence of operative biliary tract injuries, resulting in leaks and/or strictures. Such complications occur in 0.2–0.5% of laparoscopic cholecystectomies, with some relationship to the experience of the surgeon

2 Bile leaks may result in acute illness from intraperitoneal bile collections. However, the most dreaded complication of major bile duct injury is long-term obstruction of bile flow with recurrent cholangitis, liver atrophy, and/or secondary biliary cirrhosis

B Classification

1 Biliary tract injuries during cholecystectomy may result in:
- leakage of bile without interruption of ductal continuity
- injury to one or more ducts with impairment or complete interruption of bile flow but without bile leak
- combined bile leak and damage to a duct resulting in interrupted bile flow

2 A useful classification system for bile duct injuries was proposed recently by Strasberg et al. (1995)[14]

- **Type A**: bile leak from a minor duct with preservation of continuity between the liver and duodenum. Most commonly, this involves a bile leak from the cystic duct remnant. Less commonly, there can be a leak from an accessory duct connecting the gallbladder to the liver bed (duct of Luschka)
- **Type B**: occlusion of the right hepatic duct or one of its branches because it was mistaken for the cystic duct during cholecystectomy. This occurs because, in some people, the cystic duct joins the right hepatic duct rather than the common duct
- **Type C**: transection rather than occlusion of an aberrant right hepatic duct, resulting in bile leak
- **Type D**: lateral injury to an extrahepatic bile duct with preserved communication between the biliary tree and duodenum
- **Type E**: occlusive injury to the common bile duct at any level from the hepatic bifurcation to the duodenum

C   Diagnosis

1 Recognition of injury may occur intraoperatively or may be delayed for days, months, or even years

2 Bile leaks present with pain, low-grade fever, abdominal tenderness, leukocytosis, mild abnormalities of liver function tests including bilirubin (as high as 2–3 mg/dL). Overt jaundice is more common with major occlusive injuries of the bile duct. Additional features of the latter include pruritus and signs of infection

3 When a bile leak is suspected, ultrasonography or CT establishes the presence of an intraperitoneal fluid collection. The possibility of an ongoing leak is evaluated with a nuclear DISIDA scan, which may whether a leak is from the hepatic bed or the cystic duct remnant

4 ERCP is required for precise localization as well as therapy (see below)

5 Direct cholangiography by ERCP or percutaneous transhepatic cholangiography (THC) is necessary to delineate all major bile duct injuries. ERCP is the preferred modality and usually suffices, but there are two situations in which THC may be necessary:

- involvement of the biliary tree above the hepatic bifurcation, in which case delineation of the proximal extent of the injury can best be accomplished by THC
- any suspicion of an excluded segment of the biliary tree with absent communication between a portion of the liver (usually part of the right lobe) and the distal bile duct

D   Management

1 **The cornerstone of therapy for biliary leaks is to reduce outflow resistance into the duodenum, thereby minimizing flow of bile through the leak and allowing it to seal**. This can be accomplished by sphincterotomy and stent placement or even stent placement alone

2 If a leak results in a large bile collection, percutaneous or operative drainage may be required

3 Although many bile collections from leaks are uninfected, it is prudent to administer antibiotics until the leak is controlled or drained

4 Surgical treatment of major injuries usually consists of ligation of the bile duct and creation of a Roux-en-Y connection between the proximal biliary tract (common hepatic duct or left and right hepatic ducts) and jejunum. Small lateral injuries to the bile duct may be repaired by suturing the bile duct over a T-tube. In contrast, complete transection of the bile duct recognized during surgery and treated by suturing over a T-tube is rarely successful in the long term

5 There is controversy about the role of endoscopic therapy of benign bile duct strictures resulting from operative injury. Reports of successful therapy emphasize the use of indwelling stents, with exchanges every 3–6 months, for a year or more. Two large series differ on the need for balloon dilation prior to stent placement.[15,16] The two studies agree, however, that good long-term results can be achieved in 80–85% of patients. In a retrospective comparison of patients treated with surgery or endoscopy for a mean of 4 years, results were similar.[16] However, no prospective randomized trials have been conducted

4 Oriental Cholangiohepatitis

A Overview

1 A syndrome characterized by primary intrahepatic stones associated with strictures of the intrahepatic ducts

2 Seen predominantly in Far Eastern Asian populations; rare in the USA

3 Most primary intrahepatic duct stones are composed predominantly of calcium bilirubinate

B Pathogenesis

1 Although not necessarily a prerequisite for the formation of primary intrahepatic stones, bacterial infection of the bile is associated with this syndrome. Bacterial beta glucuronidases hydrolyze conjugated bilirubin. Unconjugated bilirubin binds with calcium and precipitates as calcium bilirubinate, the chief constituent of intrahepatic stones

2 Parasitic infections with agents such as *Ascaris* or *Clonorchis* have long been invoked in the pathogenesis of the syndrome, but such infections are not demonstrable in some patients

3 An excess of rural over urban patients in endemic countries has led to speculation that the low-protein diet prevalent in rural areas decrease glucurolactone, a beta glucuronidase inhibitor, in bile. This promotes enhanced endogenous beta glucuronidase activity with further deconjugation of bilirubin, leading to precipitation of calcium bilirubinate[17]

C Presentation

1 The syndrome becomes manifest at younger ages than Western gallstone disease and may affect children and young adults

2 Clinical features include abdominal pain, fever, and jaundice. The frequency with which the syndrome presents with infection has led to the common use of the term "recurrent pyogenic cholangitis." Potential long-term consequences include liver abscesses and atrophy of affected segments of the liver

3 Laboratory features include leukocytosis when infection is present and cholestatic liver function test abnormalities

D   Diagnosis

Ultrasonography and CT may reveal focal areas of dilated intrahepatic bile ducts as well as stones. Definitive diagnosis requires ERCP or THC

E   Treatment

1 Broad-spectrum antibiotics to treat episodes of acute cholangitis

2 Long-term relief involves various surgical options that must be tailored to the individual patient:

- resection of atrophic hepatic segments and the diseased ducts draining that portion of the liver
- anastomosis of jejunum to intrahepatic segments proximal to sites of obstruction, when possible
- creation of permanent access through which choledochoscopy, balloon dilatation, and stone extraction can be performed repeatedly. Such access can be provided via a T-tube tract or a loop of jejunum brought to a subcutaneous site to which the bile duct has been anastomosed

3 Endoscopic therapy of Oriental cholangiohepatitis may be difficult because of the proximal location of strictures and stones, although successful endoscopic therapy has been described.[18] Percutaneous techniques are generally preferred to an endoscopic approach

5   Choledochal Cysts

A   Introduction

1 Anomalies of the biliary tree characterized by cystic dilation of variable portions of the intra- and/or extrahepatic ducts.

2 More common in Asia; female-to-male preponderance of 3 : 1

3 Primarily a disease of children and young adults, but reported age range varies widely

4 Conservative management carries significant morbidity and mortality. With surgical management the vast majority of patients have good long-term results

B   Etiology

Proposed theories include:

- Abnormality in biliary epithelial proliferation when the fetal ducts are solid, resulting in an abnormally dilated proximal duct and a more normal or stenotic

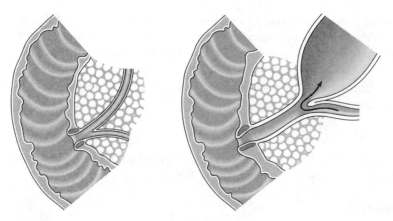

Fig. 33.1 The normal anatomy (left) contrasted with the anomalous pancreaticobiliary function (arrow) believed to be responsible for free reflux of pancreatic enzymes and choledochal cyst formation (Modified from O'Neill 1992[19])

distal portion.[20] A role for obstruction by distal common bile duct stenosis in inducing proximal cystic dilatation has been supported by other authors[21,22]

- intrinsic autonomic dysfunction, based on the finding of deficient postcholinergic neurons in some portions of the cyst wall[23]
- anomalous pancreaticobiliary junction, which is particularly common in type I cysts but not seen with types II, III and V (see below), may result in lack of normal sphincter function and reflux of pancreatic enzymes into biliary ducts causing progressive damage to, and dilatation of, the bile duct (see Fig. 33.1)[24]

C Classification

The classification of Todani et al. (1977)[25] is used most often (see Fig. 33.2):

Type I (A, B, C) – dilatation of the extrahepatic duct alone, by far the most common type of choledochal cyst

Type II – a diverticulum of the extrahepatic bile duct

Type III – choledochocele, involving only the intraduodenal duct

Type IVA – multiple extra and intrahepatic cysts

Type IVB – multiple extrahepatic cysts only

Type V – Caroli's disease – single or multiple intrahepatic cysts

D Clinical symptoms and signs

1 Right-upper-quadrant pain
2 Jaundice (often the sole symptom in infants)
3 Palpable abdominal mass
4 Fever
5 Epigastric or diffuse abdominal pain, if pancreatitis present

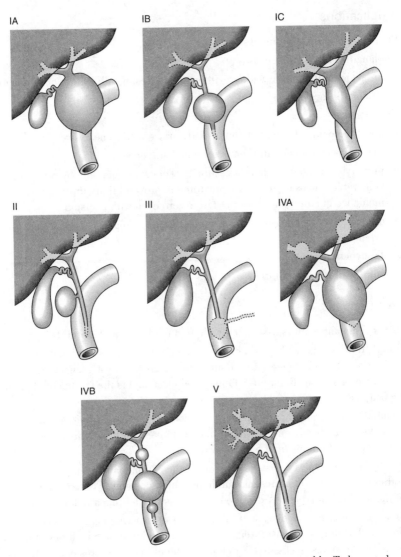

Fig. 33.2   Classification scheme of choledochal cysts suggested by Todano et al. (Modified from Savader et al. 1991[26])

E   Diagnosis

1   Noninvasive modalities including ultrasonography and CT may initially reveal or suggest diagnosis

2   Direct cholangiography by ERCP or THC is usually diagnostic, important for classification (see above) and planning therapy

3   THC may be important for delineating proximal biliary anatomy or providing drainage

4   ERCP has the advantage of evaluating the pancreatic duct and pancreatic–biliary junction, including an anomalous junction when present

F   Complications

1   Stone formation within the cysts
2   Cholangitis and liver abscesses
3   Acute pancreatitis, either with or without stones, especially with a choledochocele
4   Secondary biliary cirrhosis
5   Carcinoma
   • a well-recognized complication; usually arises within the cysts.
   • the risk is significant after nonresectional surgery[27]
   • primary excision of cysts reduces the risk of cancer not only by removing the vulnerable mucosa but also by providing improved biliary drainage. However, the incidence of carcinoma does not fall to zero even with excision
   • preoperative diagnosis of cancer is rare, and the prognosis is poor because of extensive spread
6   Portal hypertension
7   Rupture with bile peritonitis

G   Treatment

1   Medical management is associated with high morbidity and mortality
2   Simple drainage is inadequate. Excision followed by reconstruction of the biliary tree is the procedure of choice rather than simple drainage. Cyst excision with biliary tract reconstruction (Roux-en-Y hepaticojejunostomy) is the treatment of choice for types I and II cysts
3   In addition to various operations for choledochoceles, endoscopic management by sphincterotomy has been described. In one study[28] 7 of 8 patients remained symptom-free for a mean of 5 years
4   Management of type IV cysts is excision of the extrahepatic cyst, partial resection of intrahepatic cysts when present, and hepaticojejunostomy. Predominant involvement of the left lobe in type IVA disease may necessitate left hepatic lobectomy.
5   Management of type V disease (Caroli's disease) is partial hepatectomy for localized disease. For diffuse disease, Roux-en-Y hepaticojejunostomy with placement of transhepatic stents is effective[29] Recurrent stones and strictures can be treated by percutaneous techniques. Liver transplantation may be required for severe diffuse disease

References

1   Amouyal P, Amouyal G, Levy P et al. *Diagnosis of choledocholithiasis by endoscopic ultrasonography.* (Gastroenterology 1994) 106: 1062–7

2   Soto JA, Barish MA, Yucel EK et al. *Magnetic resonance cholangiography: comparison with endoscopic retrograde cholangiopancreatography.* (Gastroenterology 1996) 110: 589–97

3   Prat F, Amouyal G, Amouyal P et al. *Prospective controlled trial of endoscopic ultrasonography and endoscopic retrograde cholangiography in patients with suspected common bile duct lithiasis.* (Lancet 1996) 347: 75–9

4   Heinerman PM, Boeckl O, Pimpl W et al. *Selective ERCP and preoperative stone removal in bile duct surgery.* (Ann Surg 1989) 209: 267–72

5 Neoptolemos JP, Carr-Locke DL, Fossard DP, et al. *Prospective randomised study of preoperative endoscopic sphincterotomy versus surgery alone for common bile duct stones.* (Br Med J 1987) 294: 470–4

6 Bergman JJGHM, Rauws EAJ, Tijssen JGP, et al. *Biliary endoprostheses in elderly patients with endoscopically irretrievable common bile duct stones: report on 117 patients.* (Gastrointest Endosc 1994) 42: 195–201

7 Johnson GK, Geenen JE, Venu RP, et al. *Treatment of non-extractable common bile duct stones with combination of ursodoxycholic acid plus endoprostheses.* (Gastrointest Endosc 1993) 39: 528–31

8 Lai ECS, Mok FPT, Tan ESY, et al. *Endoscopic biliary drainage for severe acute cholangitis.* (N Engl J Med 1992) 326: 1582–6

9 Ranson JHC, Rifkind KM, Roses DF, et al. *Prognostic signs and the role of operative management in acute pancreatitis.* (Surg Gynecol Obstet 1974) 139: 69

10 Pederzoli P, Bassi C, Vesentini S, et al. *A randomized multicenter clinical trial of antibiotic prophylaxis of septic complications in acute necrotizing pancreatitis with imipenem.* (Surg Gynecol Obstet 1993) 176: 480–3

11 Neoptolemos JP, Carr-Locke DL, London et al. *Controlled trial of urgent endoscopic retrograde cholangiopancreatography and endoscopic sphincterotomy versus conservative treatment for acute pancreatitis due to gallstones.* (Lancet 1988) ii: 979–83

12 Fan ST, Lai ECS, Mok FPT, et al. *Early treatment of acute biliary pancreatitis by endoscopic papillotomy.* (N Engl J Med 1993) 328: 228–32

13 Geenen JE, Hogan WJ, Dodds WJ, et al. *The efficacy of endoscopic sphincterotomy after cholecystectomy in patients with sphincter of Oddi dysfunction.* (N Engl J Med 1989) 320: 82–7

14 Strasberg S, et al. *Biliary injury during laparoscopic cholecystectomy.* (Surg Gynecol Obstet 1995) 180: 101–25

15 Geenen DJ, Hogan WJ, Geenen JE, et al. *Long-term follow-up in endoscopic therapy of benign bile duct strictures.* (Gastroenterology 1995) 108: A415

16 Davids PHP, Tanka AKF, Rauws EAG, et al. *Benign biliary strictures: surgery or endoscopy?* (Ann Surg 1993) 217: 237–43

17 Kim MH, Sekijima J, Lee SP. *Primary intrahepatic stones.* (Am J Gastroenterol 1995) 90: 540–7

18 Sperling RM, Koch J, Harris H, et al. *Role of therapeutic ERCP in the management of recurrent pyogenic cholangitis (RPC).* (Gastrointest Endosc 1995) 41: 417 (abstract)

19 O'Neill JA. *Choledochal cysts.* (Curr Prob Surg 1992) 29: 365–410

20 Yotuyanagi S. *Contribution to aetiology and pathology of idiopathic cystic dilatation of the common bile duct with report of three cases: new aetological theory based on supposed unequal epithelial proliferation at stage of physiological epithelial occlusion of primitive choledochus.* (Gann 1936) 30: 601–50

21 Ito, et al. (Z Kinderchir 1984) 39: 40–5

22 Suda K, Matsumoto Y, Miyam T. *Narrow duct segment distal to choledochal cyst.* (Am J Gastroenterol 1991) 86: 1259–63

23 Kusunoki, et al. *Choledochal cysts: oligoganglionosis in the narrow portion of the choledochus.* (Arch Surg 1988) 123: 984–6

24 Babbitt DP, Starshak RJ, Clemett AR. *Choledochal cyst: a concept of etiology.* (Am J Roentgenol Rad Ther 1973) 119: 57–62

25 Todani T, Watanabe Y, Narusue M, et al. *Congenital bile duct cysts: classification, operative procedures, and review of thirty-seven cases, including cancer arising from the choledochal cyst.* (Am J Surg 1977) 134: 263–69

26 Savader SJ, Benenati JF, Venbrux AC, et al. *Choledochal cysts: classification and cholangiographic appearance.* (Am J Rad 1991) 156: 328

27 Flannigan DP. *Biliary carcinoma associated with biliary cysts.* (Cancer 1977) 40: 880–3

28 Venu RP, Geenen JE, Itogen WJ et al. *Role of endoscopic retrograde cholangiopancreatography in the diagnosis and treatment of choledochocele.* (Gastroenterology 1984) 87: 1177–9

29 Doty JE, Tompkins RK. *Management of cystic disease of the liver.* (Surg Clin N Am 1989) 69: 285–95

30 Freeman ML, Nelson DB, Sherman S, et al. *Complications of endoscopic biliary sphincterotomy.* (N Engl J Med 1996) 335: 909–18

31 Lillemoe KD, Pitt HA, Cameron JL. *Current management of benign bile duct strictures.* (Adv Surg 1992) 25: 119–74

32 Lopez RR, Pinson CW, Campbell JR, et al. *Variation in management based on type of choledochal cyst.* (Am J Surg 1991) 161: 612–15

Tumors of the biliary tract

KEITH D. LILLEMOE, M.D.

▼

Key Points

1 Polypoid lesions of the gallbladder larger than 1 cm should be treated by cholecystectomy

2 Carcinoma of the gallbladder, due to its late stage of presentation, has an overall 5-year survival of <5%

3 Aggressive surgical resection, including partial hepatectomy, may result in increased survival in patients with cancers limited to the gallbladder wall

4 Cholangiocarcinoma is strongly associated with cystic disease of the biliary tree (choledochal cysts, Caroli's

disease), Clonorchis infection, sclerosing cholangitis, and hepatolithiasis.

5 Proximal (hilar) cholangiocarcinomas have an overall poor survival, although aggressive resection that includes hepatectomy to achieve negative margins may improve the outcome

6 Distal bile duct tumors, which present similarly to other periampullary malignancies, have a higher rate of resectability and better long-term survival than more proximal cholangio-carcinomas

▲

1 Benign Tumors of the Gallbladder

A Pseudopolyps

- represent the most commonly observed "polypoid" lesion of the gallbladder accounting for 52% of such lesions
- not a true neoplasm but rather cholesterol-filled projections of gallbladder mucosa protruding into the lumen
- usually less than 1 cm in size; visualized on gallbladder imaging studies (ultrasound, oral cholecystogram) as nonmobile filling defects
- usually asymptomatic unless associated with gallstones
- do not have malignant potential

B Adenomyosis

- consists of a thickened gallbladder muscular layer with Rokitansky–Aschoff sinuses
- three types: fundal (most common), appearing as a hemispheric lesion with a central dimple; segmental, consisting of an annular stricture; or diffuse, involving the entire gallbladder
- may represent muscular hypertrophy secondary to biliary dyskinesia; therefore, symptoms are relieved by cholecystectomy
- may be associated with carcinoma of the gallbladder

C Adenomas

- represent true neoplastic epithelial tumors of gallbladder mucosa
- usually solitary, nonmobile filling defects seen on gallbladder ultrasound or oral cholecystogram
- premalignant with carcinoma in situ found in larger polyps
- unlikely to play a major role in the overall pathogenesis of gallbladder cancer

D Treatment

1 **since histology of polypoid lesions of the gallbladder cannot be determined nonoperatively by current methods, patients with polyps greater than 1 cm should undergo cholecystectomy**

2 Polyps 0.5 cm or less in size should be followed by repeat imaging studies every 3–6 months

3 Any patient with biliary symptoms and a gallbladder polyp should undergo cholecystectomy

2 Benign Tumors of the Bile Duct

- benign bile duct tumors are much less common than benign gallbladder tumors
- histologic types:

a papillomas

b adenomas

c cystadenomas – tumors with inner layers of mucin-secreting epithelium, a mesenchymal stroma, and an outer layer of hyalinized fibrous tissue

- may be solitary or multiple
- symptoms are usually due to bile duct obstruction: intermittent jaundice or cholangitis
- diagnosis is usually made by either endoscopic retrograde cholangiography or percutaneous transhepatic cholangiography
- treatment consists of surgical resection, most commonly with hepaticojejunostomy for reconstruction
- both benign cystadenomas and multiple papillomatosis of the bile duct can be associated with a high rate of local recurrence

3 Carcinoma of the Gallbladder

A Incidence

1 The most common biliary tract malignancy; the fifth most common gastrointestinal cancer (3–4% of gastrointestinal tumors)

2 The incidence has increased as the population has aged. Currently, 6000–7000 new cases are diagnosed each year (2.5 cases/100,000 population)

3 Female/male ratio of 3 : 1

4 Usual age of onset is sixth or seventh decade of life

5 An increased incidence is seen in southwestern American Indians, Alaskans, Mexicans, Hispanics living in the USA, and in northern Japan, Israel and Chile

6 A markedly lower incidence is seen in African–Americans and in India, Nigeria, and Singapore

B Etiology

Risk factors for gallbladder carcinoma

- gallstones
- choledochal cysts
- anomalous junction of the pancreatic and bile ducts
- carcinogens
- estrogens
- typhoid carrier
- porcelain gallbladder
- gallbladder polyps

1 **Gallstones**
- Present in over 90% of patients with gallbladder carcinoma; conversely, only 1% of patients with gallstones have gallbladder carcinoma.
- larger stones (>3 cm) are associated with a 10-fold increase in gallbladder cancer
- role of gallstones in the development of gallbladder cancer is likely related to chronic irritation and inflammation
- gallstone composition does not seem to affect pathogenesis

2 **Choledochal cysts**
- Associated with carcinomas throughout the biliary tract including the gallbladder
- risk increases with age
- risk may be related to association of an anomalous pancreaticobiliary duct junction frequently seen with choledochal cysts
- Surgical removal of the choledochal cyst and the gallbladder is recommended to prevent further reflux and stasis and to eliminate cancer risk

3 **Anomalous pancreaticobiliary duct junction**
- type 3B anomalies, with a long common channel of the pancreatic and common bile duct, appear to be associated with a significantly increased risk of gallbladder cancer
- reflux of pancreatic juice into the biliary tree or bile stasis are proposed mechanisms

4 **Carcinogens**
- industrial exposure – rubber industry
- animal studies – azotoluene, nitrosamines

5 **Estrogens**: an epidemiologic association; may simply be related to increased incidence of gallstones

6 **Typhoid carriers**: likely due to chronic irritation and inflammation

7 **Porcelain gallbladder**: calcification of gallbladder wall constitutes an indication for cholecystectomy, even in asymptomatic patients

8 **Gallbladder polyps**
- clear premalignant potential for adenomas and adenomyosis
- cholecystectomy indicated for any polyp greater than 1 cm

C **Pathology and staging**

1 **Histologic type**
- adenocarcinoma
  - scirrhous (65%) – infiltrating, 90% desmoplastic, obliterates gallbladder lumen, invades liver
  - papillary (15%) – polypoid, slow growing, late to metastasize
  - colloid (10%) – soft, gelatinous, mucinous tumors filling gallbladder
- anaplastic – 5%
- squamous (adenosquamous) – 5%

2 **Routes of spread**
- Primarily by local extension, although disseminated disease can occur.

- lymphatic drainage is first to the adjacent lymph node basins – cystic duct, pericholedochal, and hilar lymph nodes. Secondary basins include the retropancreatic, celiac axis, and periaortic nodes
- the veins of the gallbladder drain directly to the liver parenchyma and to branches of the portal vein of segments V and VIII
- direct invasion of adjacent organs including the common hepatic duct, duodenum, and colon

3 **Staging** see Tables 34.1 and 34.2 for staging systems

Stage	Extent of tumor
I	Mucosa only
II	Muscularis and mucosa
III	Subserosa, muscularis, mucosa
IV	Cystic duct lymph node involvement and all layers of the gallbladder wall
V	Distant spread

(Table 34.1: Nevin's classification for carcinoma of the gallbladder)

Stage 0	Carcinoma in situ
Stage I	Tumor confined to mucosa and muscularis
Stage II	Tumor invades perimuscular connective tissue but does not extend beyond serosa
Stage III	Tumor perforates the serosa and/or invades an adjacent organ or has metastasized to cystic duct, pericholedochal, or hilar lymph nodes
Stage IV	Distant lymph node or organ metastases

(Table 34.2: American Joint Commission on Cancer (TMN) Staging: summary for carcinoma of the gallbladder)

D Clinical presentation

1 **Symptoms** (frequency)
   - abdominal pain (80%): present in up to 80% of patients, usually of < 1 month duration, difficult to distinguish from symptoms of acute cholecystitis or biliary colic
   - nausea/vomiting (50%)
   - weight loss (40%)
   - jaundice (30–40%)
   - incidental finding at cholecystectomy for gallstones (10–20%) (incidental cancers are found at 1% of cholecystectomies for symptomatic gallstones)

2 **Physical findings** – usually represent advanced disease
   - right-upper-quadrant mass

- hepatomegaly
- jaundice

E Diagnosis and preoperative staging

1 Laboratory tests
- abnormal liver function tests when associated with biliary obstruction
- no reliable tumor marker

2 Radiologic studies
- Ultrasonography
- sensitivity of 75–80%
- findings:
  - complex mass filling the gallbladder lumen
  - gallbladder wall thickening
  - polypoid gallbladder mass
  - gallstones
  - normal in up to 10% of patients
- b Computed tomography (CT)
  - similar findings as ultrasound with respect to gallbladder wall thickening or mass
  - defines extent of disease better than ultrasound; demonstrates liver or adjacent organ invasion, liver metastases, lymph node involvement, vascular invasion, and biliary obstruction
- c Magnetic resonance imaging (MRI): little advantage over CT scan
- d Endoscopic ultrasound: preliminary investigations suggest value in determining extent of local invasion and nodal involvement
- e Cholangiography
  - endoscopic retrograde cholangiography (ERC) or percutaneous transhepatic cholangiography (THC) – indicated in patients with clinical evidence of biliary obstruction
  - the typical cholangiographic appearance is a long stricture of the common hepatic duct usually below the bifurcation
  - endoscopic or percutaneous stents can be placed for preoperative biliary decompression, to aid in surgical management, or to provide long-term palliation
- f Visceral angiography
  - can be used to assess resectability with respect to invasion of the major vessels (portal vein, hepatic artery) by tumor
  - contrast-enhanced spiral CT may noninvasively provide similar information as angiography

3 Preoperative biopsy and cytologic findings
- percutaneous fine-needle biopsy for histologic or cytologic analysis can be performed in large tumors that appear unresectable
- bile or bile duct cytology or brushings have a low diagnostic yield
- there is no indication to pursue a preoperative tissue diagnosis in patients who are considered candidates for surgical resection

F   Treatment

1   Nonoperative palliation

- Indicated in patients in whom preoperative evaluation reveals extensive local or metastatic disease that precludes resection
- obstructive jaundice can be palliated with either a silastic or metallic endoprosthesis or internal–external silastic stents changed at 2–3 month intervals
- pain, if significant, can be managed with oral narcotics or a percutaneous celiac axis block

2   Surgical management

a   Laparoscopic cholecystectomy and gallbladder carcinoma

- with the widespread use of laparoscopic cholecystectomy for symptomatic gallstones many gallbladder cancers are first encountered in this setting
- contraindicated if gallbladder carcinoma is suspected preoperatively
- if a gallbladder carcinoma is recognized at the time of laparoscopic cholecystectomy, the patient should be converted to an open procedure for resection
- if a gallbladder carcinoma is recognized pathologically after laparoscopic cholecystectomy, management is dictated by histologic findings
  - if carcinoma is limited to the gallbladder mucosa, cholecystectomy is adequate
  - if carcinoma penetrates the gallbladder wall, the patient should be re-explored for wedge resection of the liver adjacent to the gallbladder fossa plus a regional lymph node dissection. Laparoscopic cholecystectomy trochar sites should also be excised

b   Surgical management of a suspected gallbladder carcinoma

- the resectability rates for gallbladder carcinoma range from 15% to 30%
- if the tumor is comfined to the gallbladder wall, simple cholecystectomy is adequate resection
- if the tumor penetrates the gallbladder wall, resection includes the gallbladder, segment V and the anterior portion of segment IV of the liver, and a lymph node dissection, including hilar, choledochal, and retropancreatic nodes
- Japanese investigators have advocated more aggressive resection including combined hepatic resection and pancreaticoduodenectomy
- postoperative morbidity and mortality rates are directly related to the extent of resection (see Table 34.3)

3   Adjuvant therapy following resection

- a high incidence of local recurrence supports the need for adjuvant therapy
- no randomized prospective trials available
- currently no regimen, including single or multiple agent chemotherapy, with or without radiation, has been of clear proven benefit
- uncontrolled studies have reported improved survival with high dose local radiation or superselective intra-arterial mitomycin C

Resection	Operative morbidity rate (%)	30-day mortality rate (%)
Cholecystectomy	10–15	2
Extended cholecystectomy	20–25	<5
Hepatic lobectomy	45–55	5–15
Hepatopancreaticoduodenectomy	50–65	15–20

(Table 34.3: Morbidity and mortality rates for different resections)

4 Treatment of unresectable disease
- standard chemotherapy (single or multiple agent) is associated with response rates of approximately 10%
- radiation therapy, including external beam and intraoperative radiotherapy and brachytherapy, has not been shown consistently to improve survival significantly

G Survival

1 Due to the late stage of presentation, the overall 5-year survival is less than 5%
2 Survival depends on the stage of tumor
- stage I tumors result in a 5-year survival rate of 85% following simple cholecystectomy
- overall 5-year survival rates for stage II, III, and IV disease are 25%, 10% and 2%, respectively
- patients with stage II tumors treated with extended cholecystectomy may have up to a 65% 5-year survival
- patients with unresectable stage III tumors presenting with obstructive jaundice survive approximately 6 months on average
- median survival with unresectable stage IV disease is only 2–3 months
- isolated reports of improved survival with aggressive surgical resection exist, particularly in the Japanese literature

4 Carcinoma of the Bile Duct – Cholangiocarcinoma

A Incidence

- represents approximately 25% of hepatobiliary cancers
- incidence in the USA of 1.0 per 100 000 population per year
- diagnosed in 3000–4000 new patients per year in the USA
- male/female ratio of 2 : 1
- age range of 50–70 years
- an increased incidence in Israel and Japan and among American Indians

B Risk factors for cholangiocarcinoma

Strong Association:

- Caroli's disease
- choledochal cyst
- clonorchiasis
- hepatolithiasis
- sclerosing cholangitis
- ulcerative colitis
- thorotrast

Possible association:

- asbestos
- dioxin (Agent Orange)
- isoniazid
- methyldopa
- oral contraceptives
- polychlorinated biphenyls
- radionucleotides

1 **Caroli's disease/choledochal cyst** (see Ch. 33)
   - the reported incidence of cholangiocarcinonma in patients with cystic abnormalities of the biliary tree ranges from 2.5% to 28%
   - patients with cystic lesions of the bile duct tend to develop cholangiocarcinoma 2–3 decades younger than patients with sporadic cholangiocarcinoma
   - more than 75% of patients with cholangiocarcinomas associated with choledochal cysts symptoms first appear in adulthood
   - factors possibly accounting for the development of cholangiocarcinoma in patients with cystic disease of the biliary tree include:
     - reflux of pancreatic exocrine secretions as a result of an anomalous pancreatic duct–bile duct junction;
     - bile stasis;
     - chronic inflammation and bacterial infection within the cyst
     - stone formation within the cyst

2 ***Clonorchis sinensis* (liver fluke) infection** (see Ch. 29)
   - common in Asia and associated with ingestion of raw fish
   - the adult trematode resides in the intrahepatic and, less commonly, the extrahepatic bile ducts, can obstruct biliary flow, and can cause periductal fibrosis, hyperplasia, stricture, and stone formation
   - *Opisthorchis viverrini* is a second liver fluke associated with cholangiocarcinoma

3 Hepatolithiasis (see Ch. 33)

- cholangiocarcinoma will develop in 5–10% of patients with hepatolithiasis
- bile stasis, bactibilia, and cystic dilatation may all be associated with this increased risk
- cholelithiasis is seen in up to one third of patients with and without cholangiocarcinoma; therefore, gallbladder stones are not considered a risk factor for cholangiocarcinoma

4 Primary sclerosing cholangitis (see Ch. 15)

- unrecognized cholangiocarcinoma is found in up to 40% of autopsies in patients dying with and 10% of patients undergoing liver transplantation for sclerosing cholangitis
- cholangiocarcinoma in patients with sclerosing cholangitis is often manifested by rapid clinical deterioration and progressive jaundice
- prognosis in patients with cholangiocarcinoma and sclerosing cholangitis is poor, with a median survival of less than 1 year

5 Ulcerative colitis

- incidence of cholangiocarcinoma in patients with ulcerative colitis ranges from 0.14% to 1.4%, 400–1000 times that of the general population
- cholangiocarcinoma develops 20 years earlier in patients with ulcerative colitis than in others
- patients with cholangiocarcinoma and ulcerative colitis tend to have pancolonic involvement and a long duration of disease

6 Thorotrast (thorium dioxide)

- a radiocontrast agent used several decades ago which emits alpha particles and, when injected intravenously, is retained in the reticuloendothelial system for life
- cholangiocarcinoma may develop after a mean latent period of 35 years

C Pathology and staging

1 Histologic type

- adenocarcinoma accounts for over 95%
- rare histologic types include squamous and mucoepidermoid carcinoma, cystadenocarcinomas, carcinoid tumors, and leiomyosarcoma
- histologic types of adenocarcinoma include nodular (most common), scirrhous, diffusely infiltrating, and papillary (often multifocal)

2 Location (see Table 34.4)

3 Route of spread

- most commonly (70%) by direct invasion of the adjacent liver, portal vein, hepatic artery, pancreas, or duodenum
- liver and/or peritoneal metastases occur in up to 50% of patients
- regional lymph nodes are involved in 75–80% of patients

4 Staging (see Table 34.5)

Common bile duct	33–40%	Upper third (proximal to cystic duct)	56–58%
Common hepatic duct	30–32%	Middle third (cystic duct to pancreas)	13–17%
Hepatic duct bifurcation	20%	Lower third (intrapancreatic)	18%
Cystic duct	4%	Diffuse	7–13%
Diffuse	7%		

aExcluding intrahepatic cholangiocarcinomas, which account for approximately 6% of all cholangiocarcinomas

*(Table 34.4: Location of cholangiocarcinomas*a*)*

Stage 0	Carcinoma in situ
Stage I	Tumor invades the mucosa and muscular is only
Stage II	Tumor invades perimuscular connective tissue
Stage III	Regional lymph node involvement
Stage IV	Tumor invades adjacent organs or is associated with distant metastases

(Table 34.5: American joint commission on cancer (TMN) staging: summary for cholangiocarcinoma)

D   Clinical presentation

1 Symptoms
- jaundice is the most common presenting symptom and is present in over 90% of patients
- pruritus
- weight loss
- abdominal pain – vague, nonspecific, and mild – may be the only symptom with proximal tumors located above the hepatic bifurcation
- cholangitis (uncommon)

2 Physical findings
- jaundice
- hepatomegaly
- palpable gallbladder – only with distal bile duct cancers

E   Diagnosis and preoperative staging

1 Laboratory tests
- abnormal liver function tests – increased bilirubin and alkaline phosphatase levels
- prolonged prothrombin time with long-standing biliary obstruction

2 Tumor markers
- serum carcinoembryonic antigen (CEA), alpha fetoprotein, and carbohydrate antigen 19-9 (CA-19-9) individually are of limited value

- serum tumor marker index (CEA × 40 + CA-19-9) has been shown in one study to be 86% accurate in diagnosing cholangiocarcinoma. The cut-off value is 400 μ
- bile CEA levels are significantly elevated in patients with cholangiocarcinoma when compared with patients with benign bile duct strictures and may fall and rise with resection and progression of disease, respectively

3 Radiologic studies

a Ultrasonography/CT

- hilar tumors – dilated intrahepatic biliary tree, contracted gallbladder, and normal extrahepatic biliary tree and pancreas
- distal tumors – dilated intra- and extrahepatic biliary tree with a distended gallbladder
- primary tumors are seldom visualized, although newer techniques of duplex ultrasound and spiral CT may yield better results

b MRI: may be more sensitive than ultrasound or CT for visualizing primary tumor

c Cholangiography

- either ERC or THC should be performed to define the location and extent of the tumor
- THC is preferred for proximal biliary tumors because this technique better defines the proximal extent of the tumor
- cholangiographic appearance can predict resectability in proximal cholangiocarcinoma (positive predictive value of 60%)
- percutaneous placement of biliary catheters is indicated for proximal cholangiocarcinomas to help guide hilar dissection and to facilitate placement of silastic transhepatic stents used for biliary reconstruction. For tumors at the bifurcation, bilateral catheters should be placed
- either ERC or THC is appropriate for distal bile duct cancers

d Visceral angiography

- should be used to assess for major vessel (hepatic artery, portal vein) encasement or occlusion (positive predictive value 71%); include portal venous phase studies
- the positive predictive value of combined cholangiography and visceral angiography is 79%

e Preoperative biopsy and cytologic findings

- a tissue diagnosis to rule out malignancy is necessary in patients being considered for nonoperative management of presumably benign strictures or in those with sclerosing cholangitis being considered for liver transplantation
- bile cytology will demonstrate malignant cells in 30% of cases of cholangiocarcinoma
- cytologic brushings performed either via a percutaneous or endoscopic approach will yield positive results in 40–50% of patients; results improve with multiple attempts
- percutaneous fine-needle aspiration or cholangioscopic biopsies may increase the diagnostic yield to 67%

F   Treatment

1   Nonoperative palliation

- indicated in patients with extensive local or metastatic disease that precludes resection (if determined preoperatively)
- obstructive jaundice can be palliated with either silastic or metallic endoprostheses or internal–external silastic stents changed at 2–3-month intervals
- in patients with proximal (hilar) cholangiocarcinoma, percutaneous, bilateral access is usually necessary
- death is usually the result of recurrent biliary sepsis and liver abscess, which occur as tumor extension occludes proximal bile duct radicles

2   Surgical palliation

- **surgical exploration for attempted resection is indicated in all good-risk patients not determined to be unresectable by preoperative staging**
- patients with disseminated disease or extensive tumor involvement of the porta hepatis should undergo minimal intervention
  - a   preoperative biliary catheters should be left in place for palliation of jaundice
  - b   a cholecystectomy should be performed to prevent the development of acute cholecystitis
- surgical approaches for palliation of locally unresectable cholangiocarcinoma:
  - – proximal tumors – operative dilatation of the tumor with placement of silastic stents and a Roux-en-Y choledochojejunostomy, or a segment III bypass to the left hepatic duct using a Roux-en-Y limb of jejunum
  - – distal tumors – hepaticojejunostomy and gastrojejunostomy

3   Surgical resection

- approach to intrahepatic cholangiocarcinoma is similar to that for hepatocellular carcinoma, with a standard hepatic lobectomy
- perihilar cholangiocarcinomas require local resection of the hepatic duct above the level of the hepatic duct bifurcation to achieve a microscopically negative margin
  - – reconstruction is performed over bilateral silastic stents with anastomosis to a Roux-en-Y limb of jejunum
  - – extension of the carcinoma along either hepatic duct may require hepatic lobectomy
  - – many surgeons, primarily in Japan, advocate routine resection of the caudate lobe (segment I) of the liver because of direct drainage from that lobe to the hepatic duct bifurcation
  - – addition of a major hepatic resection significantly increases perioperative morbidity and mortality
- Table 34.6 shows the relative mortalities for hepatic bifurcation resection and reconstruction with and without hepatic lobectomy
- distal cholangiocarcinomas require a pancreaticoduodenectomy (perioperative mortality <4%, morbidity 30–40%)

	Operative morbidity	30-day mortality
Hepatic bifurcation resection and reconstruction	<5%	25–30%
Hepatic bifurcation resection, reconstruction, and hepatic lobectomy	15–20%	45–55%

(Table 34.6: Morbidity and mortality rates for different resections)

4 **Adjuvant therapy following resection**
   - no randomized prospective trials available
   - to date, no single chemotherapeutic agent or combination of agents, with or without radiation, has been shown to be of clear benefit
   - a large retrospective analysis from Johns Hopkins of comparable operatively staged resected patients with perihilar cholangiocarcinoma and similar Karnofsky functional scores compared external beam radiation plus iridium-192 seeds delivered through transhepatic stents with no treatment and showed no survival advantage
   - in absence of prospective data, most groups advocate adjuvant chemotherapy and radiation therapy for resected distal cholangiocarcinomas based on the results of the GI Tumor Study group's protocol for resectable pancreatic carcinoma

5 **Treatment of unresectable disease**: neither chemotherapy, radiation therapy, or any combination has been shown to be of benefit

G   Survival

1 **Intrahepatic cholangiocarcinoma**
   - usually presents at an advanced stage (15–20% resectability rate)
   - resectable: 3-year survival   45–60%
                          median survival   18–30 months
   - unresectable: median survival   7 months

2 **Perihilar cholangiocarcinoma** (see Table 34.7)

	Mean survival (months) following resection	Actuarial survival (%)		
		1-year	3-year	5-year
Hilar resection	18–21	68–76	21–30	7–11
Hilar and hepatic resection	18–24	60–65	30–40	10–15

(Table 34.7: Survival following resection for perihilar cholangiocarcinoma)

Factors influencing survival include negative surgical margins, preoperative serum albumin level, and postoperative sepsis
   - operative but unresectable
      – median survival   8 months

- – 1-year survival 27%
- – 2-year survival 6%
- unresectable: as determined preoperatively
  - – median survival 5 months
  - – 1-year survival 25%
  - – 2-year survival 5%

3 Distal cholangiocarcinoma

- best resectability rate (>50%)
- when resectable, median survival is 24 months; overall survival at 1 year of 70%, at 3 years 35%, at 5 years 28%
- factors influencing survival following resection: negative lymph node status, poor tumor differentiation
- when unresectable, median survival is 8 months

References

1 Bismuth H, Nakache R, Diamond T. *Management strategies in resection for hilar cholangiocarcinoma.* (Ann Surg 1992) 215: 31–8

2 Gagner M, Rossi RL. *Radical operations for carcinomas of the gallbladder: present status in North America.* (World J Surg 1991) 15: 344–7

3 Jones RS. *Carcinoma of the gallbladder.* (Surg Clin North Am 1990) 70: 1419–28

4 Nagorney DM, Donohue JH, Farrell MB, et al. *Outcomes after curative resections of cholangiocarcinoma.* (Arch Surg 1993) 128: 871–7

5 Nakeeb A, Pitt HA, Sohn TA, et al. *Cholangiocarcinoma: a spectrum of intrahepatic, perihilar, and distal tumors.* (Ann Surg 1996) 224: 463–75

6 Nimura Y, Hayakawa N, Kamiya J, et al. *Hepatopancreatoduodenectomy for advanced carcinoma of the biliary tract.* (Hepatogastroenterology 1991) 38: 170–5

7 Nordback IH, Pitt HA, Coleman JA, et al. *Unresectable hilar cholangiocarcinoma: percutaneous versus operative palliation.* (Surgery 1994) 115: 597–603

8 Rosen CB, Nagorney DM, Wiesner RH, et al. *Cholangiocarcinoma complicating primary sclerosing cholangitis.* (Ann Surg 1991) 213: 21–5

9 Pitt HA, Nakeeb A, Abrams RA, et al. *Perihilar cholangiocarcinoma: postoperative radiotherapy does not improve survival.* (Ann Surg 1995) 221: 788–98

10 Pitt HA, Dooley WC, Yeo CJ, Cameron JL. *Malignancies of the biliary tree.* (Curr Prob Surg 1995) 32: 1–100

INDEX

Numbers in italics refer to illustrations or tables; numbers in bold refer to color plates